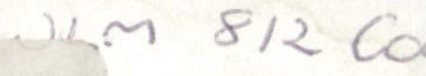

Communication Skills Training for Health Professionals

JOIN US ON THE INTERNET VIA WWW, GOPHER, FTP OR EMAIL:

WWW: http://www.thomson.com
GOPHER: gopher.thomson.com
FTP: ftp.thomson.com
EMAIL: findit@kiosk.thomson.com

A service of I(T)P®

Communication Skills Training for Health Professionals

Second edition

David Dickson
School of Behavioural and Communication Sciences
University of Ulster
Jordanstown
Northern Ireland

Owen Hargie
School of Behavioural and Communication Sciences
University of Ulster
Jordanstown
Northern Ireland

and

Norman Morrow
Formerly Director of Postgraduate Pharmaceutical
Education and Training for Northern Ireland

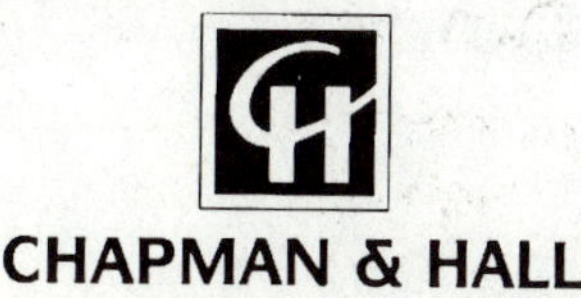

CHAPMAN & HALL

London • Weinheim • New York • Tokyo • Melbourne • Madras

Published by Chapman & Hall, 2–6 Boundary Row, London SE1 8HN, UK

Chapman & Hall, 2–6 Boundary Row, London SE1 8HN, UK

Chapman & Hall GmbH, Pappelallee 3, 69469 Weinheim, Germany

Chapman & Hall USA, 115 Fifth Avenue, New York NY 10003, USA

Chapman & Hall Japan, ITP-Japan, Kyowa Building, 3F, 2-2-1 Hirakawacho, Chiyoda-ku, Tokyo 102, Japan

Chapman & Hall Australia, 102 Dodds Street, South Melbourne, Victoria 3205, Australia

Chapman & Hall India, R. Seshadri, 32 Second Main Road, CIT East, Madras 600 035, India

Distributed in the USA and Canada by Singular Publishing Group Inc., 4284 41st Street, San Diego, California 92105

First edition 1989

Second edition 1997

Typeset in Great Britain by Saxon Graphics Ltd, Derby
Printed in Great Britain by T. J. Press (Padstow) Ltd.

ISBN 0 412 61450 2   1 56593 766 X (USA)

A catalogue record for this book is available from the British Library

♾ Printed on permanent acid-free text paper, manufactured in accordance with ANSI/NISO Z39.48-1992 and ANSI/NISO Z39.48-1984 (Permanence of Paper).

This book is dedicated to:

Kerri and Shona;
Ernest, Pat and Elizabeth;
and
Michael, Victoria and David

Contents

Preface

The importance of skilful interpersonal communication to the provision of effective health-care is now more widely recognized than when we wrote the first edition of this book some 7 years ago. In addition to the various other dimensions of expertise which health professionals draw upon, they must be able to interact successfully with colleagues and other health workers as well as patients and clients. It would still seem to be the case, however, that standards of practice in this respect frequently fall short of public expectations and levels of professional acceptability. There is evidently much ‘room for improvement’. One level at which interventions for improvement can be targeted is the training of, for instance, doctors, dentists, nurses, pharmacists, health visitors, physiotherapists, occupational therapists, speech therapists and dietitians. At present, however, those intent upon implementing such a training initiative often feel ill-prepared to do so, having little to direct them in the planning, operation and evaluation of communication skills training (CST) procedures. This book has been prepared to meet this need for information and advice by tutors faced with the task of contributing inputs in this area as part of either pre- or in-service education programmes.

The book is essentially concerned with elaborating a structured and systematic instructional procedure for enhancing skilful face-to-face communication. It is organized in four parts. Part One contributes a firm conceptual base for the rest of the text by introducing and examining the notions of communication and communicative competence. The importance of effective interpersonal communication in the health professions is assessed and contrasting approaches to facilitating performance are considered. An initial overview of CST is also given. Part Two is devoted to the content of training. Here a theoretical model of skilled communication is developed incorporating interpersonal, intrapersonal and situational determinants. A range of skills commonly documented as being relevant to health-care personnel are presented and analysed. These include non-verbal communication, questioning, listening, explaining, reinforcement and assertiveness. Furthermore, the incorporation and integration of such skills within the strategic contexts of interviewing, counselling and influencing is discussed.

The CST process encompassing preparation, training and evaluation stages is the subject of Part Three. Having established the aims and objectives of the training intervention, techniques are presented for isolating and identifying appropriate skills content. Sensitization, practice and feedback phases of training *per se* are expounded and guidelines are offered for their implementation. This section is concluded by focusing upon methods of programme evaluation.

The fourth and final part of the book brings a more integrative perspective to bear upon CST. A detailed exposition is given of the major considerations which the tutor must acknowledge in designing and implementing training and the influence of these, at different levels, on the instructional sequence formulated. Planning issues to do with the crucial matter of maximizing the transfer of training to the workplace are also brought together and addressed. Finally the impact of CST upon the communicative competence of professionals is discussed from within the institutional and organizational framework of the present health service.

As with the first edition, it has been our intention to produce a book that is fundamentally practical in orientation, containing not only information and guidance but also material that trainers can directly apply in planning, teaching and evaluating programmes. Practical exercises are inserted throughout. Some of these are intended for the reader as trainer to work through; others can form the content of CST programmes to be completed by participants. Suggestions as to how the latter may best be made use of, are offered. Material is also included that can be used to analyse performance, identify skills and present structured feedback to trainees. This can either be accepted in its present form or adapted to more fully meet particular requirements.

In outlining CST procedures and techniques we have, however, avoided a 'cook-book' approach, which merely describes a stereotypical sequence of steps to be reflexly followed on each and every occasion. This is not how we see CST. Rather we have resolved to document the underlying rationale for this type of training and illuminate the theoretical, conceptual and empirical underpinnings of the various instructional mechanisms that contribute to it. Trainers who have a firm understanding of why they are doing what they are doing are infinitely better prepared to maximize the potential which CST has to offer with different groups in disparate settings. An inevitable consequence of this stance is that the book takes on some of the trappings of an 'academic' publication. Nevertheless, no prior knowledge of CST techniques is assumed on the part of the reader, although those with a background in the behavioural sciences, particularly psychology, will be at an advantage.

Perhaps a mention should be made of the nomenclature that we have adopted. In the literature, terms including 'interpersonal skills', 'social skills' and 'interactive skills' can sometimes be found to refer to what practitioners do when they relate to others, which we have here called 'communication skills'. While not wishing to deny conceptual distinctions, in practice these terms tend to be applied interchangeably. There does seem, though, to be an emerging orthodoxy favouring 'interpersonal communication skills training', or simply 'communication skills training', in professional contexts. Throughout the book we have endeavoured to avoid sexist forms of expression. Where we have not been successful, we have tried to vary gender-specific forms in a reasonably random manner.

The second edition of this book, while retaining the basic structure and detailing the same essential approach to CST as the first, differs in a number of important respects. A new chapter, Chapter 13, is devoted to the important issue of promoting the transfer of training so that it impacts upon professional practice where it matters, in the workplace. Numerous additions have been make to chapters to take account of developments in training in this field. For example, the use of interactive video as a means of skill sensitization is outlined in Chapter 8. The literature on interpersonal communication and health has burgeoned since the first edition was prepared. Parts One and Two of this edition, in particular, have been modified to accommodate this material. Indeed the whole book has been brought up to date with developments in the broader field of training. Finally, some new exercises have been added, which the trainer can both do and use.

This book could not have been completed without the help of a great many people – we owe them all a very real debt of gratitude. We would like to acknowledge the contribution of colleagues, including Christine Saunders, Colin Hargie and Denis Tourish, whose ideas and suggestions have found their way into the book at different points. Philip Burch deserves a mention for his assistance with computer graphics. Students who have undertaken CST programmes also merit a special word of thanks – we have learned a lot from them about CST! Rosemary Morris at Chapman & Hall must not be forgotten. Her unflagging support and encouragement made the difficult bits much easier. Finally we are eternally indebted to our long-suffering wives and families for their forbearance throughout.

David Dickson
Owen Hargie
Norman Morrow

Jordanstown, Co. Antrim, April 1996

PART ONE

Background

The first part of the book introduces the topic of communication, its importance in health-care delivery and training approaches to improving its effectiveness. As such, this part is designed to orient the reader to the detailed exposition, in subsequent sections, of the content and process of CST for health-care personnel.

Part One comprises two chapters. Chapter 1 provides a firm conceptual base which is built upon and extended throughout the remainder of the text. It begins with an initial examination of the salience of effective face-to-face communication within the health-care context and continues by assessing the present effectiveness of practitioners in this respect. The bulk of the chapter, however, is given over to a detailed analysis of the concepts of interpersonal communication and communicative competence, the latter having cognitive, motivational and performative dimensions identified. Extending this theme, the notion of communication as an essentially skilful activity is introduced and elaborated.

The manner in which the nature of interpersonal communication is construed has clearly inescapable implications in respect of training. Three general approaches to instruction in this area are noted and labelled 'On the job', 'Model the Master' and 'Directed training'. Having established some of the weaknesses of the first two, 'Directed training' procedures are concentrated upon and descriptions are given of methods based variously upon 'thinking', 'feeling' and 'doing'. CST goes some way to synthesizing these three methods and the chapter is brought to a close with an overview of the CST process on which the book is based.

Chapter 2 reintroduces the issue of the importance of effective communication in the health professions and examines it more thoroughly. At the outset a skill-based model of professional competence is developed incorporating a significant communicative dimension. The promotion of professional competence must, therefore, include training in interpersonal skills in addition to the more traditional areas of the curriculum. The chapter continues by examining a number of sources of influence which have resulted in the increasing acceptance, of late, of the legitimacy of CST and the contribution which it can make in the training of health workers. The chapter finishes with a brief consideration of the outcomes of such training and conclusions are drawn concerning the efficacy of this type of intervention.

Introduction 1

1.1 INTRODUCTION

'It was just like that scene from *Doctor in the House*', she said, laughing. 'You know, the one where James Robertson-Justice plays Sir Lancelot Spratt, the surgeon in whose presence everyone trembles. Remember the bit where he is by the bed of a patient waiting for surgery, with a group of housemen and nurses standing around. In the middle of discussing all the gory details of the pending operation with the group, he turns to the patient and tells him that he won't understand any of what is being said and that in any case it has nothing to do with him!'

Most of the group had seen the film and recalled the scene. We all laughed and then she continued, 'I was recovering from a laminectomy. Each morning it was the same routine. The group would move to my bed. The surgeon would be talking to the group, ignoring me completely. Indeed they would **all** be ignoring me completely.' We all laughed again. 'He would pull down the sheet, lift my leg and let it drop. They would then discuss my progress and walk off, without even pulling the sheet back up – until one morning I made my mind up that I wasn't prepared to be dealt with like that any more.' The smile faded as she relived her anger and frustration. There was a pause.

'What did you do?' someone asked. 'Well,' she continued, laughing once more, 'as he was about to pull the sheet down, I caught hold of it. I didn't say anything, just held it. I think for the first time he looked at me. At first he seemed confused. The rest were horror-stricken. Then he smiled. "Good-morning, Mrs Dillon. Would you mind if we took a look at your leg? You seem to be getting more control back."'

'You know, he was really quite pleasant. Each morning after that he made an effort to treat me like a person, not just a laminectomy. The group seemed more relaxed as well!' she concluded.

The story was told by a nurse during an introductory group discussion on communication and health. It was only one of a number of such stories told of instances of poor communication on the part of health practitioners. No doubt there are many like Mrs Dillon who have been subjected to unnecessary feelings of humiliation and frustration under similar circumstances. Others have experienced confusion, helplessness, anger or shame due to the insensitivity and interpersonal ineptitude of some well-intentioned health professional who probably remained totally oblivious of the fact.

This book is about improving the interpersonal communication skills of health personnel through focusing upon training. It takes as its starting point the claim that effective communication lies at the heart of successful health-care delivery. Two further premises are invoked: that health practitioners' levels of work-based communication often fall short of acceptable standards of proficiency and that this state of affairs can be improved, in part, through more and better training targeted specifically on this aspect of care. To this end a systematic instructional framework is elaborated that encompasses:

- procedures for identifying aspects of communication that could most usefully be considered by particular trainee groups;
- a structured technology for training in these skills;
- a variety of approaches to the evaluation of outcome.

Procedures for maximizing the carry-over of training to the workplace are also considered. Several types of interaction that staff may be involved in and that require specialized knowledge and skill are also examined. These include interviewing, influencing and counselling. In addition, a range of specific skills that facilitate these processes are outlined. In this way it is hoped that the book will, in at least some small measure, contribute to a health service that is 'caring' in the fullest sense of the word.

1.2 THE HEALTH PROFESSIONAL'S COMMUNICATION NETWORK

It is worth pausing for a moment to remind ourselves of just how central communication is to the work of the health professional. It is so pervasive that it can, ironically, be overlooked! Interacting with patients readily springs to mind, but the health-care worker is typically at the centre of a much wider network of relationships, as depicted in Figure 1.1.

Depending upon the specific profession and the particular role played within it, some of these contacts will be more common and important than others. Taking the example of a GP, consultations with patients, without doubt, are foremost in importance. But the GP may also discuss the patient's progress with members of the family, face to face or over the telephone, as well as with colleagues and other caring professionals (e.g. community nurse, social worker), perhaps during a formal case conference. There will also be contacts with administrative staff, including receptionists and secretaries. Prescriptions will be written and read by the pharmacist. Representatives from various pharmaceutical companies may also visit. The GP could additionally be invited to speak to members of the local women's group on some aspect of health care, be interviewed on the topic on local radio or act as a practice tutor to a student undergoing training in general practice. This network could no doubt be further extended! A more systematic audit of the communication that formed part of the work of a swallowing clinic was carried out by Skipper (1992). The results make fascinating reading and underscore the ubiquity and indispensability of this type of activity in such a setting.

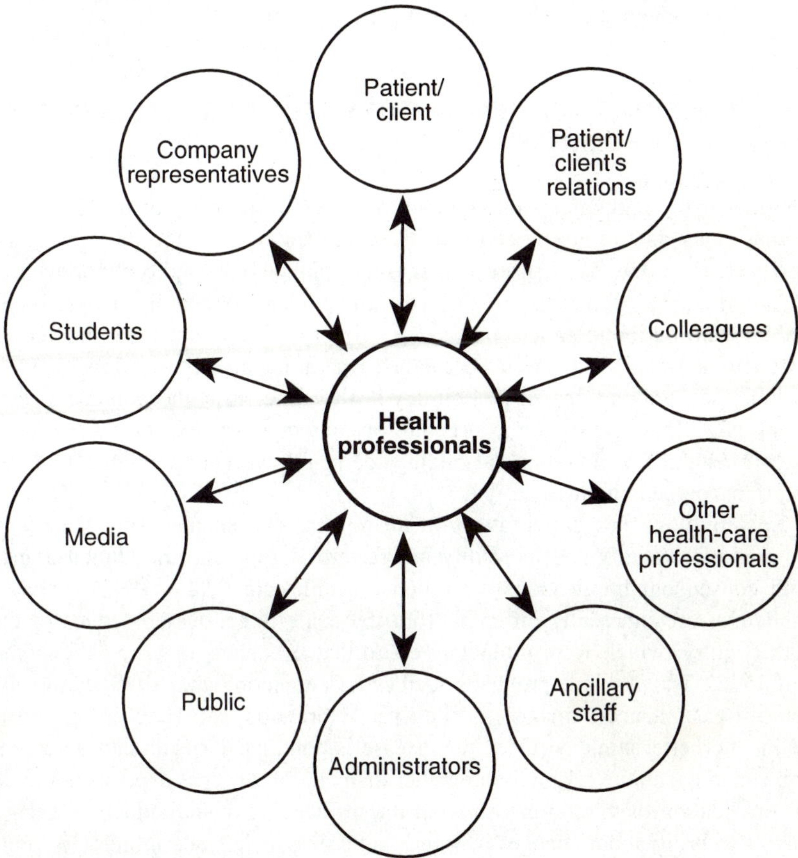

Figure 1.1 The health professional's communication network.

A useful way to commence a session on communication with students just beginning their professional training is to ask them, in small groups, and with a sheet of flip-chart paper and some felt-tips, to draw a communication network such as this, centred upon their chosen profession. The resulting networks can then be presented to the larger group and elaborated.

In unpacking Figure 1.1, we have mentioned communication in a number of guises such as via telephone, on radio, in writing, as well as face to face. To attempt a comprehensive coverage of each of these various contexts is beyond the scope of this text. We will concentrate, for the most part, on dyadic (two-person) interaction in those relationships with, for instance, patients, relatives, colleagues and other professionals, which, it could be argued, are more central to the work of the practitioner. However the general instructional mechanism, which is detailed in the following chapters and encompasses preparation, training and evaluation stages, has a much wider application.

1.3 THE IMPORTANCE OF EFFECTIVE COMMUNICATION IN THE HEALTH PROFESSIONS

The fact that communication commonly features in the work of health professionals does not, of itself, confirm its pivotal role. Over the past 15 years, however, there has been an ever-increasing appreciation of the importance of the interpersonal dimension of the work undertaken by health-care personnel and its contribution to patient well-being. Dickson (1995a) attributes this recognition to a range of interrelated factors, operating at different levels. They include the changing face of present-day health concerns, conceptualizations of health and illness, shifts in the structure of contemporary society, current policies of health care and empirical findings on health worker communication and its effects on patient outcome.

Epidemiology has drawn attention to the dramatic changes this century in patterns of mortality and morbidity in Western Europe and the United States, with consequent implications for primary health care (Clare, 1993). Today's challenges are inherently different from the acute infectious epidemics of the 19th century, which were ultimately controlled by means of vaccinations and antibiotics. They include problems such as HIV infection and AIDS, cardiovascular disease, cancer, cirrhosis of the liver, depression, etc. Here prevention is by far the better strategy. Once the disease is contracted, health-care intervention can at best hope to ameliorate rather than cure it. Success depends not upon the eradication of microorganisms but the influencing of individuals in such a way as to bring about changes in values, attitudes, beliefs and ultimately habits and lifestyles. As such, it owes more to disciplines such as communication than to chemistry or microbiology.

There are very obvious implications here for models of health care. The limitations of the traditional biomedical model, which draws its inspiration from the natural sciences, are increasingly becoming obvious. This disease-oriented 'body-as-machine' approach, with its accompanying conceptualization of the patient as damaged structure or malfunctioning system, demands no great communicative ability on the part of the 'practitioner-as-expert' since the 'client-as-person' is scarcely recognized. We saw as much from the nurse's anecdote which began the chapter. A more broadly based and holistic, biopsychosocial alternative to this model, which can additionally accommodate interpersonal and societal influences on health together with the expectations, beliefs and predispositions of the individuals concerned, is now widely accepted, if not always acted upon. Here effective interpersonal communication is unavoidable.

Changing views of health itself, from the mere absence of illness to more positive, holistic and dynamic notions of optimizing resources to maximize personal potential (Ewles and Simnett, 1992), should be appreciated as a further reason for the recent reinstatement of communication at the centre of health care. Working with those with health needs in a spirit of active cooperation and participation so that, through empowerment, they are enabled to adapt to change, more successfully meet their needs and fulfil their potential for quality life, obviously places a premium upon such communicative activities as informing, teaching, interviewing, influencing, persuading, negotiating and counselling (Seale, 1992).

Present health policy constitutes a related influencing factor in the present emphasis upon good communication in health-care delivery. Indeed the White Paper *The Health of the Nation* (Department of Health, 1992a), launched in July, 1992 was described as 'not about taking pills. It is about changing habits and behaviour – though it is stating the obvious to say that behaviour change is very much harder to achieve than taking tablets' (Bottomley, 1993, p. 1). With an increased emphasis upon care in the community, different patterns of contact with clients and families, and the often long-term involvement necessitated by chronic conditions, an added premium is placed upon effective communication. The ramifications of these policy changes in this respect, though, need to be much more extensively researched (Sharf, 1993).

Additionally, the advent of consumerism in the NHS has cast the client as the consumer of a service with a set of attendant and now formalized rights and expectations (Department of Health, 1992b). This proposes a type of relationship between provider and recipient of care that is radically different from that which has traditionally prevailed, especially in medicine, and brings the need for improvements in communication with patients sharply to the fore.

Many of these shifts in policy and attitude have taken place alongside more basic structural changes in society. A less clearly differentiated class structure, better educated population, lowering of class barriers and adjustments to established norms and values surrounding status now mean that people are more insistent that their rights be acknowledged and respected and less willing to unquestioningly acquiesce in the face of authority. Commensurably, many patients are demanding a different type of relationship with their doctor, one based upon what DiMatteo (1994, p. 154) describes as 'collaborative informed choice', rather than the paternalism that traditionally pertained. Once more, this new relationship of equality and openness is dependent upon free and full communication between professional and client/patient.

Finally, there is now a growing body of empirical evidence suggesting that patients who are dealt with by professionals with good interpersonal communication benefit in a number of respects. They tend to be better satisfied with the service which they receive (Lewis, 1994) and are more inclined to comply with medical regimens and procedures (Sherbourne *et al.*, 1992). This may be partly due to increased comprehension and recall of information received (Ley, 1988). Moreover, outcomes appear to be not only psychological (e.g. feelings of satisfaction) and behavioural (e.g. adherence/compliance) but physical, measured by improved health indices and recovery rates (Ley, 1988; Davis and Fallowfield, 1991; Ong *et al.*, 1995).

1.4 CURRENT LEVELS OF COMMUNICATION IN THE HEALTH PROFESSIONS

The establishment of facilitative levels of communication, enabling meaningful and trusting relationships with patients to be developed, is now widely accepted as fundamental to effective management and care. It would therefore be reasonable to assume that health professionals manifest particularly high levels of interpersonal skill. The facts unfortunately often fail to bear this out. Indeed this aspect of care has consistently been criticized by recipients of health services (Meredith, 1993). In the report *What Seems to Be the Matter* (Audit Commission, 1993) into communication with hospitalized patients, the conclusion was reached that 'As health care processes and organizations become increasingly more complex, so the need to communicate with patients clearly about the clinical and non-clinical aspects of their care grows. But provision has not kept up with the growing need, and lack of information and problems with health professionals usually come at the top of the patients' concerns' (p. 1).

But deficits are not confined to the hospital setting nor to medicine. The Health Services Commissioner's Annual Report has consistently identified poor or inadequate communication between patient and health professional as the source of many of the grievances dealt with. The Annual Report for 1992–93, for example, places this category of complaint highest of the 15 categories established for acute hospital outpatients and mental health (HMSO, 1993). When considered by professional grouping, Nursing, Midwifery and Health Visiting, taken together, recorded the second highest number of communication complaints of the eight service groups mentioned. Only Medical and Dental recorded a higher incidence of complaint of this type. For Nursing, Midwifery and Health Visiting, communication issues represented the second highest category of upheld complaint, being almost a quarter of the total number brought against this group. The Health Services Commissioner's conclusion was that 'Good oral and written communications are essential for the provision of a satisfactory service. Without failures in communications there would be a dramatic fall in the number of complaints to me – and to health authorities themselves' (HMSO, 1993, p. 9).

This decidedly depressing picture is made worse by those who have focused directly upon the interpersonal competence of health professionals. The interpersonal skills of students just finished medical school were found to be disappointing in a study carried out by Sloan *et al.* (1994). Even experienced hospital doctors have been accused of showing a lack of interest in patients and failing to acknowledge their needs. As a consequence, psychosocial dimensions of cases were largely neglected (Maguire, 1981). Nurses whose conversations with patients have been studied have fared little better. MacLeod Clark (1985) summarized the findings by saying that 'the overall picture was one of tactics that discourage communication rather than skills that encourage it' (p. 16). Furthermore, it seems that some nurses at least may be not unaware of a lack of skill in some of the more challengingly interpersonal aspects of their work (Noble, 1991; Greenwood, 1993).

Clearly the assertion by Argent *et al.* (1994) that the communication skills of health professionals are in need of improvement can be readily sustained. Specific features of communication which are problematic have been identified and reported (Maguire, 1984a; MacLeod Clark, 1985; Davis and Fallowfield, 1991; Abraham and Shanley, 1992). In general it would appear that problems that arise centre on deficiencies in five major areas.

- **Gathering information.** Badenoch (1986) highlighted this deficiency by relating the apocryphal story of the busy physician rapidly writing out the patient's history without looking up and blithely unaware that the patient is deaf and his questions are being answered by the blind patient in the next bed! While this may be extreme, Newell (1994) has made the comment that, while done frequently, by and large health workers interview poorly. They often neglect important areas, interview in an overly practitioner-centred way and collect detail in such a way that it is likely to be inaccurate or incomplete.
- **Giving information.** This frequently invites criticism either because the amount provided is inadequate or alternatively because it is delivered in an incomprehensible or insensitive way. The findings have been summarized by the Audit Commission (1993, p. 1) as follows: 'A common complaint is that there is not enough information. Equally, information often exists, but the quality is poor.'
- **Poor listening.** In a sense this is related to the last issue. Health-care personnel have been accused of taking little time to listen to what the patient wants to say (DiMatteo, 1994). Instead of 'saving time', which may sometimes be the motive, they frequently end up losing it!
- **Neglect of psychosocial concerns.** Communication that does take place tends to be primarily factual, addressing physical aspects of the condition. As a consequence the psychosocial needs of patients are often neglected. The

professional's role in offering comfort and emotional support is thereby neglected. Male physicians would seem to be more negligent than their female colleagues in this respect (Roter, Lipkin and Korsgaard, 1991).

- **Relationship work**. Negotiating a mutually acceptable professional–patient relationship is an important communicative function (Ong *et al.*, 1995). It can lead to frustration and difficulty when the health professional insists on operating within the terms of the traditional paternalistic arrangement that has typified health-care delivery, while the patient demands the right to a more egalitarian alternative in which a contribution to the decision-making process can be claimed. More mundanely, patients complain that health professionals often do not greet them appropriately, introduce themselves or explain what they intend to do. Techniques for improving communication in these respects will be considered in Chapters 4, 5 and 6.

1.5 CAUSES OF POOR COMMUNICATION

The causes of what would appear to be rather disappointing standards of communication in the health professions are, no doubt, multifarious. A more detailed consideration of this issue will be left to the final chapter. Attention, though, has been directed to deficiencies in the basic training received. According to Numann (1988, p. 212), 'we have failed to teach our students the interpersonal skills which will enable them to effectively communicate with the patient, to consider the patient's needs and wishes, to encourage the patient to appropriately participate in their care, and to treat the patient with respect and dignity'. The interpersonal dimension has all too frequently been ignored, underestimated or misunderstood. The archaic view still persists in some quarters that communication cannot be taught. On the one hand it is argued that it is a 'natural attribute' and that 'you either have it or you haven't'. Alternatively it is suggested that it can only be picked up 'on the job' and that intelligent individuals have no difficulty doing so. As a consequence, communication has tended to be relegated to the 'hidden curriculum', rather than being formally and explicitly addressed. More enlightened thinking, though, recognizes that 'Teaching communication skills is arguably the most important part of the medical curriculum, not an optional extra' (Sleight, 1995, p. 69). As discussed more fully in Chapter 2, the need for explicit instruction in this area is increasingly gaining acceptance.

When training has been attempted, inappropriate methods have frequently been employed, leading to largely ineffective outcomes. Many of those tutors who have been given the task of providing formal instruction in interpersonal skills are unfamiliar with the training possibilities that exist (MacLeod Clark and Faulkner, 1987; Davis and Fallowfield, 1991). Approaches which define communication skills in more explicit terms and offer a systematic and structured approach are advocated by many (Eastwood, 1985; Fielding and

Llewelyn, 1987) and are often better received by students (Bird *et al.*, 1993). The instructional procedure which we present in this book is of this type.

1.6 COMMUNICATION

What exactly is communication? We have taken the term somewhat for granted. It may be useful, therefore, to pause at this point to examine what communication actually is. As a concept, communication is notoriously difficult to pin down. Ellis and Beattie (1986) described it as 'fuzzy', with boundaries that are blurred and not altogether certain. This, understandably, has created difficulties when it comes to matters of formal definition. Holli and Calabrese (1991) attributed the problem in part to the range of disparate activities subsumed under this label. From the plethora of definitions of communication that have been mooted over the years, Hewes and Planalp (1987) distilled two central themes:

- **intersubjectivity**, which has to do with striving to understand others and being understood in turn;
- **impact** which represents the extent to which a message brings about change in thoughts, feelings or behaviour.

1.7 INTERPERSONAL COMMUNICATION

Interpersonal communication concentrates upon communication which is non-mediated (or face to face), takes place in a dyadic (one-to-one) context or small group, with participants being essentially unconstrained in the form and content of their interaction by other than normal personal characteristics and the dictates of the situation within which they find themselves (Hartley, 1993). In simple terms, it has been defined by Brooks and Heath (1985, p. 8) as 'the process by which information, meanings and feelings are shared by persons through the exchange of verbal and non-verbal messages'. Several features of interpersonal communication will now be briefly elaborated.

1.7.1 Interpersonal communication is a transactional process

The notion of process is one of the most commonly cited characteristics of interpersonal communication, accentuating the ongoing, dynamic quality of the activity. This process involves at least two participants, who individually act as source–receivers (i.e. they are simultaneously both senders and receivers of messages). Other related concepts are:

- message – the content of communication and that which communicators wish to share;
- medium – the means which they use to do so, such as touch, speech, etc.;

- code – the system of signs and symbols through which meaning is established (e.g. English language, semaphore);
- channel – that which 'connects' communicators and accommodates the medium (e.g. sound waves, light waves, etc.);
- noise – which can be regarded as any interference with the successful exchange of meaning;
- feedback – information on the extent to which a message was successfully received;
- context – all interpersonal communication takes place within frameworks which may be physical (e.g. the setting), relational (e.g. doctor–patient) or temporal (e.g. in the morning), to name but a few.

Describing the communication process as transactional implies that an alteration to any one of the components brings about corresponding changes to others and affects the system as a whole. As each participant acts and reacts to the other in a system of reciprocal influence, ongoing adjustments are made to the communication which unfolds (Burgoon, Hunsaker and Dawson, 1994).

1.7.2 Interpersonal communication is purposeful

Another commonly cited feature of this activity which should be recognized is its purposefulness. Those who enter into it, do so with some end in mind; they want to effect some desired outcome. To put it another way, communicating is a strategic act (Kellermann, 1992). It is this purposefulness which both provides impetus and gives direction to the transaction. French (1994) proposed that the nurse communicates with the patient to:

- establish and maintain a relationship;
- promote equality in that relationship;
- gather information;
- provide information;
- facilitate self-expression;
- promote recovery;
- reassure the patient;
- manage and control.

Describing communication as purposeful does not imply, however, that it must always be done with conscious awareness (Hargie, Saunders and Dickson, 1994). Messages may even be conveyed unintentionally (e.g. disgust on the face of a doctor examining an infected wound) (DeVito, 1995).

1.7.3 Interpersonal communication is multidimensional

Another significant feature of communication is its multidimensionality – messages exchanged are seldom unitary or discrete. Watzlawick, Beavin and Jackson (1967) asserted that it takes place at two separate but nevertheless interrelated levels. One has to do with substantive content, the other with relational matters, helping to determine how participants define their association in terms of, for instance, extent of affiliation, balance of power and degree of intimacy and trust. This bifurcation has been found to have broad validity in the field of health communication, where Thompson (1990) stressed its importance in understanding nurse–client interaction.

Content is probably the more immediately recognizable dimension of interpersonal communication, dealing as it does with the subject matter of talk. But familiarity should not be allowed to conceal the fact this is often problematic. Meanings belong to the people who use the words, not to the words themselves. The same word has often radically different connotations for interactors, leading to confusion, misunderstanding and possible distress. To the patient the description of a condition as 'chronic' may conjure up a whole set of quite different, possibly alarming, images from those it would for the health worker! Sutherland *et al.* (1991) produced evidence that cancer patients attach markedly differing interpretations to probabilistic information based upon words and phrases like 'common', 'occasionally', 'rarely', 'may occur', etc. Considerable diversity also appears to exist amongst health professionals in the meanings attached to psychological terms (Hadlow and Pitts, 1991)!

Through relational communication, interactors work at establishing where they stand with each other *vis-à-vis*, for instance, dominance, intimacy and liking. These matters are typically handled in an indirect and subtle way involving, although not exclusively, non-verbal behaviour such as eye contact, touch and interpersonal distance (Knapp and Hall, 1992). Forms of address and ways of conducting talk are also implicated (Hargie, Saunders and Dickson, 1994).

Elaborating upon these notions, Wilmot (1987) highlighted the complexity of the interrelationship between these two facets of communication – content and relationship. While relational issues are seldom explicitly confronted at the content level, the way in which discourse is conducted has inevitable relationship implications. This assertion was borne out in the study by Chalmers and Luker (1991) of the development of health-visitor–client relationships. Building the relationship was found to be a feature of the ongoing interactional process rather than being in some way separate and distinct from it. Even when the relationship became problematic it was uncommon for this topic to become part of the content of communication and be dealt with explicitly.

Communication has additionally an identity dimension. Personal, social and professional identities are projected, and in turn either confirmed or invalidated, in the types of topic chosen to form the content of talk, the linguistic codes used, accents revealed, along with non-vocal features of dress and general deportment.

In addition to the projection of an image of self, the health worker can propose, affirm or deny a particular patient identity in the ways in which the latter is related to. This may be grossly at odds with the 'face' being presented by the patient, reflecting a personal sense of self. Simplified addressee registers, including 'secondary baby talk', are sometimes a feature of helper conversations with the elderly (Caporael and Culbertson, 1986) and people with learning disability (Sines, 1988).

Finally, interactors can, in part, create the situation which they share in communicating. An assessment interview, for instance, can take on the trappings of a relaxed, friendly chat or something approaching an interrogation depending upon, amongst other features, the amount and type of questioning featured.

1.7.4 Interpersonal communication is inevitable

This is a contentious claim made by some theorists (e.g. Watzlawick, Beavin and Jackson, 1967; Scheflen, 1974) who hold an extremely broad view of what constitutes communication. It is represented in the often-quoted maxim that under circumstances where people are aware of the presence of others in a social situation, 'one cannot **not** communicate' (Watzlawick, Beavin and Jackson, 1967, p. 49). All witnessed behaviour is communicative. Others, including Ekman and Friesen (1969) and Burgoon, Hunsaker and Dawson, (1994), restrict communication to a particular subset of human behaviour on the basis of several criteria including intention. Interpersonal communication presupposes some degree of intentionality, they hold. It is argued that while some behaviours (e.g. blushing, spontaneous yawning, etc.) might be expressive of bodily or psychological states and thereby informative, they are not strictly speaking communicative. This conceptual distinction makes informing but not necessarily communicating inevitable. The implications are significant. As we shall see, intentionality and control are entailed when referring to communication as a skilled activity. (A fuller discussion of the issue can be found in Hargie, Saunders and Dickson, 1994.)

1.7.5 Communication is irreversible

Simply put, when something has been said it cannot be taken back. A junior doctor begins to discuss with the patient how a cancer is reacting to treatment, unaware of the fact the patient has not been informed that a treated 'mole' was malignant! But it must not be overlooked that the personal and relational consequences of such actions can sometimes be retrieved. 'Accounts', which can be thought of as explanations for troublesome acts, are one communicative device which is often used to this end. We explain why we acted in the way that we did to make the action more acceptable and/or ourselves less culpable.

1.8 COMMUNICATION COMPETENCE

Communication that is consistently and inclusively effective invokes the idea of competence. Arriving at a commonly accepted defining of communication competence, however, is a daunting task. Many possibilities abound (Kreps and Query, 1990). Part of the inconsistency resides in how the relationship between notions of **competence** and **performance** is construed. According to Chomsky (1965) competence can be thought of narrowly as knowledge: the knowledge that an individual has of a language and the rules which govern it. As such, it is quite distinct from performance, or what a person might or might not do. Further differentiations have been made between, as Fillmore (1979) puts it, 'knowing that' and 'knowing how'. (A medical student may know about epidurals, their effects and when they should be used, but not know precisely how to perform one.) Certain theorists, therefore, define competence to include both of these types of knowledge while still excluding actual behavioural aspects (e.g. Cooley and Roach, 1984). Others go a step further to incorporate both knowledge and performance in their conceptualization of communication competence. Parks (1994, p. 591) asserted that 'to be competent therefore we must not only "know" and "know how", we must "do" and "know what we did"'. This more inclusive way of thinking is endorsed by, for example, Rubin (1990) who argued for the concept having cognitive, behavioural and affective/motivational dimensions. It is this broad view that will be adopted in this book.

Several additional features of communication competence are worth highlighting. Spitzberg and Cupach (1989) pointed out that two attributes seem to feature in most deliberations on the topic. They are **effectiveness** (i.e. being successful at achieving a set goal or completing a task) and **appropriateness** (i.e. avoiding contravening norms, rules or expectations about interpersonal conduct). In relation to the latter, it should be appreciated that much of what is accepted as being socially competent is very much culturally determined. Thus what constitutes competent behaviour in one context may not do so in another (DeVito, 1995).

Communicative competence is circumstantially determined in another sense. As noted by Rubin (1990), it is really an impression or judgement based upon inferences made from observations and experiences. The values, beliefs, attitudes and standards observers reflect in their customary ways of relating must not be overlooked in establishing which performances warrant this label. In a sense, a communicator is only socially recognized as competent when judged to be so by another, no doubt based upon criteria such as effectiveness and appropriateness.

Three other features of communicative competence that Parks (1994) regards as pivotal, which will also be taken up again when we turn our attention to the notion of communication skill, are **control**, **adaptability** and **collaboration**. Being socially competent presupposes the successful exercise of a measure of control over one's interpersonal environment. Adaptability entails making behavioural choices on the basis of an ongoing monitoring of outcomes. It is the opposite of rigidly pursuing fixed courses of action. Finally, social competence requires the collaboration of others.

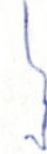

1.9 COMMUNICATION AS SKILL

The distinction between communication competence and communication skill is often blurred in the literature (Spitzberg and Cupach, 1989). In some cases, 'skill' has been used to refer only to the strictly performative aspects of competence and separated from knowledge and motivational dimensions in this way. While acknowledging the unavoidably action-based connotations that surround the term, regarding 'skill' as such is overly simplistic. After all, behaving in a truly skilful way in a social setting commonly requires considerable knowledge about routines, conventions and such like. Likewise, it depends upon potentially dysfunctional emotions being held in check. The stance taken here, therefore, approximates that which Rubin (1990) described as the communication skills approach to communication competence. As such, 'skills typically represent the specific components that make up or contribute to the manifestation or judgement of competence' (Spitzberg and Cupach, 1989, p. 8). In so doing, the concept of skill, while narrower than that of competence, shares many of the same attributes, as we shall see.

The scientific study of skill has a long and illustrious pedigree within psychology. The possibility of 'skill' being applicable to what takes place during an interpersonal exchange is less immediately evident. Crossman (1960) is generally credited with having first drawn parallels between perceptual–motor skill performance and the processes underpinning social interaction. The analogous nature of social and motor skills was further elucidated by Argyle and Kendon (1967). Both types of activity, it was argued, are carried out with the intention of achieving some end-state; both rely upon a complex system of perceptual, central and motor mechanisms; and in both cases purposive actions are associated with commensurate environmental changes the careful monitoring of which enables decisions to be taken as to goal achievement. Limitations of the analogy were also recognized. These are taken up in Chapter 3.

But what exactly is communication skill? Again there is no single, commonly accepted answer to this question. Dimbleby and Burton (1985, p. 58) define it as 'an ability to use means of communication effectively, with regard to the needs of those involved'. It is therefore accomplished within the parameters of communicative competence as already explained. Acknowledging the needs and rights of all concerned is another feature strongly endorsed by many. Skilled communication, therefore, involves much more than the mere encoding, transmission and decoding of a message in such a way that it is understood.

The main defining feature of communication skill offered by Dimbleby and Burton would appear to be the effective use of available means, once more in keeping with one of the features of competence already introduced. This criterion is also encompassed within the comprehensive definition of skill given by Hargie, Saunders and Dickson (1994, p. 2) as 'a set of goal-directed, interrelated, situationally appropriate social behaviours which can be learned and which are under the control of the individual'. Here, six separate components of skilled performance are stressed.

- **Goal-directed.** The purposive nature of communication has already been highlighted. But 'skill' implies not only that acceptable intentions have been successfully actualized but that they have been actualized in a particular way. There is a connotation of efficiency in the manner in which the goal state is attained. It has sometimes been described as obtaining the maximum effect from the minimum of effort. Along these lines, Dickson, Saunders and Stringer (1993) refer to skilled performance as having 'utility'.
- **Inter-related.** Elements of communication, both verbal and non-verbal, must be closely synchronized in order to bring about a desired consequence.
- **Appropriateness.** It has already been mentioned that appropriateness of use is a prerequisite of communicative competence. This applies both to the goals striven for and the manner in which they are pursued during skilled action.
- **Behaviours**. Dickson, Saunders and Stringer (1993) refer to the 'behavioural facility' of skills. Skills involve identifiable units of behaviour which the individual displays. But this does not mean, however, that such actions have a mystically inherent quality by dint of which they are skilful in some absolute sense. What makes them 'skilled' is their use within the framework of characteristics of skilful performance already identified. Perceptual, affective and cognitive elements will be introduced in Chapter 3.
- **Learned.** It is widely accepted that most forms of behaviour displayed in social contexts, apart from basic reflexes, are learned by the individual. Verbal and non-verbal communication peculiar to a culture is a very obvious case-in-point. This fact, of course, makes CST a viable proposition.
- **Control.** To be considered skilful, communicators must have a measure of control over actions and outcomes.

1.10 APPROACHES TO TRAINING

Since communication skills are essentially learned entities they must be amenable to training. Several broad approaches to this task will now be considered.

1.10.1 'Doing the job' training

The 'logic' behind this strategy is that, having been successful in obtaining a certain job, one then begins to train oneself to do it, while doing it! Argyle (1994), in reviewing research conducted into on-the-job learning, concluded that while this method is probably the most common, it 'seems to be a very unreliable form of training. A person can do a job for years and never discover the right social skills' (p. 290).

Yet this approach is the one that has traditionally been employed in the health professions in respect of the interpersonal parameters of the work undertaken. It is still invoked by those who view communicative competence as something that will 'come with experience' being essentially 'caught rather than taught'. The available empirical evidence would seem to offer scant support for the comfortable assumption that this aspect of the professional role is gradually but inevitably acquired through increased experience (Maguire, 1986).

There are a number of inherent weaknesses of this method of training.

- Learning is predominantly by trial and error.
- The learner may develop habits of 'survival' rather than situationally appropriate strategies and skills.
- The learner may be unable to cope in certain situations or cope at the expense of the patient.
- It raises profound ethical issues.

It does have one advantage, however, in that issues of transferring learning outcomes from the training setting to the work-place are, of course, redundant.

1.10.2 'Model the Master' training

This technique consists of a learner being assigned to an experienced professional. The rationale would appear to be that, through observation of 'the Master' at work, the skills displayed will be grasped by the novice. This, of course, is the philosophy underpinning the apprenticeship system of vocational training. Indeed elements of it can be found in most courses incorporating periods of practical placement or clinical experience. Many medical schools and postgraduate training programmes continue to rely upon it. But when exclusive reliance is placed upon this technique, training can be limited, as Maguire *et al.* (1978) discovered in relation to the history-taking skills of medical students.

Again there are problems surrounding this mode of instruction.

- The notion of the 'master practitioner' is contentious. Even experts have bad habits and can make mistakes.
- There is no guarantee that the neophyte will identify the subtleties of effective performance and discriminate between those and inappropriate ways of relating.
- Particular difficulties may occur in modelling when there are marked differences between the experienced professional and the student in, for instance, cultural background, attitude, personality, age, sex and behavioural style.
- It promotes conservatism and militates against innovation, given that experts may not be aware of the considerable literature on, for instance, factors that enhance patient comprehension, recall, satisfaction and adherence/compliance.

1.10.3 Directed training procedures

This rubric includes disparate techniques for providing instruction prior to job experience. They are all classroom-based and explicitly directed to the furtherance of interpersonal functioning. While sharing this general aim, marked differences exist in relation to the formulation of specific training objectives and, more evidently, the procedures implemented in order to achieve them. We can typify them as methodologically based on 'thinking', 'feeling' or 'doing' (Phillips and Fraser, 1982; Laird, 1991; Irving, 1995).

'Thinking'-based methods of training

This approach tends to favour more traditional, didactic techniques. The emphasis is upon providing information and effecting conceptual learning by means of, for example, readings, formal lectures, seminars, group discussions, films and case studies. Throughout, trainees are expected to be essentially passive and receptive. They are required to assimilate content and thus further their knowledge and understanding of interpersonal communication and its various facets, but to do little else. In relation to the different dimensions of competence it is, therefore, knowledge about communication that is, primarily, targeted.

While this approach is non-threatening and safe, familiar and, if well done, intellectually satisfying, Phillips and Fraser (1982) highlighted some of its weaknesses.

- It provides little opportunity for skills to be developed.
- Trainees may fail to personalize the knowledge.
- Too great a dependence upon the trainer is often fostered.
- It fails to adequately address the complementary dimensions of communicative competence.

'Feeling'-based methods of training

Here training concentrates upon the affective component of social functioning and the illumination of interpersonal operation is achieved by this means. Approaches that can be grouped under this heading rely upon experiential learning afforded by some sort of small group participation such as a T-group or sensitivity training group.

Broadly speaking the aim of this type of training is to increase awareness and sensitivity. At the end of the experience members should be more aware of themselves, their needs, motives and feelings, together with the impact that they have on others. They should also be more sensitive to those with whom they may come in contact. This is achieved through the process of group involvement – the group itself is the learning resource. The group contemplates itself and what is happening within it. Participants, therefore, share perceptions of each other and what is taking place and by so doing exchange feedback. A corollary of this is that the group is responsible for its own learning, making it much more difficult for the trainer to specify pre-determined learning objectives.

In addition to utilizing the group as a vehicle for learning, T-groups share several other features. They tend to have a 'here-and-now' orientation: discussion is based upon what is being experienced at that time in the group. They are less structured than many of the 'thinking' and 'doing' approaches; are typically process-directed; and explore the internal and external bases of various happenings in the group.

Advantages of this method are in providing trainees with total involvement in, and responsibility for, training; increasing awareness of self and others; and heightening appreciation of the role of the affective domain in interpersonal relationships.

Among the disadvantages, on the other hand, can be included the fact that they:

- may be threatening especially for the more shy, introverted, timid and serious participant;
- can prove damaging for some trainees;
- have little conceptual framework given for what takes place;
- pose difficulty in setting precise training objectives;
- may seem to bear little obvious relevance to the job;
- place more emphasis upon increasing interpersonal awareness than on the various other parameters of communicative competence.

'Doing'-based methods of training

These techniques rely upon action as a means of bringing about learning. Trainees undertake practical tasks of different kinds necessitating interpersonal communication with one or more others. The task may be a simulated exercise or could involve role-play (e.g. counselling a 'patient'). Throughout, training is closely related to what takes place during the task – with the performative aspects of the encounter. Practice opportunities can be built in to enable trainees to identify and implement various ways of dealing with the situation. Encouragement is often given by the trainer to try out different interpersonal skills and strategies. Based upon feedback provided, decisions can be reached as to those which are most comfortable and seem to work best. This is undertaken within the context of a tightly structured and controlled programme derived from clearly articulated learning objectives.

A positive feature of this approach is that it focuses directly upon what individuals actually do when they communicate. There are drawbacks nevertheless.

- Little insight may be gained into why what took place happened if exclusive emphasis is placed upon behaviour.
- Feelings may be neglected.

- Trainees may be more concerned with performing well and not making mistakes than with learning.

Rather than being thought of as inherently diverse and incompatible, a more fruitful framing of these three approaches acknowledges their unique contributions, complementing each other in a comprehensive training framework. Such a framework is reflected in the instructional procedure outlined in this book, which utilizes a variety of techniques, including lectures, readings, group discussions, videotape displays, role-play, simulation exercises and games, *in vivo* practice and focused feedback. In so doing, the complex and multifaceted nature of communication is respected.

While training must, accordingly, be concerned with behaviour, it must not be so to the exclusion of, for instance, the underlying needs and motives, feelings and emotions, perceptions and sensitivities of the individual. Consonant with the conception of communicative competence and skill already presented, effective instruction must provide knowledge, enable that knowledge to be used appropriately and ultimately make possible successful performance.

1.11 COMMUNICATION SKILLS TRAINING (CST)

In the view of Anastasi (1987, p. 740–741), 'Good communication training should conform to two principal criteria. It should be simple and it should be skill-oriented'. Thinking of communication in terms of skill has profound implications for training. In keeping with other examples of skill, what transpires when two (or more) people interact can be reduced to a set of subprocesses and constituent elements. An encounter with a patient may comprise greeting, getting information, giving information and parting. But analysis can take place at different levels within a hierarchical structure of performance (French, 1994). At the broad level of strategy the health worker could, perhaps, be interviewing, counselling or indeed influencing the patient to follow some course of action (Chapter 6). Each of these procedures is, in turn, capable of further analysis. At a more fine-grained level we can view the process as comprising molecular elements such as questioning, listening, explaining, asserting and so on. Each of these skills is amenable to further reduction (Chapters 4 and 5).

A corollary of this way of thinking is that the resulting subskills can usefully form the content of training. Trainees undergoing CST are typically not expected to attempt a full-blown performance, be it interviewing or counselling, from the outset. Instead the programme is organized in such a way that, in the early stages, isolated components are concentrated upon. A session, for instance, may be given over to questioning, another to non-verbal behaviour, the next to explaining and so on. Beginning training by concentrating upon these simpler task units has been endorsed with counsellors (Dryden and Feltham, 1994) and nurses (Faulkner, 1993). Because of the progressive and systematic nature of instruction, by the end of the programme the repertoire of skills practised should be synthesized into a complete and effective performance of the communicative task. This is brought about in a number of ways and alternatives for structuring training will be presented in Chapter 12.

Regarding communication as skill implies not only that instruction can be planned, executed and evaluated but points the way to the sorts of training method that may prove suitable. CST, as elaborated in the chapters to follow, is procedurally based upon fundamental concepts of learning theory including modelling, practice and feedback. Its origins reside in 'microcounselling', or to use the more generic label, 'microtraining', a technique pioneered by Allen Ivey to offer training in the skills of interviewing and, more particularly, counselling (Ivey and Authier, 1978). Reviews of research have attested to its general effectiveness (Baker, Daniels and Greeley, 1990; Dickson and Mullan, 1990; Irving, 1995).

The three key phases of the CST process are **preparation**, **training** and **evaluation**.

1.11.1 Preparation

An initial starting point with any training endeavour lies in identifying the needs of the trainees. The objectives of the devised intervention accrue from these. This entails establishing the specific skill requirements of the group. Some of the techniques available for unearthing precisely what health professionals do when they relate to others in particular situations will be outlined in Chapter 7. The outcome helps shape the content of training. Advantages of involving both participants and their managers in this process are discussed in Chapter 13, from the point of view of enhancing the transfer of learning outcomes to the work setting.

1.11.2 Training

The training process combines sensitization, practice and feedback components. During the sensitization stage, the student is presented with an analysis of the skill under consideration by means of a lecture, perhaps with group discussion and readings. This, it will be recalled, is very much a 'thinking'-oriented facet of the procedure, designed to contribute the necessary knowledge base. Skill discrimination also forms part of sensitization training. Practical examples of the skill in use, typically presented on video or audiotape, facilitate a more concrete appreciation of what is involved and promote modelling. The emphasis here is on fostering the ability to make appropriate use of the knowledge acquired as a result of skill analysis (Chapter 8).

The next stage of training requires that ability to be put to use. Trainees are given the opportunity to practise the skill in an interactive context. Chapter 9 examines this part and outlines some of the modes of practice available, together with their advantages and disadvantages. The reader will recognize this as very much a 'doing' form of training, which addresses the performative dimension of communicative competence. Following on from practice is feedback. Here participants are made more fully aware of what they did during practice in relation to what they were striving to achieve and the effects it had on the other party. This is a particularly important stage for promoting greater awareness of self and others, if properly handled by a skilful trainer. It forms the content of Chapter 10.

The rationale underlying this sequence has been characterized as 'telling them what to do, having them do it and telling them how well they did it'. While this is a crude oversimplification and mistakenly depicts an extremely trainer-centred operation, it does reflect the three essential training components outlined above.

1.11.3 Evaluation

The final phase of CST has to do with evaluation. This can be more or less formal and may be instituted for a number of reasons, including student assessment and programme evaluation. At the very least it should ensure a more successful intervention next time around. Chapter 11 is devoted to these issues.

In sketching this operational framework, we may have unintentionally created the impression of CST as an extremely fixed and inflexible procedure, uncompromisingly adhered to on each and every occasion. Nothing could be further from the truth. While accepting the basic tenets of this approach (namely that communication can rightly be construed as skilful, that analysis can reveal constituent elements and subprocesses, and that these skills can be systematically taught), trainers have modified and adapted the *modus operandi* of instruction just outlined to meet the needs of specific groups of trainees more fully and/or accommodate exiguous resources and limiting circumstances (see Chapter 12 for more detail).

This reflective strategy is strongly recommended. It has, nevertheless, spawned a plethora of idiosyncratic programmes, each representing something of a 'variation on a theme'. Inconsistencies in nomenclature also abound. While not wishing to deny that subtle conceptual distinctions exist between social, interpersonal and communication skills, in practice these terms tend to be used interchangeably (Hewitt, 1984), with essentially similar training procedures masquerading under different labels. This confusion is compounded by the fact that skills training of this genre has been implemented in remedial and developmental contexts in addition to that of professional education. As far as the latter application is concerned, though, there would seem to be an emerging orthodoxy favouring the adoption of the term 'communication skills training' or, more long-windedly, 'interpersonal communication skills training'. Our choice of title was made essentially on this basis.

1.12 OVERVIEW

In this chapter the concepts of communication and communicative competence were introduced and examined. Furthermore communication was presented as skilled activity and its associated characteristics expounded. One significant implication countenances the possibility of interpersonal improvement through training and contrasting approaches were considered. The particular training procedure featured in this book, communication skills training (CST), was identified and briefly outlined.

The importance of effective communication in the health professions and the extent to which practitioners manifest it were also introduced. It is to these fundamental matters that we return in the following chapter.

The importance of effective communication in the health professions

2

2.1 INTRODUCTION

The foundations of a case advocating a place for CST in the training of health professionals were laid in Chapter 1. Some of the issues introduced there are taken up again in this chapter and further developed. The notion of professional competence is examined in accordance with a model depicting the integration of several sets of subskills. Communication skills are identified, together with those of a technical and cognitive nature which have more commonly been associated with effective health care. A corollary of this extended view of professional competence is the acknowledgement of the necessity for instruction to be targeted on all its facets.

Continuing this theme, several major sources of influence which have resulted in the increasing acceptance of CST procedures as part of training courses for health workers are highlighted. These influences include a growing realization, in many quarters, of the traditional neglect of the social and behavioural sciences in the preparation of health professionals and the contribution of these disciplines to health care. Secondly, bodies within the different professions charged with the responsibility of maintaining standards of training and practice have begun to recognize a need for improvements in practitioner communication. Thirdly, this need has been underscored by research outcomes into what actually takes place at the patient–practitioner interface and its potential ramifications for patient satisfaction and well-being. Linked to the latter is a fourth factor, taken up in Chapter 7, to do with the consequences of appraisal- or accountability-focused audits of communication.

The extent to which CST currently features in the medical curriculum is surveyed to underscore some of the key issues relating to the place of CST in pre-qualification training. Some of the empirical work that has been conducted into the assessment of training outcomes is also examined and conclusions are reached as to the efficacy of this type of intervention.

For the present, though, we continue with a more fundamental consideration of the concepts of health and health need.

2.2 HEALTH AND HEALTH NEEDS

It was Voltaire who said that 'Doctors pour drugs of which they know little, to cure diseases of which they know less, into patients of whom they know nothing'. Clearly, at the receiving end of any therapeutic intervention is a person. The concept of a person rather than a patient is not often fully appreciated by health-care personnel, and is an issue largely neglected in professional training. Thus, the delivery of care is frequently conducted at an impersonal or functional level, reminiscent of a production line approach, with little attention being devoted to the interpersonal dimensions of practice, or indeed to the individual's behaviour and attitudes towards health and illness. It is, therefore, often a salutary lesson in interpersonal communication for the health professional to experience being a patient and thereby subjected to the realities of the health-care system.

Moreover, within the health professions the concept of health is often viewed within narrow limits, the focus of attention being on the physical well-being of the individual. However, it is important to understand that being 'healthy' can and does mean different things to different people. Ewles and Simnett (1992) have presented several practical exercises designed to help health practitioners examine their attitudes to, and concepts of, health in relation to their own lifestyle and practice, and the reader is referred to this resource material. These authors indicate that health needs to be understood not only in physical terms but also embracing mental, emotional, social and spiritual domains. The physical aspects of health relate to the mechanistic functioning of the body; mental health to the ability to think clearly and coherently; emotional health to the recognition and appropriate expression of emotions and also the ability to cope with stress, tension, anxiety and depression; social health to the initiation and maintenance of relationships with other people, and spiritual health to religious beliefs and ethical and moral codes, the keeping of which may be a means of achieving peace of mind.

These five aspects obviously apply at an individual level. However, the concept of health must also be viewed at a societal level in that health is related to society at large. This means that the idea of being truly healthy in a holistic sense must be questioned in societies where there is oppression, violence, famine, racial prejudice, or mass unemployment. Thus, at the practitioner–client level it will be important to recognize and perhaps relate across a much broader framework of health needs in order to provide effective health care within the context of a helping relationship. Exercise 2.1 can be used with students to stimulate thought along these lines.

Exercise 2.1 The helping relationship

Instructions

Divide the training group into small subgroups of three or four people. Give each member a copy of the case study and the questions for discussion. Each group should appoint a secretary and/or a spokesperson to feed back the group's response to the tutor. The responses should be tabulated and the main issues to emerge from the discussion should be highlighted.

Case study

Jane is a 19-year-old single parent living in a council flat with a 6-month-old baby. She has no family support but is visited regularly by a social worker, whom she views as interfering in her affairs. The baby has been very irritable recently and hard to manage although Jane has not expressed this difficulty to the health visitor. To ease her own tension Jane has taken up smoking again which she had stopped during her pregnancy. She asks a health professional for advice to help her stop smoking.

For discussion

- What factors are affecting (1) Jane's health, (2) her baby's health?
- Analyse these factors within a holistic approach to health.
- What communication problems/dilemmas/issues would you envisage in dealing with Jane?
- What actions or strategies would you employ to help Jane?
- What behaviour would be consistent with the helping relationship?

Thompson (1994) has highlighted the uniqueness of the health-care context, claiming that 'few other interpersonal contexts are characterized by the urgency and life-and-death nature that can exist in health care interactions'(p. 698). Health communication is also characterized by frequent interaction among those with pronounced status differences, for example, doctors being accorded high status in most societies. In a review of the clinical and social scientific research allied to doctor–patient communication, Waitzkin (1984) indicated that in regard to the sociolinguistic structure of communication, doctors often maintain a style of high control, involving many doctor-initiated questions, interruptions and neglect of patients' real 'life world'.

In contrast, the practitioner–patient consultation, when conceived as a helping relationship, is by definition different. Here a co-operative communication process exists in which the patient's needs and wishes are expressed and responded to by the practitioner. It is the adoption of a holistic approach to patient care that acknowledges and addresses not only physical needs but psychological and social needs, among others, that will result in greater patient satisfaction and more effective and comprehensive health care. Indeed Davis and Fallowfield (1991), in an extensive review of the literature, have demonstrated the positive health outcomes, both physical and psychological, that have resulted from counselling approaches to care.

Unfortunately, in communicating with patients the tendency of the health practitioner is to do what has been learned, that is to teach, to sell or to tell. Such behaviours are more likely to serve the professional than the patient, to the extent that the patient may be disadvantaged in negotiating his/her own needs. Thus, it must be recognized that patients are not products but people, deserving of their place, not to be manipulated or controlled by those in a position of power. While Thompson (1994) has shown that the bulk of the research evidence points to a negative evaluation of provider (practitioner) control of interactions, she argues for a balance of control in that patients want some, but are not comfortable having too much control in the consultation process.

The equilibrium that is required may well be achieved through recognition and application of Newell's (1994) critique of patient characteristics that are based on a humanistic account of human experience (Table 2.1).

Table 2.1 Assumptions about the patient (Source: adapted from Newell, 1994)

Each patient is unique	Emphasizes the individuality of the patient
Each patient has skills	Emphasizes the abilities of the patient, which can be utilized in a consultation
Each patient interacts with the environment	Emphasizes the situational aspects of the patient
Patients are like us	Emphasizes similarities that can be used to form therapeutic alliances
Patients are honest	Emphasizes patients' desire to give the best information they can
Each patient sincerely desires success	Emphasizes the positive goals and aspirations of patients
Each patient shares responsibility with the carer	Emphasizes the partnership within the consultation
Patients desire interaction and negotiation	Emphasizes the two-way exchange of information on a consultation
Each patient knows what the problem is	Emphasizes patient awareness of his/her 'situation'
Each patient knows when success has occurred	Emphasizes patient judgement regarding outcomes

2.3 PROFESSIONAL COMPETENCY

This book is premised on the assertion that any conceptualization of professional competence in the health setting must make reference to the inevitable communicative dimension of the job. Health practitioners comprise a number of professional groups, who are related not only on the grounds of health as a common focus but also by the fact that their activities involve pre-eminently face-to-face interaction and whose objectives, in terms of service, are largely effected through this means.

The notion of interpersonal competence has already been introduced and discussed in the preceding chapter. Professional competence is a wider concept. In relation to physiotherapy, Caney (1983) formulated a homoeomorphic model of the competent practitioner, which featured the integration of skills involved in communication together with those, traditionally recognized, of a more cognitive and technical nature. Similarly, Bensing (1991) classified the quality of practitioner (physicians') conduct along three lines:

- a traditional technical dimension, involving knowledge and technical skills;
- a non-traditional dimension involving concern for the psychosocial aspects of care;
- an 'art' dimension involving the interpersonal behaviour of practitioners, their personal qualities and how the care is delivered.

Applying these approaches on a wider basis, professional competence involves the ability to execute three main sets of subskills: cognitive, technical or psychomotor and social or communicative.

Cognitive skills

This represents the knowledge base of the profession, the body of knowledge that characterizes it and makes it unique from other groups of professionals. Obviously, within the health-care field there will be some overlap in the knowledge base because of similarity to, and complementarity of, practice activities. Cognitive skills enable informed judgements to be made and decisions taken in relation to assessing and meeting need.

Technical or psychomotor skills

This relates to the manipulative skills inherent in the profession. This is quite obvious within the physiotherapy discipline but is also exemplified by surgical and palpable techniques, blood pressure measurements, the application of dressings and analytical skills in other health professional domains.

Communication skills

This refers to the ability of the individual to interact effectively with others in the professional context. It represents the aspect of health practice concerned with practitioner–patient relationships, inter- and intra-professional relationships, attitudes and behaviour to the delivery of health care and compliance with therapeutic management. It is also the area which historically has received least attention in the curricula of the various health professional groups. Recently, the General Medical Council has gone some way to rectifying this situation in its recommendations for revising undergraduate medical training. In the new curriculum, communication skills is acknowledged as a central theme (General Medical Council, 1993).

While it is clearly acknowledged that it is important to be competent in each of these areas, the demonstration of one's competence to practise is, in reality, primarily based on assessment and appraisal of cognitive and technical skills. Communication skills are not subject to the rigorous scrutiny demanded in knowledge/problem-based or technical/manipulative tests. The challenge to assess seems too difficult and too inconvenient and, where there are communicatively poor students, refuge is taken in the view that 'a few months in practice will soon sort them out!'

2.4 IMPETUS FOR SKILLS TRAINING WITHIN THE HEALTH PROFESSIONS

In relation to communication in the medical context, Waitzkin (1984) has stated:

> Communicating well is an important part of practising medicine. Previously, practitioners have often paid lip-service to doctor–patient communication, have felt that it is someone else's problem, and have immersed themselves in the technical challenges of practice. The common assumption has been that communication is either too obvious or too mysterious to justify much detailed attention.
>
> *Waitzkin, 1984, p. 2446*

Applied to other health disciplines the statement is equally true for, as has been previously indicated, CST has been largely neglected in health professional training. Within the professions themselves there has been the feeling that the interpersonal dimensions of practice are naturally and automatically understood and acted upon and that socially skilled action is not amenable to training and education. Furthermore, research within this area has been met with a considerable degree of scepticism and resistance by those committed to traditional scientific investigation. Indeed, the viability of some university departments is seen to be dependent upon being able to attract significant amounts of external funding for 'scientific' research. It must also be recognized that part of the justification of this is that the end product from scientific research is also much more easily quantifiable than a 'better' practitioner. Resistance to change is also evidenced by the conservatism that exists in various health disciplines, where the form and structure of education is very similar to that which existed some 30 years ago or more and which produces the attitude 'what did for me then is good enough for you now!'

In addition, and also summary to the above, the development of CST within the health professions has been strongly influenced by a number of factors:

- the need to clearly identify and define interpersonal skills pertinent to particular contexts of practice;
- the lack of training or experience of teaching staff to actually teach communication skills;
- the lack of facilities and resources required to teach communication skills;
- the limited time available in already crowded curricula;
- the hidden curriculum syndrome – that communication is dealt with as and when it arises in the teaching of other topics;
- the lack of commitment from educators to introduce new areas of training;
- the limited cross-fertilization of teaching and research by the behavioural sciences to the health disciplines;
- the need for more evidence of benefit of CST courses in terms of patient outcomes;
- the need for a better understanding of the social and psychological contexts of health-care practice;
- the need to ensure an integrated form of CST.

Against this background it is important to highlight the major factors that have contributed to the increasing interest in the behavioural aspects of health-care practice and the development of communication skills programmes in particular. Among these can be identified the recognition of the neglect of the social and behavioural sciences in traditional training, the outcomes of reviews of professional practice, and research into patient–practitioner communication. These sources of influence will now be examined in turn.

2.4.1 The contribution of the behavioural and social sciences

There has been a move to redress the imbalance in training through neglect of the behavioural and social sciences in their contribution to health care. It may be argued that the relevance and success of these sciences in the education of health personnel will depend largely upon the multidisciplinary context in which they are presented, the degree to which they are considered as basic to the delivery of effective health care, their teaching and reinforcement throughout an individual's training both at pre- and post-qualification stages, the extent to which humanization occurs within the learning experiences of these personnel, and the degree to which the teaching and learning of the social and behavioural sciences result in improved patient care.

The Audit Commission (1993) has pointed to the difficulty of designing studies that test the relationship between communication and clinical outcomes, noting that the 'topic is both under-researched and poorly researched' (p. 3).

Yet, the Commission concluded that, 'there is increasing evidence of a positive relationship between communication and clinical outcomes across a range of clinical conditions and types of treatment'(p. 3). Thus, as a contribution to producing positive health gains, the application of the behavioural and social sciences to health professionals' training must be pursued. This will address the complexities of the individual, not only in chemical and biological terms, but emotionally, intellectually and socially.

2.4.2 Professional review of practice

Various reports following reviews of professional practice have strongly endorsed the need for better communication at the practitioner–patient interface.

Pharmacy

This is perhaps best exemplified by reference to the pharmaceutical profession within both the USA and the UK. In the USA, the Dichter Institute for Motivational Research reported in 1973 that many of the pharmacist's problems could be traced back to his/her failure to adequately communicate the value of his/her services to the patient. The pharmacist was stereotyped as the hidden practitioner closeted in his/her dispensary, typing labels and putting pills in little bottles, but who did not see, speak with or touch the patient. Furthermore, the report indicated that patients expressed the desire that pharmacists should communicate with them. Two years later, the Millis Commission (1975) gave strong emphasis to the need for good communicative ability among pharmacy practitioners and called for increasing the training of pharmacy students in communication skills.

Later the Association of Colleges of Pharmacy Study Committee (Chalmers, 1983) on the preparation of students for the realities of contemporary pharmacy practice addressed, among others, the issue of deficiencies in communication training and abilities. The report stated that 'the core and elective courses throughout the curriculum should include instruction, guided experience, and formal evaluation and feedback to students regarding their written and oral communications' (p. 398).

This recommendation would appear to have been heeded. Billow (1990) in a survey of US Colleges of Pharmacy reported that approximately 90% of respondents indicated that they offered a course specifically on communication skills. The remaining respondents reported that it was integrated into other study modules. However, the approaches to training were quite variable and individualized to a particular institution's curriculum.

In the UK, the Working Party report on pharmaceutical education and training (Pharmaceutical Society of Great Britain, 1984) stressed the importance of developing the interpersonal skills of students and graduates. It was pointed out that without such skills pharmacists would not have an adequate basis for the provision of the full range of professional services that should be available in community practice. Indeed, a satisfactory level of communication skills was suggested as a criterion for graduation and professional registration.

Perhaps more importantly the report of the Nuffield Inquiry into Pharmacy (Nuffield Committee of Inquiry, 1986) clearly identified 'pharmacy's neglect of its own social context, and social science's neglect of pharmacy' (p. 98). The report advocated that the pharmacy curriculum should be restructured to include the behavioural sciences to involve the teaching of 'social psychology especially in relation to the behaviour of health-care professionals and patients' (p. 104). Specific attention was also drawn to the importance and need to develop CST as part of both undergraduate and postgraduate education. Further, the Inquiry Committee recommended that 'research into pharmacy practice in co-operation with social and behavioural scientists should be increased' (p. 139).

The importance of these issues was also highlighted by the Government's discussion paper on Primary Health Care (Department of Health and Social Security, 1986), which pointed out the importance of ensuring that pharmacists' training supplements their scientific training with skills relevant to their wider roles, i.e. skill in communication, counselling and behavioural science.

More recently, the report of the Joint Working Party on the Future Role of the Community Pharmaceutical Services (Royal Pharmaceutical Society of Great Britain, 1992) emphasized the importance of the development of both clinical and communication skills and the provision of appropriate training at undergraduate and postgraduate levels. Furthermore, the Royal Pharmaceutical Society of Great Britain has required UK Schools of Pharmacy to include CST in their undergraduate programmes, in order for their degree to be recognized by the Society. This commitment to CST is also reflected in the Society's Code of Ethics, where the development of interpersonal skills forms part of a continuing education syllabus (Royal Pharmaceutical Society of Great Britain, 1995).

Medicine

It is possible to trace similar sources of influence from within other health disciplines. One good example of this at a national level was the Law Reform Commission's recommendation that the National Health and Medical Research Council in Australia formulate guidelines for the medical profession on the provision of information to patients about proposed treatment and procedures. Part of the impetus for CST here came from the recognition that patients should be given more information to enable them to better understand and make decisions about their treatment. In attempting to set out the content of communication, reference was clearly made to the way that information should be communicated, so prompting the training requirement. Interestingly, much emphasis was placed on respect for patients.

In 1993, guidelines were published and circulated among health professionals and public (National Health and Medical Research Council, 1993). Underpinning these guidelines was a set of general principles:

- Patients are entitled to make their own decisions about medical treatment or procedures and should be given adequate information on which to base those decisions.
- Information should be provided in a form and manner which would help patients to understand the problem and treatment options available, and which is appropriate to the patients' circumstances, personality, expectations, fears, beliefs, values and background.
- Doctors should give advice but not coercion.
- Patients should be free to make their own decisions.
- Patients should be frank and honest in giving information about their health, and doctors should encourage them to be so.

Paralleling the guidance about the nature of the information to be given was a clear directive as to how that information should be conveyed.

- Communicate information and opinions in a form the patient should be able to understand.
- Allow the patient sufficient time to make a decision. The patient should be encouraged to reflect an opinion, ask more questions, consult with the family, a friend or advisor. The patient should be assisted in seeking other medical opinion where this is requested.
- Repeat key information to help the patient understand and remember it.
- Give written information or use diagrams, where appropriate, in addition to talking to the patient.
- Pay careful attention to the patient's response to help identify what has or has not been understood.
- Use a competent interpreter when the patient is not fluent in English.

In its report on improving patient information and education on medicines, the International Medical Benefit/Risk Foundation (1993) concluded that one of the reasons why health care professionals have been ineffective patient educators is that 'insufficient attention has been given to the training of communication skills of health care professionals, and to retuning these skills in continuing education programmes' (p. 14).

Further, the report recommended that 'practical education on patient communication should be fostered in undergraduate curricula and postgraduate training for doctors, pharmacists, nurses and other health-care professionals. It should also be incorporated into mid-career and recertification programs' (p. 20).

Nursing

Within the UK, the Nurses, Midwives and Health Visitors (Training) Amendment Rules 1989 18A(2) state the need for nurses to learn the skills of communication in association with an understanding of the nurse–client–family relationship, and to function effectively in a team and participate in a multiprofessional approach to the care of patients and clients. The teaching of these skills is mandated in the *Curriculum Requirements and Guidelines* issued by the National Board for Nursing, Midwifery and Health Visiting for Northern Ireland (1990).

Dentistry

In respect of dentistry, Furnham (1983a) has provided compelling reasons why social skills training is important to dentists, in terms of improving patient satisfaction, compliance and attendance, as well as possibly reducing occupational stress and improving job satisfaction. However, despite the fact that dentistry, like the other health professions, is an 'interpersonal profession', social skills training occupies no part of the formal curriculum of training institutions in the UK but is supposed to occur in the 'hidden curriculum'. Interestingly, however, the training syllabus for dental hygienists in the UK includes requirements in the behavioural sciences, including communication issues (Collins, Slater and Smart, 1993).

2.4.3 Practitioner–patient communication

The findings of research into the patient–practitioner interface have had substantial effect on the development of skills training programmes in the health professions. Indeed, Eastwood (1985) suggested that the need to improve nurse–patient communication is supported from three distinct sources:

- patient opinion studies which show social need;
- expressed needs within the profession to improve communication performance;
- nursing research into the clinical needs of patients particularly in respect of reducing patients' anxiety.

Research evidence from the dental field indicates that the attributes that patients seek in their dentists concern:

- the dentist's ability to perceive and cope with patient anxiety;
- the dentist's ability to establish and maintain rapport with patients;
- the dentist's ability to inform patients and provide explanations (Furnham, 1983a).

At the heart of this issue is 'What matters most to patients or clients?' It is, of course, well accepted that the quality of the practitioner–patient relationship is extremely important to the outcomes of treatment. Within the context of a consumer service, Parasumaran, Zeitholm and Berry (1986) have suggested that the behaviours that affect perceptions of service quality include reliability, responsiveness, competence, access, courtesy, communication, credibility, security, understanding and tangibles. A number of these issues are intrinsically linked to the communicative process and in their appropriate application inspire confidence in the client (Drummond, 1992). Exercise 2.2 can be used to bring this message home to the training group.

Exercise 2.2 Health professionals' communication behaviour

Instructions

Make out the matrix below on a worksheet and distribute to each member of the training group. Ask each person to complete the exercise individually before gathering feedback to record the range of responses for subsequent group discussion.

Reflect on your experiences (direct or indirect) with members of the health professions. List those communicative behaviours which for you were (1) positive and (2) negative.

Positive communicative behaviours	*Negative communicative behaviours*
e.g. Personal greeting	e.g. Lack of privacy

Ross, Bower and Sibbald (1994), commenting upon the research into practitioner–patient communication, have indicated that 'patients rate communication skills as the most sought after quality of the primary health care provider' (p. 17). Thus, practitioners need to be aware of their own behaviours and how they are perceived and interpreted by patients. Secondly, they need to be able to recognize, interpret and respond appropriately to patient behaviours. Thirdly, they need to be fully aware of patient expectations in order to begin to satisfy expressed and unexpressed needs. If, then, quality is meeting client needs and by implication contributing to positive health outcomes, this final element is of crucial importance. This is well reflected in the Toronto Consensus Statement on doctor–patient communication. Here quality is related to the freedom of patients to express their concerns without interruption, explaining and understanding patient concerns, greater participation by the patient in the encounter and the receipt of what is perceived as adequate information (Simpson *et al.*, 1991).

More specifically the results of research at the patient–practitioner interface can be summarized under six headings as follows.

Patient dissatisfaction with advice and information received

Among early studies, McGhee (1961) in a survey of 490 patients discharged from hospital reported that 65% of them saw communication with medical personnel as the least satisfactory part of their hospital stay. In a similar study, Cartwright (1964) showed that 60% of 739 patients recently discharged from hospital reported difficulty in getting the information they required about their illness, treatment, progress and tests. Their levels of dissatisfaction were strongly linked to their 'need to know'. Interestingly, they expressed difficulty in knowing whom to ask. Only 11% of patients said that the nurse was the main source of information, with 70% reporting that they received no information from nurses. Korsch, Gozzi and Francis (1968) in a study of child care referrals showed 40% of mothers highly dissatisfied with the consultation with the doctor as a whole. The overall evidence suggests that on average 35–40% of patients are dissatisfied with communications with their doctors (Ley, 1982a) and that the aspect of medical care that gives rise to greatest dissatisfaction is the amount and form of information received (McKinlay, 1972).

In a recent analysis of paediatric consultations Street (1992) showed that less satisfied parents received more directive and proportionally less patient-centred communication than did more satisfied parents. In addition, doctors' use of patient-centred statements correlated with parents' perceptions of doctors' interpersonal sensitivity and partnership building. Bensing (1991) identified particular behaviours as being most important in delivering patient satisfaction. In consultations where GPs were positively rated, they were observed to show more interest in the patient, had more eye contact, demonstrated more empathy and used more vocalizations of encouragement.

Recent reviews of research in this area are provided by, for example, Thompson (1994) and Lewis (1994). The latter concluded that the general practitioner's communication skills are a fundamental contributory factor in accounting for patient satisfaction. The giving of information is an important aspect given that 'people are driven by uncertainty to see their doctor and a requirement for information is high on their agenda. How this information is imparted is also of considerable importance' (p. 667).

Non-compliance with advice

Non-compliance with medical advice is a widespread, multivariate phenomenon. Crichton, Smith and Demanuele (1978) presented three primary factors that influence patient compliance with medication instructions. Firstly, the credibility of the information as viewed by the patient is an integral aspect of compliance. Here the patient must believe that the psychological, financial and physiological costs of taking the prescribed medication are less than the perceived benefits. Secondly, compliance is a feature of behavioural modification in the patient, and as such is a series of trade-offs by the patient between the normal daily routine and the restrictions imposed by the drug regime. Thirdly, the knowledge of the patient concerning his medications is important, in that if instructions are not understood medication errors and defaulting occurs. With regard to this latter aspect, Berger and Felkey (1989) have indicated that higher compliance rates are demonstrated among patients whose physicians give explicit and appropriate instructions, and more and clearer information, and where patient feedback is encouraged.

Against this background, decisions have to be made regarding what information should be given. Ley (1982b) listed three basic criteria that may be used to establish the information needed by patients, namely behavioural objectives, rationality and empirical criteria. The first is primarily knowledge-related, in that it is concerned with information about the disease itself, recognition of drug effects, etc. The second criterion demands that a patient is given sufficient information to make rational decisions about treatment (e.g. to weigh up the risks-to-benefit ratio). The third depends on having established a correlation between the provision of certain information and particular outcomes. Thus, effective explaining skills will be a fundamentally important part of the health practitioner's interpersonal communicative ability.

Patient satisfaction and compliance are related

In an analysis of patient non-compliance, Ley (1988) showed that almost 50% of patients were non-compliant not only with their medication but with other forms of medical advice. At a more specific level non-compliance was viewed as being related to a number of discrete variables:

- duration and complexity of regime;
- patients' levels of satisfaction;
- influence of family and friends;
- patients' perceptions of their vulnerability to the consequences of the illness;
- the seriousness of the illness;
- the effectiveness of the treatment;
- the level of supervision provided;
- patients' expectations.

Indeed, Becker and Rosenstock (1984) stated that 'compliance is greatest when patients feel their expectations have been fulfilled, when the physician listens and respects patient concerns and provides responsive information about their condition and progress, and when sincere concern and sympathy are shown' (p. 197). Correlations between satisfaction and compliance have also been made with the patient's perceptions of convenience and waiting time before and during appointment (Becker and Maiman, 1975).

A final aspect of the satisfaction–compliance relationship is the fact that it can be linked to the provision of information by the practitioner. For example, a meta-analysis of a large number of studies related to health-care communication indicated that compliance was positively associated with information-giving and positive talk, but where question-asking and negative talk were the norm the association was negative (Roter, 1989).

Patients often forget or fail to understand what they are told

Failures of comprehension are related to at least three factors:

- oral or written material is too difficult in terms of vocabulary, terminology, etc. for some patients (Becker and Maiman, 1980);

- patients often lack elementary technical medical knowledge such as the position of vital organs (Ley, 1977);
- patients are often reluctant to ask their doctor for more information (Maguire, 1984a).

Ley (1988) has summarized those studies into patient recall of medical information. What these showed was recall levels ranging from 40–88% in both hospital and general practice patients. However, these studies need to be interpreted against the background of the amount of information to be remembered, the delay before recall and the method of assessment of recall, whether free, cued, written or probed.

Cassata (1978) has made a number of other observations in relation to patient distortion and forgetting of medical recommendations.

- Instructions and advice are more likely to be forgotten than other information.
- The more a patient is told the more he/she will forget.
- Patients will remember what they are told first and what they consider most important.
- Intelligent patients do not remember more than less intelligent patients.
- Older patients remember just as much as younger ones.
- Moderately anxious patients recall more of what they are told than highly anxious patients or non-anxious patients.
- The more medical knowledge a patient has the more he/she will recall.

This leads to the fifth aspect of patient–practitioner communication.

Patient understanding and recall can be improved though better instructional technique, which will enhance patient satisfaction and compliance

A number of factors pertain to this issue. Firstly, patients remember best the first instructions presented (Podell, 1975; Cassata, 1978). Secondly, instructions that are emphasized are better recalled. Ley *et al.* (1973) used the term 'explicit categorization' to refer to attempts by the communicator to emphasize and label the message given to the patient. For example, a doctor, nurse or pharmacist may tell the patient that he/she should be aware of three things – the drug dose, how it should be administered and potential side effects – and then go on to give specific information on each point. Thirdly, repetition of instructions aids recall. Fourthly, the fewer the instructions given, the greater the proportion of remembered information (Podell, 1975). Fifthly, simplification of information aids recall (Ley *et al.*, 1972; Bradshaw *et al.*, 1975). Finally instructions should be concrete and specific. An explanation or instruction that employs vague indeterminate words and expressions is not as clear as one that employs concrete and specific information (Hargie, Saunders and Dickson, 1994). This is particularly true of situations where a helper is giving directions to a client. (See Chapter 5 for further information on the skill of explaining.)

It should be pointed out that the above factors are important for both vocal and written communication. The research evidence going back some 20 years clearly demonstrates that written information reinforces oral messages and that patient understanding and retention of information is improved by such provision. Unfortunately, routine provision of written information to complement the verbal message is not the norm, such that the Audit Commission (1993) has explicitly recommended that patients be provided with good-quality written clinical information.

Practitioners often ignore or fail to fully attend to the psychosocial needs of patients, which in turn leads to alienation from, and dissatisfaction with, medical care

Patient satisfaction, as a fundamental aspect of quality, is multidimensional. For example, Lochman (1983) suggested that patient satisfaction is a factor of the organization in which care is provided (accessibility, mode of payment, treatment length), the perceived competence of the practitioner and the relationship elements within the consultative episodes. DiMatteo and colleagues have argued that patient satisfaction is related to the emotional tone of the interaction, the transmission of information and the patient's confidence in the practitioner's expertise (DiMatteo and Hays, 1980; DiMatteo *et al.*, 1980; DiMatteo, Hays and Prince, 1986). Street (1992) indicated that 'patients' satisfaction with care and evaluations of physicians diminish when doctors are overly directive and rarely exhibit behaviour reflecting sensitivity to or interest in the patient's feelings, concerns and opinions' (p. 987). Maguire, Fairbairn and Fletcher (1986), in a study of 40 young doctors, concluded that most of them were extremely incompetent in giving information and advice to patients. In addition, few obtained and took any account of patients' views or expectations of their own predicament. There was also a tendency to avoid social and psychological aspects within the consultation.

In an effort to link the issue of satisfaction to communicative competence, Evans, Stanley and Burrows (1992) conducted a study of patient satisfaction relative to consultations with a control group of medical students and a group who had been exposed to specialized skills training. This study demonstrated superior satisfaction associated with the trained group across a wide range of behaviours including patients' psychosocial care, expressing warmth and caring and interview skills.

Epstein *et al.* (1993) described three core functions of the medical interview:

- gathering data to understand the patient;
- developing rapport and responding to the patient's emotions;
- patient education and behavioural management.

On this basis these authors argued the case for 'listening with both ears', one for biomedical information, the other for psychosocial information. However, because teaching is centred on the former there is the tendency to listen only with that ear. Thus the concept of 'double listening' needs to be given more emphasis, listening concerned with facts and listening with feelings (see Chapter 4 for further discussion of listening).

Overall then, the patient–practitioner focus provides compelling reasons why CST is, and indeed must be, incorporated into the education and training of health personnel. Such training of necessity has to consider not only models of the communication process but the range of social skills required to interact effectively at the practitioner–client interface.

2.5 COMMUNICATION SKILLS TRAINING IN THE HEALTH PROFESSIONS

Within the health professions medicine has had the longest tradition of CST. The refinement and development of interpersonal skills training in dentistry followed that of medicine, certainly within the USA (Jackson and Katz, 1983). Within the last 10–20 years skill-based training has become a more central part of nursing and pharmaceutical training. Individual initiatives within other health disciplines have also been described, including occupational therapy (Furnham, King and Pendleton, 1980), physiotherapy (Dickson and Maxwell, 1985; Maxwell, Dickson and Saunders, 1991), health visiting (Crute, 1986), psychiatric nursing (Hargie and McCartan, 1986) speech therapy (Saunders and Caves, 1986) and radiography (Makely, 1990; Hargie, Dickson and Tourish, 1994).

The first edition of this book traced the development of CST in various health disciplines. In the intervening years there is little doubt that CST has obtained a firmer foothold in the curricula of many health disciplines. At the same time CST does not receive universal acceptance as a fundamental area of training and is often relegated to the 'hidden curriculum', being dealt with as and when it is deemed appropriate. Wrate and Masterson (1990) wryly comment that 'Communication skills training being in the curriculum may seem like Banquo's ghost making an appearance; impossible to ignore but certainly not especially welcomed'. The following update on the medical situation serves to illustrate key issues in the development of CST in the health disciplines.

Two recent surveys in the UK have attempted to chart the development of CST in undergraduate medical education. In the first, Whitehouse (1991) surveyed departments in 26 medical schools. A total of 25 schools responded, covering 79 departments of which 44 (56%) were involved in teaching communication skills. Most medical schools appeared to have communication skills teaching in their curricula. However, considerable variation existed in terms of course objectives related to knowledge, skill and attitudes and in the detail and depth of their expression.

Based on the survey returns, Whitehouse estimated that communication skills' teaching averaged no more than 20 hours/year and accounted for less than 2% of curricular time. Group teaching was common practice and video recording with feedback was used in the majority of schools, although there was limited exposure to this training method. Evaluation of CST showed little standardization of assessment procedures, with more emphasis placed on subjective assessment by tutors than on the use of rating scales.

Although progress has been made in this area, variability of teaching practice was a dominant theme to emerge from the survey. Why this was so is perhaps partly answered in the assertion by Whitehouse that there is a 'tension between a perception of communication skills as fundamental to our role or function as doctors, or as a skill fundamental to our relationship with patients' (p. 316).

In the second study, Frederikson and Bull (1992) reflected many of the observations made by Whitehouse. The purpose of their survey was to examine CST (1) as a factor in selecting candidates for medicine; (2) as part of the total curriculum offered; and (3) in the manner, purpose and evaluation of training in communication. Again from the responses to the purposes of CST there was a clear dichotomy between 'medical function' purposes (i.e. communication skills to be used in a professional interaction) and the 'relational function' concerned with meeting patient needs and providing satisfaction. It is not then surprising that the authors concluded that CST is a relatively minor, low significance subject deprived its proper place in the medical curriculum, pointing out that 'medical education pays lip service to communication and interpersonal relations while remaining disease oriented in its approach' (p. 520).

The fact that only 25% of schools formally assessed communication skill competence was interpreted as failure in communication not being critical – desirable, yes! – but not essential. If true, this has far-reaching consequences, not least problems of litigation. In one report, Nesbitt (1990) quoted 59 complaints made in one month to the Medical Defence Union related to practitioner inability to communicate. Indeed, Frederikson and Bull (1992) concluded that 'the patient's problem ultimately becomes the doctor's problem and unless the issue of communication is adequately and appropriately addressed at the level of basic education, doctors will have to labour on with a disappointing legacy of dissatisfaction' (p. 521).

Against this background, the recommendations made by Carroll and Monroe (1980), following a review of 73 studies of the teaching of medical interviewing, are still pertinent today. In concluding that instruction in clinical interviewing had generally promoted significant gains in students' interview skills, they suggested four principles for designing instructional programmes:

- the provision of direct observation and feedback on students' interviewing behaviour;
- the use of standardized presentations of illustrative patient interviews;
- the explicit stating of the skills to be learned and evaluated;
- the provision of sufficient time to undertake small group or individualized instruction.

This approach has been followed by Morrow and Hargie (1988a) in the provision of a national communication skills training package related to pharmacist–patient communication, incorporating both video and written training formats.

2.6 EDUCATIONAL AND EVALUATIVE ISSUES

As has been previously stated there is a body of evidence to indicate that good communicative technique enhances patient satisfaction, aids compliance and improves recovery. But does training improve performance? What happens to performance over time? Are there any differences in specific outcomes? Do skills become habituated and do they become generalized across different situations? What objective criteria can be established to measure performance and to what extent can reliability and validity be built into evaluation scales?

The Toronto statement raised three important areas where questions remained unanswered in respect of doctor–patient communication (Simpson *et al.*, 1991). These concerned questions about clinical encounters, questions about education issues and questions about research methods.

Within the area of education the following queries were posed.

- Which are the most effective and efficient methods for teaching which skills and strategies?
- How does the stage of training or clinical experience of the learner effect optimal teaching methods and sequencing?
- How can teachers help learners to identify their resistances to encounter the full extent of their patient's problems?
- How can such resistance be overcome?
- Are all communication skills teachable?
- Which skills are most and least teachable?
- How can students' learning styles be best assessed so that training individuals can be appropriately tailored to understand needs?
- How can educational, health care, and reimbursement systems be best adapted so as to motivate and reward faculty or trainers and practitioners to learn and teach their skills?
- How can doctors continue to develop and apply their skills?
- How can persistent behavioural, perceptual and personal changes be produced?

2.6.1 The need for training

That there is a need for training is clear. Some 30 years ago, Byrne and Long (1976), in a study of over 2000 audio recorded doctor–patient consultations, concluded that the preferred focus of attention of the practitioner was an organic illness, with a neglect of emotional or social problems. Furthermore, there was little attempt to clarify that they had correctly identified or understood the patient's problems, and little opportunity was given to patients to ask questions.

Rees (1993) has drawn attention to the often communication mismatch between the patient's version of his/her medical story and the account constructed by the physician from selected augmented parts of the patient's narrative and from the signs of illness in the body. Rees argued in favour of patient-centred cure instead of a one-sided, physician-dominated relationship. Such incongruity can compromise mutual understanding and jeopardize effective communication. Because physicians too easily regard the medical version as reality, the re-presentation of the clinical picture to the patient may not be meaningful.

Maguire (1985), in analysing the key communication deficiencies among nurses, described their tendency to use closed or leading questions, so biasing the response made by the patient. In addition, reflective questioning skills among nurses have been found to be lacking (Faulkner, 1980), thereby closing down any extension or development of particular themes. Both authors also cited the poor ability among nurses to pick up cues covertly given off by patients. Lubbers and Roy (1990) have argued the case for CST in the nursing field, with particular emphasis on a range of skills to be trained and reinforced in continuing education programmes.

Morrow *et al.* (1993), in a microanalysis of questions asked in pharmacist–patient consultations, found that 98% of all questions asked by pharmacists were closed in nature, over two-thirds of which simply required a 'Yes' or 'No' answer, while 24% were phrased in a leading fashion. Those relating to psychosocial matters only accounted for 2%, the vast majority of questions being directed to clinical issues. The results suggested a controlling/directive style of interviewing that has inherent dangers, in that the information gathered may be incomplete or inaccurate, resulting in potentially compromised advice or action. Similarly, Morrow and Hargie (1987a; 1992) have identified a wider range of critical interpersonal factors in the pharmacist–patient consultation that have important implications for CST.

Further features of communication that are problematic and should be the focus of training have been identified by, for example, Dickson (1995a) as centring on 'inaccurate perceptions of patient needs leading to failure to detect or deal with psychosocial concerns, the adoption of an overly socially dominant position, and failure to show respect for persons. The greatest bone of contention, however, would appear to revolve around information-giving or rather lack of it!' (p. 65–66)

2.6.2 Improvements in skilled performance

In a comprehensive review of the teaching of clinical interviewing in the health professions, Carroll and Monroe (1980) concluded that 'instruction in clinical interviewing has generally promoted significant gains in students' interview skills, as measured by various cognitive tests, affective instruments and observed behaviours' (pp. 35–36). Evans, Stanley and Burrows (1992) have stated that 'students given such training subsequently display significantly improved interpersonal skills in their interviews with patients, compared to their traditionally trained counterparts' (p. 157). Such beneficial outcomes include eliciting more information, and more relevant information, the ability to communicate warmth and rapport to patients, and increased ability to detect and respond to patients' verbal and non-verbal cues.

Maguire (1984a) indicated that the most promising results would seem to follow training that has involved audio or television feedback. Using these feedback techniques, improved skills in empathy, responding to patients' feelings, covering psychosocial aspects and taking clinical histories have been demonstrated. Other evaluative studies within medicine have shown similar improved performance (Evans *et al.*, 1991; Gask, Goldberg and Boardman, 1991; Bowman *et al.*, 1992; Evans, Sweet and Coman, 1993; Kendrick and Freeling, 1993) but it is of interest to note that the majority of published reports relate to students in training.

Part of the reason is obviously that this is a 'captive' group who often have little alternative but to participate in evaluative procedures as part of their course assessment. It may also reflect the difficulty of carrying out similar studies in the real practice environment because of a reluctance or fear among practising doctors to submit to an audit of their communication performance. Where it has been carried out the interviewing skills of doctors who received feedback training were superior to those of doctors who had undergone conventional training in interviewing skills (Maguire, Fairbairn and Fletcher, 1986).

Within the pharmaceutical profession a similar situation exists where the majority of evaluative studies of CST occur in the undergraduate curriculum (Morrow, 1986). Again, the findings support the notion that training actually promotes skill performance in both content and process skills. Where assessment of CST among practising pharmacists has occurred it has been limited to self-reported methodologies the results of which suggest changes in attitudes, abilities and actual behaviour at the pharmacist–client interface (Hanson, 1981; Morrow and Hargie, 1987b, 1995; Hargie and Morrow, 1995).

In the nursing situation evaluation of skills-based programmes has been carried out during the training and postqualification stages. For example, Menikheim and Ryden (1985) described a self-reported methodology to assess skill development. Here students expressed a significant increase in their communicative competence following training. Davis and Ternuff-Nyhlin (1982) outlined a more controlled study using observer ratings of performance and also patient feedback to assess the impact of CST. The results suggested that in relation to interviewing technique the training produced positive outcomes at attitudinal, intentional and behavioural levels.

Exercise 2.3 Predicted outcomes of improved communication

Instructions

Prepare a worksheet with the following information. Trainees may complete it individually or as part of a group exercise. Take feedback and record the range of responses. This exercise may be also used to identify targets for evaluative procedures.

As a result of improved communication competence among practitioners what would you predict would be the positive outcomes for (1) practitioners, (2) patients and (3) the health organization?

Positive outcomes
Practitioners
Patients
Health organization
Specific outcomes

Davis and Fallowfield (1991), predicting the outcomes of improved communication and counselling, suggested several areas where changes could be expected to occur. These include professional satisfaction, diagnostic adequacy, patient satisfaction, treatment adherence, psychological consequences, patient understanding, memory and skills, improved physical outcomes and prevention. These authors traced the literature accumulating evidence to support each of the predictions. For example, Roter's work, particularly her meta-analyses of studies linking communication to outcomes, is particularly illuminating (Roter, 1989). Similarly, Mullen, Green and Persinger (1985), in a meta-analysis of 70 studies relating to treatment adherence (compliance) across a range of disorders, showed that various forms of behavioural intervention, including counselling, produced a significant decrease in drug utilization errors. It may be further postulated that there are other wider service benefits in terms of, for example, shorter hospital stays, decreased hospital admissions due to adverse drug reactions, reduced consultation rates, less frequent changes in treatment and the competitive advantage that could flow from competent communicative performance.

Maguire *et al.* (1980a) demonstrated the ability of nurses to acquire, through training, key social and assessment skills necessary for monitoring patients who had undergone mastectomy. In a further study Maguire *et al.* (1980b) showed that in a follow-up of these patients those who had been seen by the specially trained nursing staff had a more favourable outcome than those continued at the usual level of care.

In the psychiatric context, Goldberg *et al.* (1980) indicated that those doctors who establish good eye contact, pick up verbal leads and clarify key complaints while at the same time exercising appropriate control in the consultation are more likely to identify problems than doctors who do not have these skills. Moreover surgical patients have been found to rate students who possess good interviewing skills as more understanding and empathic than those who lack them (Thompson and Anderson, 1982).

In dentistry, Corah, O'Shea and Bissell (1985) reported that those dental behaviours associated with patient satisfaction included having a calm manner, providing reassurance, taking seriously what the patient has to say, telling the patient what is to be done and encouraging patients to ask questions. With regard to pain management, Johnston (1990), following an extensive review of 35 controlled trials, concluded that psychological methods 'have been shown to be effective in reducing pain, reducing analgesic use, reducing patient distress and increasing patient satisfaction with care' (p. 8).

2.6.3 Duration of effect and generalization of training

As mentioned earlier the Toronto consensus statement (Simpson *et al.*, 1991) posed the question: 'How can persistent behavioural, perceptual and personal changes be produced?' That question could be extended to ask: 'Are skills trained in one situation applied in another?' Maguire, Fairbairn and Fletcher (1986) demonstrated the greater clinical competence of doctors who had received feedback training on communication skills than those who had not. Their findings also suggested that the level of skilled performance decreases with time and this fact is also supported by other findings (Poole and Sanson-Fisher, 1981; Kauss *et al.*, 1980; Morrow and Hargie, 1987b).

That the influence of training diminishes with time suggests that generalization of the effects of training have a temporal dimension. However, in relation to the degree to which generalization of effects occurs, other factors such as tasks and persons involved may play a significant part (Mullan, 1986). Interestingly, Maguire, Fairbairn and Fletcher (1986) suggested some degree of generalization of interview skills training, in that the skills trained in a psychiatric setting were successfully applied to interviews with physically ill patients. More recently, however, Thompson (1992) has shown that in the evaluation of communication skills, performance was judged to be context-specific, thus demonstrating that such specificity is not purely knowledge-related. Techniques for improving generalization of training effects will be detailed in Chapter 13.

2.6.4 Assessment procedures

In relation to objectivity, reliability and validity of assessment procedures, a wide range of measurement strategies have been employed. These will be considered in Chapter 11.

2.7 OVERVIEW

This chapter has outlined the importance of adopting a holistic approach to patient care. Furthermore, it has identified the communicative competence of the practitioner as a fundamental part of the effective delivery of care. Historically, however, CST has been a neglected part of the training of health personnel and to date is still inadequately addressed within training curricula. Yet the evidence suggests that skills training is effective in improving communication performance, clinical practice and patient satisfaction.

PART TWO

Content of Communication Skills Training

A distinction commonly made by curriculum theorists is that between the subject matter to be taught and the methods and techniques that are utilized to do so. Part Two, which subsumes three chapters, is concerned with the former; the content of CST. Chapter 3 extends some of the notions of communication as skill introduced in the first chapter of the book. Here a theoretical model of the communicative process is developed which highlights its transactional nature. It is important for those undergoing CST to be made aware of the nature of communication and the underlying mechanisms by means of which it is effected.

The performative dimension of communication – what practitioners actually do when they communicate with patients or significant others – is concentrated upon in Chapters 4 and 5. A pervasive stylistic feature of interaction would seem to be that of directness. Health workers adopting a less direct style when interacting tend to make greater use of responding skills such as reflecting, reinforcement, listening and self-disclosure. These skills form the subject matter of Chapter 4. A number of initiating skills including questioning, explaining, opening and closing interactions, and asserting, which suggest a more direct style of relating, are explored in Chapter 5. There will be occasions, of course, even within the same consultation, when skills of both types are called for. Taken together, these two chapters present a set of what could be regarded as key basic skills of communicating, which should be part of the interpersonal skills repertoire of all health workers.

What transpires when two people interact can be analysed at a number of different levels. We can think of the doctor producing phonetic segments, morphemes, saying a word, asking a question, putting the patient at ease or conducting a consultation, depending upon the degree of resolution we bring to the analysis of communication. The last chapter of Part Two adopts a much more holistic perspective than that which identified the skills detailed in the two preceding chapters, by examining broad strategies which practitioners characteristically employ in order to achieve desired outcomes. Accordingly, the processes of interviewing, influencing, negotiating and counselling, together with their central features and functions form the content of Chapter 6. Responding and initiating skills already examined are reintroduced and synthesized within each of these strategic contexts.

Communication as skilled performance

3

3.1 INTRODUCTION

This chapter details a theoretical model of interpersonal communication, which provides a conceptual framework for programmes of CST. It develops and extends the analysis of communication skill presented in Chapter 1, where the analogy between social skills and motor skills was introduced.

In noting the similarities between motor and social skills, Argyle (1972) put forward a model of motor skill operation, which he claimed could usefully be applied to the analysis of interpersonal behaviour. As outlined in Figure 3.1, this model has five main components, namely goals, translation, motor responses, feedback and perception.

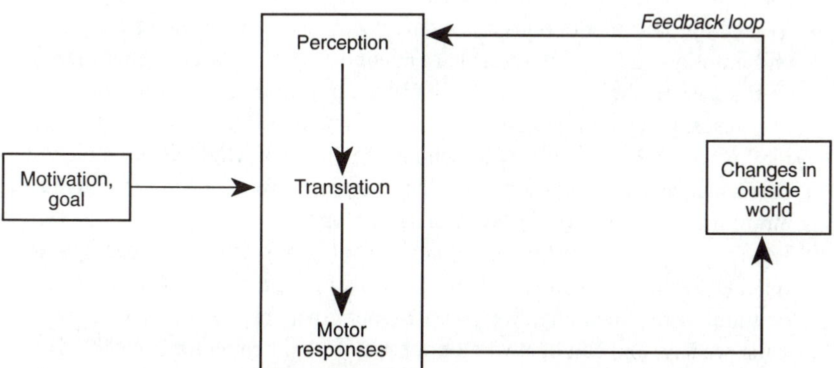

Figure 3.1 Argyle's motor skill model.

In relation to motor performance, an example of this model in practice would be someone sitting in a room where the temperature has become too cold (**motivation**) and therefore wanting to warm up (**goal**). This can be achieved by considering various alternative plans of action, such as putting on extra clothing, closing a window, turning on a heater, etc. (**translation**). Eventually one of these plans will be decided upon and executed. For example, a heater is turned on (**response**). The temperature in the room is thereby increased (**change in outside world**). This change in temperature will be **perceived** by the individual, and the goal will be deemed to have been achieved.

With regard to social performance, an example of the model in action would be a female at a party seeing a male to whom she is attracted (**motivation**) and whom she would therefore like to get to know (**goal**). In order to do so, she can **translate** various plans of action (look at him and smile, move close to him, introduce herself etc.). Eventually, she will decide upon one of these plans and execute it (**motor responses**) by, for example, saying 'Hello, my name is Joan; I don't think we've been introduced'. As she does so she will receive feedback from the male in the form of his reactions to her (**change in the outside world**), will **perceive** this feedback and, on the basis of this perception, decide upon her future course of action.

As these examples illustrate, there are clear parallels between motor and social performance in terms of the main processes involved. However, in exploring this issue Hargie (1997a) also noted the following important differences between these two sets of skills:

- Social performance always involves other people, whereas certain motor skills do not. One can eat, walk, type, swim, etc. without other people being present. However, by definition, other people must be involved during interpersonal interaction, so it is necessary to consider the goals of all those involved, as well as their actions and reactions towards one another. In this sense, social performance is often more complex than motor performance.
- The motor skill model does not satisfactorily account for the role of feelings and emotions during interpersonal encounters. Yet, it is clear that the affective state of the interactors will have an important bearing upon their responses, goals and perceptions. In addition, we often take into account the feelings of other people with whom we interact, whereas in motor skill performance this is not typically the case (e.g. we do not worry about the emotional state of a word processor we are operating!)
- Person perception differs in a number of ways from the perception of objects. Firstly, we perceive the responses of the other person with whom we communicate. Secondly, we perceive our own responses, in that we hear what we say, and can be aware of our non-verbal behaviour. Thirdly, there is the process of metaperception, which can be defined as the perception of the perception process itself. Thus, we make judgements about how other people are perceiving us and also attempt to ascertain how they think we are perceiving them. The process of attribution, wherein we attribute reasons or causes to the actions of others, is also important. Such judgements influence our behaviour and our goals during social interaction.

- The nature of the social situation in which interaction occurs has an important bearing upon the responses of those involved. The roles which people play, the rules governing the situation and the nature of the task all affect the behaviour of the interactors.
- Personal factors pertaining to those involved in the interaction also have a significant influence upon their responses. Such factors include age, gender and appearance. Thus there will be differences in the behaviour of a nurse towards a 4-year-old child, a 15-year-old male and an 80-year-old female. Recently, there has been a movement towards encouraging trainees to refer to patients by their first name. However, it may be the case, especially with more mature patients, that they do not wish such familiarity and prefer to be addressed more formally.

Having distinguished these important differences between social and motor skills, Hargie and Marshall (1986) put forward a revised model of dyadic interaction to take account of all of these facets. This model was further modified by Hargie, Saunders and Dickson (1994). As presented in Figure 3.2, this extended model takes into consideration the goals of both parties involved in interaction.

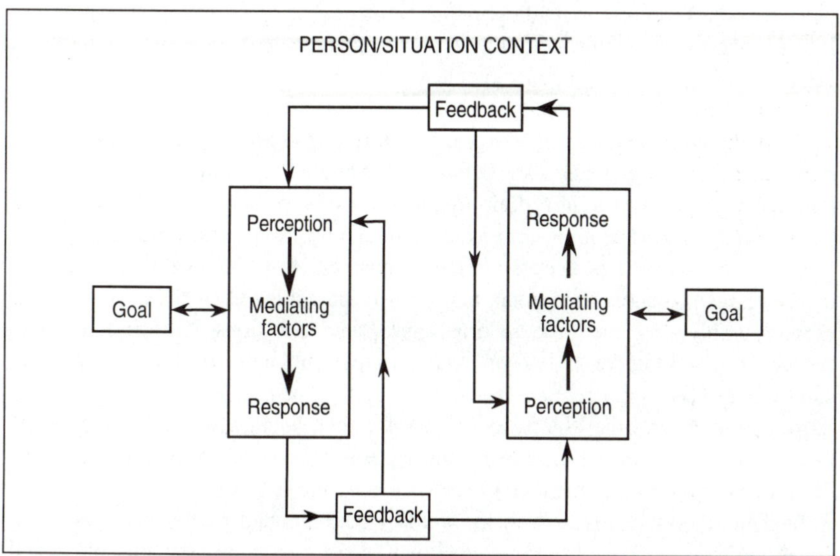

Figure 3.2 Extended model of interpersonal interaction.

It also recognizes the more complex nature of person perception as emanating both from one's own responses and from the responses of the other person. The term 'mediating factors' is introduced to encompass the role of feelings and emotions, as well as cognitions, during interpersonal communication. Finally, the importance of both personal and situational characteristics is recognized. The remainder of this chapter is concerned with an evaluation of each of the processes outlined in Figure 3.2. This model can usefully be presented to trainees at the outset of a CST programme.

3.2 GOALS

A central feature of the extended interaction model is the goal of the interactors, since behaviour is usually carried out in order to attempt to achieve certain predetermined objectives. Mulholland (1994, p. xiii) underlined the fact that each social encounter in which we engage 'is done with some purpose in mind, and that each person involved is trying to achieve a goal'. A goal can be defined as 'a desired place toward which people are working, a state of affairs that people value' (Johnson and Johnson, 1987, p. 132). Goals therefore both give incentive for behaviour and act as guides to provide direction (Locke and Latham, 1990). However, the individual may not be consciously aware, moment by moment, of the goals being pursued. Thus, just as a skilled car driver does not have to consciously think 'I want to switch on the engine, therefore I must insert the key into the ignition', so a skilled doctor does not consciously think 'I want to obtain an accurate diagnosis, therefore I must question this patient'. Indeed, one of the features of skilled performance is that once well honed it is carried out largely at a subconscious level, thereby enabling the individual to act in a smooth, skilled fashion.

A distinction also needs to be made between long-term (or primary) and short-term (or secondary) goals. Our behaviour is guided by short-term goals, with long-term goals being achieved through a subset of short-term ones. For example, a nurse may have the long-term goal of obtaining an accurate medical history from a patient who has been admitted to hospital. In order to do so, however, there are several short-term goals that need to be achieved, such as establishing rapport, explaining the task, asking appropriate questions, ensuring accurate responses are obtained, and so on. Indeed, these subgoals could also be further subdivided. Thus, in order to establish rapport, the nurse needs to effect a smooth introduction, ensure that the patient is comfortable, adopt appropriate non-verbal behaviours, etc. If any of these subgoals are not achieved, then the long-term one of obtaining an accurate medical history is made much more difficult.

In their review of research in the field of goal-directed performance, Weldon and Weingart (1993, p. 316) concluded that 'attractiveness of goal attainment and beliefs that the goal can be met are the immediate determinants of goal commitment'. Goals are selected on the basis of our degree of motivation to pursue them, while motivation, in turn, is influenced by needs. There are a large number of human needs that must be satisfied to enable us to obtain maximum satisfaction from life. Some of these are more important than others, and several different need hierarchies have been put forward by psychologists. The best known probably remains that proposed by Maslow (1954) as exemplified in Figure 3.3.

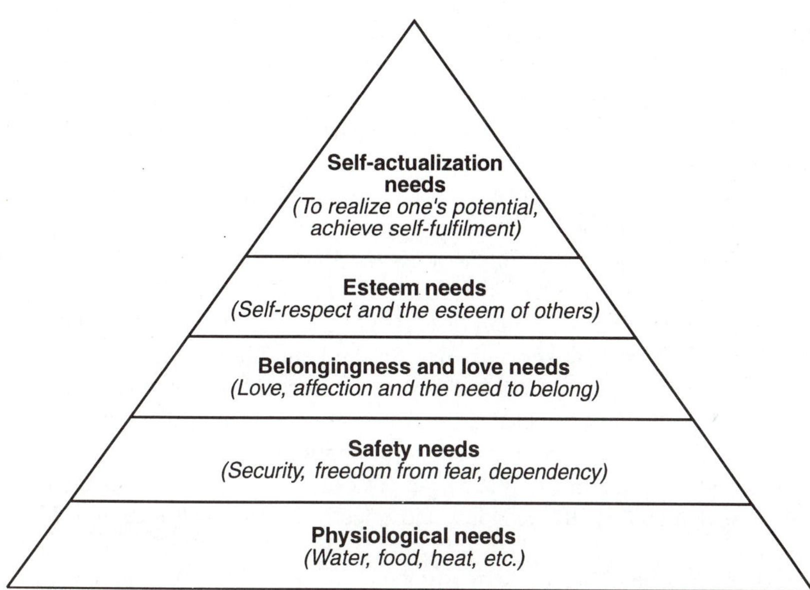

Figure 3.3 Maslow's hierarchy of human need.

At the bottom of Maslow's hierarchy, and therefore the most important, are physiological needs, concerned with the survival of the individual, including the necessity for food, water, heat and pain avoidance. Unless these needs are secured, the individual will not be particularly concerned with those at a higher level. Health professionals often deal with patients who are concerned with physiological needs and who will therefore have a strong motivation to ensure that these are satisfied. Patients who are in severe pain or who, for example at the preoperative stage, are worried about survival, will want the professional to deal directly with these concerns.

The second most important level relates to the safety of the individual and includes protection from physical harm, freedom from fear and the need for security. Thus, someone who has developed a serious illness may be worried about the possibility of being able to work again and, if not, how financial security can be achieved. At the next stage are belongingness and love needs, including the wish for love, affection and the desire to be part of a group. One of the problems with hospitalization, of course, is that the individual is cut off from friends and family who usually satisfy these needs. As a result, it is important that the health professional should be sensitive to feelings of loneliness or isolation in patients. Nurses, particularly, have an important befriending role to play in this respect. It is also interesting to note that patients often befriend one another, and this is an important process in itself. In addition, hospital visits by friends and family are crucial in maintaining belongingness and love bonds.

Esteem needs are also important. Maintaining self-respect, dignity and the esteem of others can be difficult, for example, in the case of patients who have become bedridden, are incontinent or can no longer feed themselves. Equally, an attractive individual who suffers severe facial lacerations, a woman who has a mastectomy or someone who has a limb amputated can all suffer from loss of esteem. Thus, sensitivity, patience and counselling skills are required when dealing with such patients. The final type of need is concerned with higher-order aspects, including the desire to achieve one's true potential.

As French (1994) pointed out, Maslow's hierarchy raises two important guidelines for health professionals. The first of these is concerned with the principle of meeting the lowest needs first. Severe pain in a patient requires to be dealt with before belongingness and love needs. Secondly, once lower needs are met, others further up the hierarchy will emerge and the professional has to monitor such changes and respond accordingly. In this way, the goals of patients will be influenced by their level of needs and an important goal for the professional should be to recognize and effectively deal with their immediate concerns.

The goals of the interactors in any situation are important determinants of behaviour. It is for this reason that we attempt to determine what the goals of other people with whom we interact might be. In fact, we are usually fairly accurate in making judgements about these, and this is why we are shocked if we discover that someone, whom we trusted as having honourable goals, turns out to have been deceiving us. In the health context it is important for the professional to explain as fully as possible any actions taken with a patient. Within the hospital setting, where patients are especially vulnerable, it is necessary to answer overt or covert patient questions such as: 'Why is this happening to me?' 'Why is she asking me this?' or 'Why do I need this medication?' In other words, the professional should pay attention to the important goals of the patient. Research in nursing has shown that mutual goal-setting (which involves identifying patient goals, developing goal-planning statements and evaluating patient goal progress) between nurse and patient results in increased satisfaction for both parties and facilitates patient well-being (Brearley, 1990).

However, on many occasions there may be goal conflict between practitioner and patient. As highlighted by DiMatteo and DiNicola (1982):

> Sometimes this conflict is explicit, such as when the patient wants a prescription and the clinician is unwilling to give it. . . . In other cases, however, the conflict and negotiation may be much more subtle and remain unstated. . . . An excellent example of this difference in perspectives is the interaction in the emergency room between a physician and a patient complaining of abdominal pain. Until the diagnosis is made, the practitioner must withhold pain-relieving medication in order to chart the course of the pain. The patient does not know this (and the practitioner does not explain it). The patient believes that the physician is withholding

medication out of cruelty, and is withholding communication (of diagnosis and prognosis) out of secretiveness.

DiMatteo and DiNicola, 1982, p. 74–75

Such goal conflicts need to be overcome before effective interpersonal communication can take place.

Goals, therefore, represent an essential starting point in the interaction model. Once appropriate goals have been decided upon, they will have an important bearing upon our perceptions, responses, and on intervening mediating factors.

3.3 MEDIATING FACTORS

Mediating factors are the internal states, activities or processes that mediate between the goal being pursued, the feedback that is perceived and the responses to be made. These factors influence the way in which people and events are perceived, and determine the capacity of the individual to assimilate, process and respond to the information received during interpersonal interaction. This process of mediation is important, since it allows individuals to evaluate to what extent their goals can be achieved, or whether new goals need to be adopted and different action plans implemented. In terms of such decision-making the two main mediating factors are cognitions and emotions.

3.3.1 Cognitions

This is an important area since, as Greene (1988, p. 37) noted, 'social scientists have come to recognize the central role of cognitive processes in social interaction'. Cognition can be defined as 'all the processes by which the sensory input is transformed, reduced, elaborated, stored, recovered and used' (Neisser, 1967, p. 4). From this definition it can be seen that cognition involves a number of important processes. These include **transforming** or decoding the information received from the sensory channels. Since there may be a large volume of such information it is necessary to **reduce** this in order to cope effectively. Paradoxically it is sometimes also necessary to **elaborate** upon minimal information by making interpretations, judgements or evaluations (e.g. she is not speaking to me because she is a shy child, is upset at being in hospital and is missing her mother). It is also necessary to **store** information in memory in order to cope successfully in social interaction. In particular, social information is dependent upon the effective use of a short-term memory store, so that individuals who suffer impairments in this facility find difficulty during social encounters (Antaki and Lewis, 1986). This is quite common among some elderly patients, who may have a very good long-term memory and can vividly recall the names of schoolfriends or teachers yet, because of impairment in short-term memory, forget the health professional's name seconds after being told it. Information that is stored can be **recovered** and **used** by the individual to facilitate the processes of decision-making and responding. Existing circumstances are compared with previous knowledge and experience in making decisions about action plans.

The development of conceptual schemas, or schemata, facilitates the process of problem-solving during social encounters, so that 'people acquire schemata that they use before, during, and after interactions to obtain information and make sense of it' (Heath and Bryant, 1992, p. 216). For example an experienced nurse will have a number of schemas such as: 'patient looks distressed', 'patient getting agitated', each with accompanying action plans – 'spend some time with him and provide reassurance', 'calm him down to prevent the agitation escalating and upsetting other patients on the ward'. There are four different types of schema (Saks and Krupat, 1988).

- **Person schemas** contain our knowledge of the goals, traits and actions of particular types of individuals (e.g. 'extrovert'; 'trustworthy').
- **Self-schemas** refer specifically to the set of person information we possess about ourselves – the beliefs we hold about our own personality, values and how we are likely to respond in any context.
- **Role schemas** involve the ideas and expectations we hold of people in certain social categories (doctor, patient, etc.).
- **Event schemas** are the knowledge structures we hold about certain situations and how to behave therein (e.g. the hospital ward, the canteen).

Schemas are formulated and developed primarily through experience, although one of the advantages of CST is that is can 'short-circuit' the time needed for their development (Crute, 1986). By providing college-based skill learning with related practical experience, in advance of actual clinical practice, it is possible to contribute to the schematic development of trainees.

Such schematic development will enable the practitioner to respond quickly and confidently in the professional context. This ability to respond rapidly and appropriately is in turn a feature of skilled performance (Hargie, 1997b). Thus, the skilled professional has developed a cognitive ability to analyse and evaluate available information and make decisions about how best to respond. A number of contingency plans, which can be implemented immediately should the initial response be ineffective, will also be formulated. The skilled individual, in addition, has a greater capacity for what Snyder (1987) termed 'self-monitoring', which is the ability to monitor and regulate one's own responses in relation to the responses of others. This process of regulation necessitates an awareness of the ability level of the person with whom one is interacting and of 'the way they think', since 'in order to interact successfully and repeatedly with the same persons, one must have the capacity to form cognitive conceptions of the other's cognitive conceptions' (Wessler, 1984, p. 112). This process of metacognition is therefore also an important component of social skill.

Thus, cognitions play a central role during social encounters. The skilled professional will have developed a wide range of cognitive schemas to facilitate problem-solving and decision-making during interpersonal interaction, together with the ability to make rapid, accurate, judgements about people and situations.

3.3.2 Emotions

As mentioned earlier in this chapter, the role of emotions in social interaction needs to be recognized. Gallois (1993, p. 3) has illustrated how, 'feeling, mood, and affect are central to most aspects of social life'. Izard (1977) identified three specific components of emotion: firstly, the direct conscious experience or feeling of emotion; secondly, the physiological processes that accompany emotions; and thirdly, the observable behaviours that are used to signal and express emotions. In noting these processes, he further claimed that 'virtually all of the neurophysiological systems and subsystems of the body are involved in greater or lesser degree in emotional states. Such changes inevitably affect the perceptions, thoughts and actions of the person' (p. 10). Our emotional state therefore influences how we 'see' the world, think about what is happening and respond. Thus, a depressed patient will tend to pick up negative cues and ignore positive ones, be pessimistic about the future and typically adopt a slouched posture with lowered head, avoid eye contact, speak in a dull, flat monotone and generally avoid interacting with others. Conversely, a happy person will focus upon positive cues, be optimistic and display signs of happiness by smiling, looking at others, adopting an attentive posture and engaging in conversation.

There is considerable debate about the exact nature of the relationship between cognitions and emotions (Forgas, 1994). Some theorists argue that the latter are caused by the former, so that, for example, fear or anxiety can be caused by irrational beliefs. In discussing this issue, Mathews (1993, p. 493) concluded that most clinical psychologists now believe 'cognition not only precedes emotional reactions, but is the principal agent in bringing them about'. Such a perspective is, however, regarded by others as being an oversimplification of the nature of the relationship between these phenomena, arguing in favour of reciprocity between cognition and affect. For example, it is pointed out that emotional states can have a direct influence on thought processes, so that people may be so worried that they can no longer 'think straight'. As Forgas (1983, p. 138) noted: 'We not only differentiate between, and represent social episodes in terms of how we feel about them, but mood and emotions also play a crucial role in thinking about and remembering such events'. Thus, it would seem that the way we feel can have a direct bearing on the way we think, and *vice versa*.

Emotions are therefore very important determinants of behaviour. During social interaction it is important to be aware of the emotional state of others. In many health contexts, patients may be highly emotionally charged. The curve of the relationship between emotional arousal and performance takes the form of an inverted 'U' shape so that high levels of arousal are dysfunctional in that performance is severely impaired. Thus, trainee doctors or nurses, on occasion, faint when observing their first surgical operation. Similarly, health professionals need to be aware of the level of arousal of patients, and take steps to reduce it where necessary (by providing reassurance, giving careful explanations of what the patient will experience, etc.).

The above mediating factors are operative at the decision-making stage of interpersonal interaction and play an important role in determining social responses.

3.4 RESPONSES

When a goal has been decided upon, and a response plan formulated, the next stage is to implement this plan in terms of direct action. It is the function of the response, or 'effector', system to implement the translated strategies mentioned above into appropriate behaviours.

Social behaviour may be categorized as follows:

- **Verbal** – the purely linguistic message, i.e. the actual words used.
- **Vocal** – the paralinguistic delivery of the verbal message (pitch, tone, accent, etc.), i.e. **how** something is said as opposed to **what** is said.
- **Non-verbal** – the use of posture, gestures, facial expressions and other forms of body language.

It is at this level that skills become manifest. Someone who can give a detailed description of how to behave effectively during social interaction but who cannot put this knowledge into practice would not be described as socially skilled. In this sense, skilled performance depends upon the ability to **perform** tasks effectively and efficiently. (See Chapters 4, 5 and 6 for further information on skilled responses.)

3.5 FEEDBACK

Following the response stage, feedback will be available to the individual. Such feedback allows performers 'to monitor their progress towards the goal and adjust their behaviour when monitoring suggests that the goal will not be met' (Weldon and Weingart, 1993, p. 329). Indeed, in order to carry out any task effectively, it is essential to receive such feedback in terms of **knowledge of results** of performance (Annett, 1969). The crucial role of feedback has been noted by Bilodeau and Bilodeau (1961, p. 250) who viewed this as 'the strongest, most important variable controlling performance and learning'.

Thus, it is necessary to receive feedback in order to behave in a skilled, efficient manner. We could not ride a bicycle, play tennis or perform numerous other tasks if we were unable to perceive the results of our actions. Similarly, in interpersonal interaction we require feedback in order to make judgements about the effectiveness of our communications. Such social feedback takes the form of the verbal and non-verbal reactions of others. In situations where we receive little feedback from those with whom we interact, we are generally discontented, since we are unsure about how we are 'being received'.

As illustrated in Figure 3.2, during social interaction we receive feedback not only from others but also from our own responses. When we interact we hear what we are saying and, if we are highly skilled, may be aware of our non-verbal responses (hand movements, posture, etc.). This is part of the process of self-monitoring mentioned earlier, which includes the ability to monitor one's own behaviour and take corrective action based upon this feedback. High self-monitors control and regulate the images of self they project in social interaction and adjust their behaviour to meet the requirements of particular people or situations in which they interact. This is clearly an attribute that is important for health professionals, who have to deal with a wide range of patients and other professionals, and need to adapt their skills and strategies to suit the particular context in which they are involved.

During interpersonal encounters a constant stream of feedback impinges upon the individual, both from the stimuli received from other people and from the physical environment. In order to avoid overloading the system, the individual must selectively filter this information either into the conscious or the subconscious. As Barnlund (1993, p. 31) put it: 'each person stands at the centre of his or her own universe of meaning, transforming the flow of sensations into organized and intelligible events. Each of us views the world selectively and fits it to our past experiences and changing purposes'. This selectivity means that only a certain amount of incoming information will be consciously perceived. Evidence that subconscious perception occurs can be seen during hypnosis, when individuals can recall information of which they were not consciously aware. The extent to which such subconscious information guides behaviour is unclear, although it may well be the basis for judgements such as 'There was something about him I didn't like'.

The difference between feedback and perception is that in many contexts there will be a huge volume of feedback available but only a small amount will be consciously perceived. For example, within the physical environment the ticking of clocks, the pressure of one's feet on the floor, the hum of central heating systems, etc. are usually filtered into the subconscious. However, if we are bored during an encounter then these items may intrude into our awareness.

Perception is therefore an active, selective process. For this reason it is important for practitioners to be aware of the need to pay attention to important cues from others while filtering out only the less essential information. This is especially important in busy environments such as the hospital ward, where the sensory input available to the professional may include visual and auditory stimuli such as the patients, other professionals, visitors, catering staff, beds, magazines, extraneous noises, bright lights and so on. In such contexts, concerted perceptual focus is essential.

3.6 PERCEPTION

Our perceptual system enables us to acquire information about our environment through our five senses: sight, sound, taste, touch and smell. We use these senses to accumulate information both about physical objects and about other people. As expressed by Zebrowitz (1990, p. 3): 'the study of social perception has important implications for understanding and predicting our own and others' social behaviour. Effective action in interpersonal relationships requires a sensitive understanding of the covert psychological processes that underlie people's overt behaviour.' Thus, an awareness of some of the facets that influence the way in which we perceive others is of vital importance in the study of social interaction.

3.6.1 Perceptual accuracy

One important feature here is that 'research on person perception has clearly demonstrated that people are willing to make sweeping (and sometimes detailed) assessments of other persons based on observations of brief and limited samples of their behavior' (Riggio, 1992, pp. 10–11). Such judgements are frequently inaccurate and our appreciation of many situations can often therefore be distorted. For instance, in Figure 3.4 the impossible figure seems like three parallel tubes at one end but a magnet-like object at the other although, when viewed as a whole, it is neither.

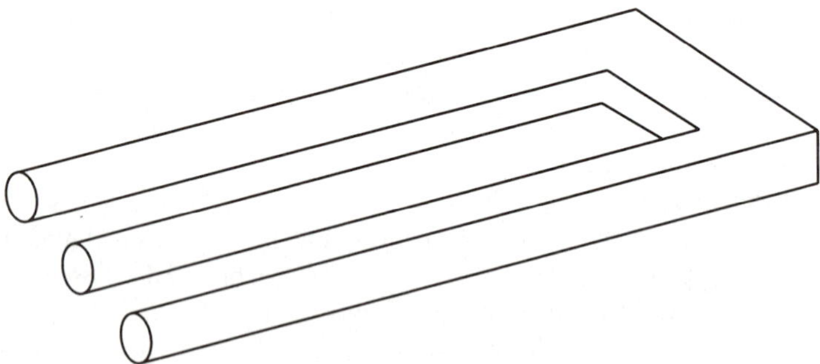

Figure 3.4 Impossible figure.

A similar phenomenon occurs in clinical practice when a patient presents in an apparent state of well-being yet the medical record indicates an emotional or personality disorder. Again, like the impossible figure, it is difficult to relate to the overall picture.

Our perceptions are also influenced by the context in which they are received. For example, there is a tendency for people with physical disabilities to be mistakenly viewed as being mentally less able – the two forms of disability being somehow associated in the mind of the observer (Herman, Zanna and Higgins, 1986). Thus, people confined to wheelchairs may be viewed as being somehow less mentally capable. Similarly, bedridden patients, particularly geriatrics, are often treated as having some degree of senile impairment regardless of their true mental state.

Misperception may not always be the fault of the practitioner. Our perceptions can be inaccurate because some patients deliberately aim to deceive. Indeed, cases have been documented in terms of clinical conditions such as Münchausen's syndrome, where the patient describes and enacts textbook symptoms of a disease state and even undergoes investigation and/or treatment, yet in fact has no such illness.

One investigation illustrated how the perceptions of doctors and patients of the same consultation can be at variance. Martin *et al.* (1991) carried out a study in four general practices in England in which one male GP in each practice assessed 500 consecutive consultations. Patients completed a questionnaire before and after the consultation and doctors completed a questionnaire after the consultation. The findings demonstrated how 'Doctors' perceptions of the consultation emphasized listening, supporting, and giving advice. Patients' perceptions emphasized prescribing, reassuring, and referring to a consultant' (p. 289). Also, doctors perceived patients to be less ill than patients did themselves, and this discrepancy was most marked among younger patients.

3.6.2 Interpreting perceptual information

There are several related processes that need to be taken into account when considering the role of perception during social interaction.

Attribution

This refers to the process whereby we attribute reasons or motives to the behaviour of others. When attempting to interpret the behaviour of other people we take into consideration situational and dispositional causes. What is known as the 'fundamental attribution error' occurs through 'the tendency to overestimate the role of dispositional factors and to underestimate the role of situational factors when judging the causes of behaviours' (Kleinke, 1986, p. 193). Interestingly, we tend to emphasize dispositional causes when interpreting the negative behaviour of others, but highlight the importance of situational factors when explaining our own poor performance (Feldman, 1985). We are also much more willing to claim personal contribution to positive outcomes and reject responsibility for negative ones. For example, Gamsu and Bradley (1987) found that medical staff and diabetic patients were both keen to take the credit for success and equally unwilling to take any responsibility for failure in controlling the diabetes. It is likely that such **self-serving bias** prevents our sense of self-worth being called into question. Negative self-inferences can be unpleasantly ego-threatening, leading in the longer-term to poor self-concept and diminished levels of self-esteem. Under such circumstances feelings of self-efficacy may suffer as the individual begins to lose faith in personal ability to achieve desired goals. In making judgements about our own and other people's behaviour, it is therefore important to carefully consider both situational and dispositional factors.

Kelley (1971) highlighted the importance of three main variables during attribution. Firstly, the **consistency** of the observed behaviour, i.e. how often the person displays this behaviour in this situation; secondly its **distinctiveness**, which refers to whether or not the behaviour is commonly displayed in different situations; and thirdly the **consensus** in terms of whether the behaviour is typical of how other people behave in this situation. These three variables can best be represented by considering a situation where a nurse bursts into tears when dealing with a particular patient (Table 3.1). As this example illustrates, when interpreting the behaviour of others in any situation, we make decisions based upon how they have behaved in the past, and how other people behave in the same situation.

Table 3.1 Example of the attribution process

	Consistency	Distinctiveness	Consensus	Attribution
1.	High. She has often cried with this particular patient.	High. She has never cried when dealing with other patients.	High. Other staff on the ward were also very upset.	To this particular patient
2.	High. She has often cried with this particular patient.	Low. She has often cried when dealing with other patients.	Low. No other members of staff were upset.	To the nurse
3.	Low. She has never cried with this patient before.	Low. She has never cried when dealing with other patients.	Low. No other members of staff were upset.	To the situation or to prevailing circumstances

Labelling

We use labels to enable us to categorize and deal with people more readily. These labels may be influenced by an individual's age, physical appearance, dress, gender and aspects of verbal and non-verbal behaviour. Such labelling is an integrated process derived from past experiences, expectations and interpretations of the situation. The function of labelling is to simplify complex information that would otherwise become unmanageable. One type of label is that of the social **stereotype**, which is an attempt to force people into certain categories or 'pigeonholes' without paying attention to how they actually are. In this way, set patterns of behaviour are anticipated in someone belonging to a specific group (racial, class, religious sect, etc.) and behaviour is interpreted in the light of preset expectations about the stereotype. This can often result in a **self-fulfilling prophecy**. For example, person A may believe that coloured people are aggressive and unfriendly. A then meets coloured person B and reacts as if B was unfriendly and aggressive, with the result that B is likely to respond in a less friendly manner. In this way, the stereotype is strengthened.

Another example of labelling in the health field occurs when patients are referred to as illnesses (e.g. 'the hysterectomy in bed 5'). Here, the result is to deindividualize patients, and treat them as medical or technical problems. Other common examples of labels include 'hypochondriac', 'malingerer', troublesome patient'. The danger with all such labels is that the professional may respond to the label rather than to the person.

Implicit personality theory

People seem to have 'implicit personality theories' (Bruner and Tagiuri, 1954), which they employ to make judgements about others. This refers to the way in which we associate certain characteristics of an individual with a range of other characteristics. For example, in the following instances judge the characteristic in parentheses that best seems to complete the sentence.

Alan is conscientious, industrious, lively and (fat, thin).
Patricia is vivacious, attractive, stylish and (young, old).

In the first instance Alan will be more likely to be judged as 'thin' and in the second case Patricia as 'young'. These are two simple examples of how we associate characteristics. This process causes a **halo effect** in that, if someone possesses a number of positive characteristics, we are more likely to infer other positive qualities. Likewise, a negative halo effect can occur, with people who display a number of negative characteristics being perceived as possessing a range of other negative qualities.

In an early study, Rosenberg, Nelson and Vivekanathan (1968) found that university students used two major dimensions along which people were differentiated, intellectual good–bad and social good–bad. Certain traits were clearly associated with one another along these two dimensions. Thus, people viewed as warm were also perceived as sociable, popular, happy, good-natured and humorous. Interestingly these traits were perceived as good socially but as indicators of less intellectual individuals. In fact, the traits 'warm' and 'cold' have been shown to be **central traits** and of crucial importance in that, once a judgement is made as to whether a person is warm or cold, a large number of other positive or negative judgements respectively are inferred.

Primacy and recency effects

The primacy effect refers to the way in which information we receive initially can affect how we later interpret further information. In person perception, the first impressions we make of others can influence how we respond to them. However, a recency effect would also seem to be operative, in that the final information perceived is also influential in making judgements (Millar, Crute and Hargie, 1992). This suggests that health professionals should pay particular attention to the way in which they greet, and part from, patients. (Chapter 5 has further information on opening and closing interactions.)

Metaperception

This refers to our perception of the perception process itself. As mentioned earlier in the chapter, when we interact with others we attempt to ascertain how they are perceiving us and try to evaluate how they think we are perceiving them. Both of these facets play an important role in interpersonal interaction.

Summary

Person perception is clearly a crucial element of social interaction. Professionals need to develop an ability to perceive accurately the cues being emitted by others while also being aware of their own responses. They also need to be sensitive to the range of factors that can cause distortion or inaccuracy during the perceptual process.

Perception is the final central process involved in the interaction model presented in Figure 3.2 and, together with goals, mediating factors, responses and feedback, comprises the core of dyadic interaction.

3.7 THE PERSON–SITUATION CONTEXT

In order to gain a fuller understanding of social interaction, we need to consider what Hargie, Saunders and Dickson (1994) termed the **person–situation context**. In other words, the situation in which behaviour occurs and the nature of the person displaying the behaviour are both important contributing factors. What is known as the person–situation debate within psychology has investigated whether behaviour is a function of the personality of the individual, the situation in which the individual is located or a combination of the two. Research has shown that indeed both the person (P) and situation (S) have a part to play, but also that the interaction of $P \times S$ is central (Phares, 1988). It is therefore necessary to examine both situational and personal factors.

3.7.1 Situational factors

As discussed earlier in this chapter, attributions about the behaviour of others are based upon dispositional and situational factors. For example, someone who gives a large sum of money to a charity collector may be seen as generous (dispositional) or alternatively as showing off or trying to impress onlookers (situational). It is therefore necessary to be aware of the influence of a range of situational factors in determining the behaviour of people during social encounters.

Cultural background

One key feature of interaction is the cultural background of the interactants. This is especially important in multicultural settings. Culture has been defined by Kreps and Kunimoto (1994, p. 1) as the system of 'shared beliefs, values, and attitudes that guide the behaviours of group members'. They illustrate how practitioners and patients approach consultations with their own set of health beliefs, customs and practices based upon their cultural backgrounds. These, in turn, influence how they perceive the encounter and the treatment.

In her review of many of the cultural factors that impinge upon practitioner–patient communication, Rasinski (1993) illustrates how members of the Chinese community are more likely to favour parenteral than oral medications, while many Native Americans believe that if medicine is really 'magic' it can work anywhere and need not be taken by the patient – so it may be placed in a 'mummy bundle' in the corner of a room. She also illustrates how in certain Arabic and Semitic cultures the doctor is regarded with unquestioning respect, such that if the physician were to ask the patient or family for an opinion about the condition this would raise serious doubts in their minds about the diagnosis and treatment. A knowledge of where the other person is 'coming from' is therefore essential, and indeed 'an important challenge to the development of effective health care relationships is the ability to bridge cultural differences between health care providers and their clients' (Kreps and Kunimoto, 1994, p. 38).

Goals

The goals that we seek are influenced by the situation in which we are interacting while, conversely, the goals that we seek also influence the situation in which we choose to interact. Thus, the nurse on the ward will have goals directly related to dealing with patients. However, if the nurse is hungry, situations will be sought where food is available. In this way, goals and situations are interdependent.

Rules

An analogy is often made between social interaction and games, in that both are governed by rules that must be followed if a successful outcome is to be achieved (Hargie, Saunders and Dickson, 1994). Rules can be explicit or implicit. For example, while there are explicit rules forbidding sexual relationships between doctors and patients, it is an implicit rule that the doctor will provide a chair for patients to sit in. Professionals need to be aware not only of the rules of the situations that they will encounter, but also how to deal with patients who break the rules (e.g. aggressive patients).

Roles

In any social situation, people play a variety of roles. Each role carries with it a set of expectations about behaviour, attitudes, feelings, beliefs and values. Indeed, an important aspect of training has to do with learning how to effectively play the role of the professional. Thus, a nurse is expected to be concerned about the well-being of patients, to behave in a caring manner, to dress in a certain fashion and so on. The trainee nurse who fails to learn these role responsibilities will not be allowed to register. As we move from one situation to another, our roles often change, e.g. from doctor in the hospital to girlfriend on a date and to daughter at home. Problems can arise, however, where there are conflicting expectations about how a role should be played. Thus, a nurse may expect patients to respond in a certain way, whereas a particular patient may not 'see' the patient role in that light. In such instances, communication problems are very likely to emanate.

In a detailed examination of the communication processes in a hospital swallowing clinic, Skipper (1992) found that the patients' perceptions of the role of various health professionals differed from the role views held by the latter. This illustrates a need for clear role explanation to patients early in a consultation. Indeed, Schommer (1994), in a study of pharmacist–patient communication, found that role congruence was an important feature, since 'quality communication is more likely when pharmacist and patient role orientations are congruent than when they are incongruent' (p. 299). In consultations with high role congruence, the patient asked more questions and the pharmacist gave more information about the purpose of medication, its side effects and contraindications. To improve communication, Schommer therefore recommended that pharmacists take steps to ensure that the role expectations of patients are compatible with those of the pharmacist.

Lambert (1995) has also illustrated how the roles of health professionals are changing. In particular, he cites the example of how pharmacists are moving beyond the traditional dispensing role to a new philosophy of practice termed 'pharmaceutical care', which includes clinical consultation with doctors, counselling of patients and responsibility for patient outcomes. However, he illustrates how this expansion of pharmacy's professional role has met with resistance from physicians and nurses, who see this as an infringement on their 'patch', and even from practising pharmacists, who are not comfortable with a new patient-oriented role. As the focus of patient care has moved from hospital to the community, many professionals have had to adapt to a change or a refocus of role. Such role-change can often be difficult both for the person and for the other professionals involved.

Behavioural sequence

In most social situations there is a particular behavioural sequence which should be followed by those taking part. Argyle, Furnham and Graham (1981) argue that many encounters can be accounted for in terms of the following five-episode progression:

1. Greeting
2. Establishing the relationship and clarifying roles
3. The task
4. Re-establishing the relationship
5. Parting.

It is important for professionals and patients to be aware of the expected sequence of interaction episodes in consultations, to ensure a smooth communicative encounter.

Physical environment

The nature of the physical environment, in terms of the layout of furniture and fittings, lighting, heating, colour, etc., can have a distinct influence upon the behaviour of individuals. For example, people feel more comfortable and tend to disclose more about themselves in 'warm' environments (soft seats, concealed lighting, carpets, etc.). Furthermore, individuals feel more secure on 'home territory' than in unfamiliar environments. Doctors, health visitors and district nurses find patients more at ease in their own homes than in the health clinic. Hospitals can be particularly disturbing for some patients, owing to the nature of the ward environment, with little personal space or privacy, bright lights, intrusive noise and few personal possessions. In such situations, the patient is likely to feel a sense of loss of control and this can cause further distress.

Concepts

In every social situation there is a range of concepts that must be understood by the interactors if the encounter is to be successful. For example, a visit to the cinema may entail a knowledge of the concepts 'queue', 'ticket', 'usherette' and 'interval'. Similarly, a patient visiting a dentist may need to be aware of the concepts of 'filling', 'plaque', 'crown' or 'bridge'. However, a common error made by some professionals is to wrongly assume that patients have a knowledge of all the concepts necessary for understanding an interaction. Furthermore, health professionals have developed a jargon of specific terminology for various concepts and need to ensure that such jargon is avoided, or fully explained in appropriate language, when dealing with patients.

One investigation revealed how the meaning of concepts can differ. In the Martin *et al.* (1991) study described earlier, the doctors reported 'examining' 70% of the patients while only 45% of patients reported being examined. It was clear that the concept of 'what comprised an examination varied according to the doctors and patients. . . . For example, many patients did not perceive measuring blood pressure to be an examination' (p. 291).

Linguistic variations

The final dimension of social situations relates to the degree of linguistic variation concerned. Certain situations require a higher degree of formality of language than others. Giving a lecture or addressing a committee meeting involves a more formal, elaborate use of language than, for example, having a chat with a colleague over coffee. Equally, changes in tone, pitch and volume of voice occur across contexts. Professionals, therefore, need to be capable of varying their language and speech patterns to meet the needs of particular situations.

These components of social situations play an important role in interpreting the behaviour of individuals during interpersonal encounters and they should therefore be taken into consideration during CST programmes.

3.7.2 Personal factors

The final element of the interpersonal interaction model outlined in Figure 3.2 concerns the personal factors of the individuals involved. Before we actually interact with others we make judgements about them based upon various features of their appearance. There are four main personal factors that are immediately available to us when we meet other people: age, gender, dress and physical appearance.

Age

The importance of the ageing process in interpersonal encounters has attracted increasing research attention (Hummert, Wiemann and Nussbaum, 1994), and indeed the study of gerontology has developed at a rapid pace (Aiken, 1994). Generally, we hold stereotypes about individuals, based upon their age, which can quite often be very inaccurate (Hummert, 1994). For example, Wolinsky (1983) illustrated how some elderly people categorized as irreversibly senile may actually be suffering from short-term depression, which can be alleviated by psychotherapy. Feldman (1985, p. 163) further reported that 'even some physicians, who might otherwise be expected to be sympathetic to the elderly, use the terms "crones" or "trolls" when talking about their elderly patients'.

Health professionals, therefore, need to be careful to avoid treating elderly patients on the basis of negative stereotypes. They also should be sensitive to possible negative changes in their interactional style. Available evidence indicates that there is a tendency for physicians to exert greater control over the content of consultations, focusing primarily on medical issues and with little attempt to explore the 'personhood' of the elderly patient (Greene *et al.*, 1994). The use of patronizing speech (Hummert, 1994) or 'baby talk' (Edwards and Noller, 1993), with older patients has also been well documented.

The age of the practitioner is also an important factor. In some contexts older professionals may be viewed as being more experienced and competent than younger colleagues. However, in other situations, younger professionals may be preferred by patients. Thus, the ages of both the professional and the client are important considerations which can affect expectations and behaviour during interpersonal communication.

Gender

During interpersonal encounters, we tend to respond differently to and hold differing expectations of others depending upon their gender. As Eckes (1994, p. 107) put it: 'Gender is one of the most important categories – if not **the** most important category – in human social life. The dichotomy between female and male is of crucial relevance to virtually every domain of human experience. . . . All known cultures . . . associate men and women with different sets of characteristic features and with different sets of behavioural expectations.' Such differences are emphasized from an early age, since male and female infants are dressed and responded to differently. These early experiences undoubtedly contribute to later differences in behaviour patterns, attitudes and values between males and females. However, the extent to which such differences are learned or innate is as yet unclear, although it seems likely that both nature and nurture play an important part in shaping later gender patterns of behaviour (Jacklin, 1992).

In terms of non-verbal communication, females tend to smile more, require less interpersonal space, are touched more, use more head nods and engage in more eye contact than males. These gender differences were exemplified in a study by Whitcher and Fisher (1979) into the reactions of males and females to preoperative therapeutic touch. It was found that one single touch by nursing staff produced a positive, significant effect upon females' response to surgery, whereas it had the reverse effect for males. Gahagan (1984) interpreted such findings in terms of dominance signals, in that high-status individuals initiate and control their touch patterns with low-status individuals. Her suggestion was that males may therefore interpret touch in terms of dominance, rather than affiliative, signals.

In terms of interpersonal skill, 'numerous studies have established women's superior abilities as both decoders and encoders of non-verbal messages when compared with men' (Borisoff and Merrill, 1991, p. 65). Gender differences have also been found in the way male and female doctors interact, with female physicians being more attentive and less directive (Meeuwesen, Schaap and van der Staak, 1991), conducting longer consultations and receiving more patient communications in the form of questions, opinions and information (Roter, Lipkin and Korsgaard, 1991), and negotiating more with patients about the topics to be discussed (Ainsworth-Vaughan, 1992).

Stereotyped images of sex roles can still be found within the health field, in that the vast majority of nurses are female and senior positions in most professions still tend to be held by males. However, in recent years the numbers of females entering what were formerly the male-dominated professions of medicine, dentistry and pharmacy have markedly increased to the point where in many institutions female entrants to courses outnumber males (Bottero, 1994). Previously, there was a tendency to perceive those health professions with a preponderance of females (e.g. nursing or the therapies) as jobs requiring 'caring' skills or needing 'a woman's touch' (Kaufman, 1984). It will therefore be interesting to chart how a changing gender balance will affect both the attitudes of and attitudes to these professions.

At a more specific level, the gender of both the professional and the patient clearly needs to be taken into consideration when evaluating interpersonal communication episodes.

Dress

Although one of the prime functions of clothing is to protect the wearer from cold or injury, it is clear that dress also serves a number of important social functions. The clothes we wear can signify group membership, gender, status, occupation, personal identity and personality. We carefully select our apparel when preparing for social encounters in order to portray a certain type of image to others. In professional contexts, however, this choice is often removed, so that in hospitals different professions are required to wear different types of uniform in order to portray a more corporate, neutral image. In other settings, however, the professional has more control over personal dress. For example, a doctor has to dress in such a way as to appear competent and efficient without being unapproachable. Likewise, a community pharmacist needs to appear professional and identifiable, and indeed one survey revealed that well over 70% of consumers expressed the view that pharmacists, irrespective of gender, should wear a white coat (Hargie, Morrow and Woodman, 1992).

Physical appearance

The final personal factor to be considered is the physical appearance of the individual, in terms of body size, shape and attractiveness. Physique can influence how people are perceived and responded to. For example, endomorphs tend to be viewed as warm-hearted, agreeable, good-natured, sympathetic and dependent on others; ectomorphs as quiet, tidy and tense; and mesomorphs as adventurous, forceful, self-reliant and healthy (Argyle, 1988). Height is also a significant element in judgements of males. Taller men tend to achieve more in our society in terms of occupational status and social opportunities such as dating. Furthermore, males of higher status tend to be perceived as taller.

Attractiveness would seem to be a crucial feature in interpersonal communication. People who are rated as physically attractive are also seen as more popular, friendly and interesting to talk to (Kleinke, 1986). Thus, individuals rated as highly attractive tend to receive more eye contact, smiles, closer bodily proximity and body accessibility (openness of arms and legs), than those rated as low in attractiveness. However, attractiveness involves more than mere physical make-up, since factors which are relevant here include dress, cleanliness, personality and competence (Dickson, Saunders and Stringer, 1993). This would indicate that less physically attractive practitioners may be successful and popular with clients by ensuring they have good interactive style and a competent, professional approach.

Summary

These four factors related to the appearance of individuals need to be borne in mind in any evaluation of interpersonal interaction. Finally, the disposition of the individual is an important facet in determining responses in social situations. Factors such as whether the practitioner is shy, outgoing, competitive, affiliative, dominant or submissive influence behaviour. The values and beliefs systems held by practitioners will also be important. For example, a devout Catholic may find difficulty in advising patients about the procedures for obtaining an abortion. Our political, moral and religious beliefs influence our attitudes towards other people, which in turn affect our thoughts, feelings and behaviour as we interact with them. The attitudes we have towards others are also influenced by our previous experiences of the person with whom we are interacting, and of similar people.

3.8 OVERVIEW

This chapter has been concerned with an examination of a theoretical model (Figure 3.2), which can be directly applied to the analysis of interpersonal communication. This model highlights the importance of a number of interrelated processes, each of which contributes to an understanding of the nature and function of social behaviour. The central processes in this model are:

- the goals of the individuals involved and their motivation to pursue them;
- a range of mediating factors including cognitions, emotions, values and beliefs;

- the responses of both parties;
- the feedback available during interpersonal encounters;
- the ability of the individuals to perceive important cues from others, while being aware of their own behaviour.

In addition, the role of various situational and personal factors was also emphasized.

While, for the purposes of description, analysis and evaluation, each stage of this model has been studied separately, it will be apparent that in reality the processes involved do not occur in isolation, but rather overlap, and are interrelated and interdependent. As described in Chapter 1, in any encounter communication is an ongoing two-way process of mutual influence, in which actions and reactions are regularly monitored and evaluated in order to guide future actions and reactions. As a result, communication is a complex process involving a myriad of impinging variables, some or all of which may be operating at any particular time. In order to attempt to interpret and make sense of this process it is necessary to systematically study the central components involved.

The model presented in this chapter provides a conceptual framework for interpreting face-to-face interaction and offers a necessary theoretical underpinning for programmes of CST. It represents a broad-based foundation upon which can later be built specific communication skills such as those presented in the following chapters of this section. Furthermore, it provides a wider perspective within which each of these skills can be evaluated. Skipper (1992) applied this model directly to the health context in her in-depth investigation of the communication patterns involved in the operation of a swallowing clinic in a large hospital. She concluded that the model was a valuable 'tool for the examination of communication in a health setting' (p. 579).

Responding skills

4

4.1 INTRODUCTION

In this chapter and in Chapters 5 and 6 a range of interpersonal skills and strategies pertinent to the needs of health professionals are examined. Given the vast literature in the field of communication skills, it is clearly beyond the scope of this text to incorporate a comprehensive review. Rather, a summative overview of the core skills will be provided, and their application to health contexts will be exemplified. The trainer is therefore recommended to pursue some of the references employed throughout the chapter for further information on each of the areas covered.

The selection of the skills and strategies included in this chapter and in Chapters 5 and 6 has been based upon an analysis of investigations into communication within different health professions (e.g. Byrne and Long, 1976; MacLeod Clark, 1982; Saunders and Caves, 1986; Hargie, Morrow and Woodman, 1993; Adams *et al.*, 1994), coupled with a review of the recommendations contained in various texts on interpersonal communication for health professionals. Methods that can be followed in identifying such skills will be dealt with in Part Three.

The skills presented in this chapter are essentially responsive in nature in that they are usually employed in reaction to the behaviour of others rather than as a means of initiating and directing interaction. The responding skills incorporated here are non-verbal communication, reinforcement, reflecting, listening and self-disclosure. Information on each and their functional significance in interaction will be outlined, together with associated exercises that the trainer can use during training.

4.2 NON-VERBAL COMMUNICATION

During the past three decades, increasing attention has been devoted to the field of non-verbal communication (De Paulo, 1992). This has resulted in a voluminous literature in the form of books, book chapters and research papers. Books on this topic have also been applied directly to the health professions (e.g. Blondis and Jackson, 1982; Blanck, Buck and Rosenthal, 1986). Given this vast array of publications, it is only possible in this chapter to present a brief overview of the topic in terms of the main components involved.

Although some theorists have argued strongly for the concept of non-verbal behaviour as skill (Friedman, 1979), others have purported that non-verbal communication *per se* is not strictly speaking a separate skilled area. As Riggio (1992, p. 6) pointed out, while 'the communication skill framework separates skills in verbal and non-verbal communication, in reality, verbal and non-verbal skills are complexly intertwined'. Non-verbal behaviour is certainly a distinct and extensive mode of communication, which can be employed when utilizing a range of other skills. For example, a nod of the head can be used as one element of a reinforcing response, or an upright posture – when coupled with other relevant behaviours – can help to convey assertiveness. However, it is essential for the professional both to display skilled use of non-verbal behaviours and to be able to interpret accurately the non-verbal signals of others.

Non-verbal communication is important in health-professional–patient encounters for four main reasons (Buller and Street, 1992). First, the patient's treatment or condition may interfere with the ability to communicate verbally. Second, their subordinate role makes patients less verbal during consultations (e.g. reluctant to ask questions) and thereby affords them more time to focus upon the non-verbal behaviour of the practitioner. Third, fear and uncertainty about the illness increase the need in patients for social comparison and reliance upon subtle cues (usually non-verbal) from practitioners that indicate how and what they should be feeling. Fourth, patients may not fully understand the verbal message, or believe it not to be wholly truthful, and will hence focus upon accompanying non-verbal cues for further information. For these reasons, practitioners need to be introduced to the concept of bodily communication as a separate and crucial field of study.

Non-verbal communication can be defined as all forms of human communication apart from the purely verbal message. Thus the term 'non-verbal' encompasses both what is referred to as **body language**, i.e. movements of the head, hands, feet, etc., as well as vocalizations associated with the verbal messages, such as tone, pitch, volume, speed, accent, etc. This latter aspect is usually referred to as **paralanguage**. Both of these dimensions will be examined briefly in this chapter.

Since *Homo sapiens* is the only species to have developed a systematic language, we tend to concentrate primarily on the verbal messages which we convey. For example, we are taught from childhood to 'watch what we say', but are not really taught to monitor our body language. The result is that we generally have much greater control over the verbal than the non-verbal channel. One implication of this is the fact that when the verbal and non-verbal messages are contradictory, we tend to believe the non-verbal aspects. Thus, if someone yawns, looks at a clock and says in a bored tone 'That's very interesting', the listener will not believe the verbal message. In this sense, 'actions speak louder than words'.

While there is information concerning deception cues in a range of fields, little work has been conducted in the health context. As Trimboli and Walker (1993) noted, we know many of the non-verbal leakage cues involved in the game of poker, yet we do not have similar knowledge concerning deception by patients during consultations! This is part of a wider dearth, since 'unfortunately, non-verbal communication in medical consultations has received less direct analysis than verbal communication' (Buller and Street, 1992, p. 120). Yet there are many occasions when health practitioners will have to make important decisions about the truthfulness of information presented, ranging from a parent explaining how a child was injured to a possible abuser requesting and explaining the need for a particular type of cough medicine.

In their analysis of this area, Burgoon, Callister and Hunsaker (1994) summarized the main reasons why patients may be deceptive as including avoidance of social disapproval, not wishing to receive bad news or be subjected to further clinical scrutiny, establishing and maintaining a favourable interpersonal relationship with the health professional, or because of their own beliefs about what should be kept private and personal. They identified five types of deceptive acts:

- **fabrication** – supplying false information;
- **concealment** – withholding truthful information;
- **exaggeration** – embellishing truthful information;
- **mixing** – including both truthful and deceptive information within the same message;
- **obfuscating** – implying false conclusions or misdirecting attention away from the issue at hand.

In a sample of 754 adults in the USA who completed questionnaires, Burgoon, Callister and Hunsaker found that 85% admitted having used concealment and one-third admitted outright lying to their physicians. In discussing this issue, they review literature to indicate that deceivers are less complete in their descriptions, tend to shy away from precise responses and give little detail, are less personalized and more reticent, and equivocate more. They therefore recommend that health professionals should force patients to be direct, explicit and complete in what they say, and to personalize or 'own' their messages.

Indeed, several meta-analyses of research studies on deception have indicated that the following non-verbal behaviours are consistently associated with deception: increased pupil dilation and blinking; more self-manipulations and gestures unrelated to the speech content; speaking at a higher pitch; greater number of speech errors and hesitations; and a shorter response length (Ebesu and Miller, 1994). However, research in the field of deception also indicates that verbal behaviour may be the most potent indicator of deceit (Hughes,

1994). Deceptive statements are more general (contain fewer specific references about people, places and temporal ordering of events), use more irrelevant information unrelated to the central theme and involve considerable 'levelling', which is the tendency to use terms such as all, every, none or nobody. Their review of this field led Miller and Stiff (1993, p. 66) to conclude that 'visual cues are not the most useful and reliable indicators of veracity . . . future studies should concentrate on verbal and vocal correlates of deception'.

Clear non-verbal patterns of behaviour have also been associated with various clinical states (Feldman and Rime, 1991). Depressed people demonstrate a lack of eye contact, eyes looking down and away from the other person, downturned mouth, downward angle of the head and absence of hand movements. Anxious patients are distinguishable by more self-stroking, twitching and tremor in hand movements, less eye contact and fewer smiles. Autistics display extreme gaze aversion, which may be employed in order to avoid any communication with others. Schizophrenics tend to look less when discussing personal matters, although they display normal gaze patterns when discussing neutral material. They also tend to be poorer at displaying emotional information non-verbally. In relation to psychopathy, it has also been shown that violent male offenders prefer greater interpersonal distance from others, use more hand gestures, look more and smile less than the norm. This behavioural pattern, in turn, probably increases the likelihood of violent encounters with other males.

These findings indicate the importance of an understanding of non-verbal behaviour in terms of evaluating the behaviour of patients in a clinical setting. However, this aspect of communication serves a number of other important functions.

4.2.1 Functions of non-verbal communication

There are six main functions of non-verbal communication.

- **Replacing speech**. This happens in various situations, the prime example being sign language among the deaf and dumb. However, in many contexts a meaningful glance, a caring touch or a deliberate silence can substitute adequately for any verbal message.
- **Complementing the verbal message**. In most instances this is the main function of non-verbal behaviour. For instance, if we say we are happy, we are expected to **look** happy. Likewise, a practitioner will use hand movements, facial expressions, etc. to facilitate verbal explanation.
- **Regulating and controlling the flow of communication**. Turn-taking during social encounters is controlled, in part, by non-verbal signals. We do not say verbally 'I am now finishing. You can take over.' Rather, we indicate this non-verbally by raising or lowering the final syllable as we stop speaking, pausing, and looking directly and expectantly at the listener. Similarly, dominant individuals maintain their dominance by speaking more loudly,

engaging in continuous eye contact, choosing a position of control (e.g. the top end of a table as with the board chairperson) and interrupting others.

- **Providing feedback**. As discussed in the previous chapter, during social encounters it is necessary to monitor the reactions of others to determine whether they are still listening, are worried, have understood what has been said and so on. Health professionals should be sensitive to non-verbal forms of feedback, and during CST should be encouraged to develop their ability to interpret this information from others, while being aware of the non-verbal feedback they themselves are providing. This latter dimension has been shown to be of crucial importance in health contexts. Patients often know little about their condition and fail to fully comprehend the technicalities of explanations they receive. As a result, they place great importance upon the non-verbal cues emitted by practitioners in order to deduce information.
- **Helping define relationships between people**. This can be clearly observed in the hospital setting where uniforms are used to indicate the role, function and status of various professionals. This is often a useful dimension, since it facilitates identification and circumvents role confusion between professionals, although at times it can also cause misunderstanding, as, for example, when a hospital pharmacist wearing a white coat is 'seen' by patients to be a doctor.
- **Conveying emotional states**. Emotions are recognized primarily on the basis of non-verbal behaviour. It is generally agreed that what is referred to as **social meaning** (attitudes, emotions, etc.) is conveyed non-verbally (Hargie, Saunders and Dickson, 1994). This is an important function, since saying verbally to someone 'I dislike you' may lead to overt aggression, whereas this message can be conveyed by more subtle non-verbal methods (looking less, orienting the body away, etc.) with less likelihood of a confrontation. Males need to be more sensitive to the affective domain, given 'the very robust research finding that women are better encoders and decoders of the non-verbal communication of emotion' (Gallois, 1993, p. 7).

Buller and Street (1992) identified three over-arching purposes of non-verbal behaviour in medical consultations.

- **Relational communication**, particularly the expression of affiliation and affect; affiliation is communicated through a close conversational distance, direct body and facial orientation, forward lean, increased and direct gaze, smiling and pleasant facial expressions, head nodding, postural openness, frequent gestures and touch. Buller and Street (1992) reported that physicians with the ability to express appropriate emotions accurately receive higher satisfaction ratings from patients. This was confirmed in a study by Bensing (1991), in which 12 experienced GPs rated 103 videotaped consultations on the quality of psychosocial care displayed by doctors. It was found that 'the **non-verbal** aspects of affective behaviour (eye contact and showing interest) had a strong predictive power on the quality rating of psychosocial care' (pp. 1307–8).

- **The enhancement of message comprehension and recall**: this is facilitated by the use of emblematic gestures (which have specific semantic meaning – such as raising three fingers to signal 'three' of something), closer interpersonal distance, direct gaze and a facing orientation.
- **Persuading patients to follow recommended actions**: once a relationship has been developed, it seems that the communication of **negative** affect is related to greater patient compliance. Such negative affect may communicate concern that the malady is more health-threatening and may also motivate patients to please the practitioner by following directives and thereby maintain the positive relationship.

4.2.2 Components of non-verbal communication

The above six functions can be achieved by coordinating a range of non-verbal behaviours. The main elements of non-verbal behaviour are as follows:

Touch

In health settings, two different types of touch can be distinguished: firstly, **instrumental touch**, in which the professional has to make physical contact with the patient in order to carry out a particular task (giving an injection, taking blood pressure, etc.); secondly, **expressive touch**, where body contact is employed to comfort or console a patient. Research into the use of these two types has produced equivocal findings. For example, the use of expressive touch by nursing staff at the preoperative stage has been shown to be effective in producing a positive response to surgery among female but not male patients (Whitcher and Fisher, 1979). In another study it was discovered that the more often physicians touched their patients during consultations the less satisfied the patients were with the doctor and the less they understood what they had been told (Larsen and Smith, 1981). This latter study focused upon initial doctor–patient contacts and this may partly have accounted for the findings. Touch tends to increase as a relationship develops and thus the use of this behaviour from an unfamiliar doctor may well be off-putting and distracting for patients.

These findings emphasize the importance of a consideration of the context in which the touch occurs, when evaluating its appropriateness. The accompanying verbal message should prepare the patient for, and complement, the type of touch given. In addition, the gender of the recipient needs to be considered, since males may perceive touch as an indicator of status or dominance, whereas females are less likely to construe it in this way (Knapp and Hall, 1992). The advice given by Buckman (1992, p. 38) about use of touch is simply to 'be sensitive to the patient's response. If the patient is comforted, continue: if the patient is uncomfortable, stop.' The form of touch employed also is of importance, since it has been found that a light 'incidental' touch, where the recipient is unaware of being touched, can produce more positive perceptions of the environment in which this behaviour occurred and can also increase the compliance of the recipient to a request (Dickson, Saunders and Stringer, 1993).

Proximity

This refers to the interpersonal distance which people maintain when interacting with one another. In Western society there are four main proximity zones: the intimate zone (0–50 cm); the personal zone (50 cm–1.2 m); the social/consultative zone (1.2–3.5 m); and the public zone (3.5 m+). These distances relate to direct face-to-face interaction, so that we might be sitting beside a stranger at a lecture and yet not feel 'too close for comfort' due to the absence of eye contact. Large variations from proximity norms can cause discomfort, as exemplified by descriptions of individuals at opposite ends of the interpersonal distance continuum as either 'pushy' or 'stand-offish'.

During social encounters we do not like others to invade our personal space without permission. This space enables us to maintain our personal dignity, respect and independence. However, there is a status difference with regard to interpersonal distance, in that high-status individuals can approach low-status individuals quite closely, but low-status individuals will usually seek approval before closely approaching people of higher status. (Another example of status differences and personal space can be seen in the fact that higher-status people occupy larger offices!)

Interestingly, in hospitals, patients on general wards often have their personal space invaded, in that practitioners can, and do, come within their intimate zone without seeking permission. This, in turn, may increase patients' sense of vulnerability and disempowerment. Professionals need to be aware of this and, where possible, seek permission from patients before actually entering their personal zone. As a rough guide, French (1994) suggested that 'An area of 2 feet [60 cm] around a patient's bed and bedside locker could be viewed as his or her personal space' (p. 46). Furthermore patients can suffer distress through being moved from a bed and ward with which they have become familiar to another ward area. Humans, like all animals, become familiar with a particular territory and feel more secure there. Thus, where movement is essential the patient should be prepared for this well in advance.

Orientation

This refers to the spatial positions that people adopt when interacting. For example, in Figure 4.1, position (b) would be the most appropriate seating position for a doctor–patient consultation, since it is friendlier than (a) yet maintains a degree of formality, which most patients will expect, as opposed to (c), which is more informal. However, if a doctor is explaining a detailed procedure the patient may be placed in the (c) position.

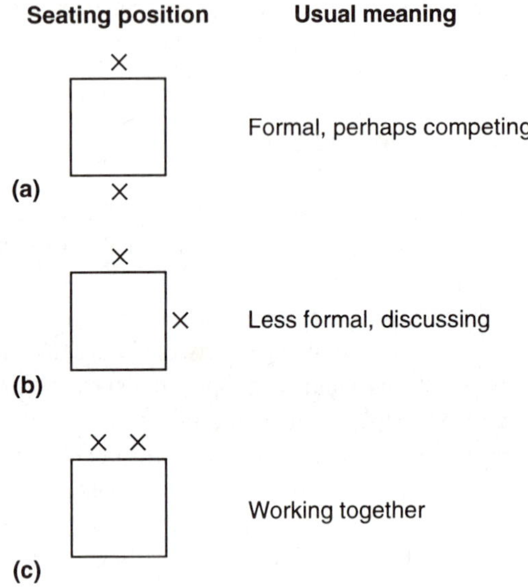

Figure 4.1 Seating orientation.

Height is another important aspect of orientation, in that it is usually associated with dominance. Hence, expressions such as 'He is above him at work', 'She is high up in the organization', 'He is someone to be looked up to' reflect the link between status and height. In hospitals, patients can feel particularly vulnerable when confined to bed, especially if staff with whom they interact remain standing. This can be overcome quite simply by sitting down on a chair beside the bed, especially if the interaction is more than just a fleeting visit. Similarly in paediatric contexts it is important for practitioners not to tower over children but rather to come down to their level when interacting.

Posture

The posture we adopt when sitting or standing can convey information about our attitudes, emotions and status. Interestingly, at staff meetings, higher-status individuals often adopt the most relaxed postures, indicating that they are confident and in control of the situation, while new staff sit bolt upright! When seated, a forward leaning posture by doctors has been found to be associated with higher patient satisfaction than a backward lean, with the head tilted back (Larsen and Smith, 1981).

Estimates of whether other people like us, or are interested in what we have to say, are influenced by their posture. A closed posture (arms and legs crossed) often signals that the person is defensive or does not wish to become too involved in an interaction, whereas an open posture tends to be interpreted as a signal of warmth, acceptance and willingness to participate (Millar, Crute and Hargie, 1992). Furthermore, when two people are getting on well together they often adopt identical postures, a process known as posture-mirroring. Such mirroring can be employed by professionals to convey to patients that they are 'with' them.

Body movements

This encompasses movements in three main regions of the body.

- **Hands and arms**. Movements here, commonly referred to as gestures, can be either communicative or self-directed. Communicative gestures serve a useful function during social encounters, since they facilitate the transmission of messages from one person to another. Indeed, when people are not permitted to use gestures when giving explanations, their speech patterns tend to be affected in terms of an increase in speech hesitancies and pauses (Hargie, Saunders and Dickson, 1994). Self-directed gestures, on the other hand, can be distracting for others and are often a sign of tension. Such gestures include ring-twisting, hand-wringing, nail-biting or self-stroking. People who display extremes of self-directed gestures tend to be viewed as anxious or neurotic.
- **Head and shoulders**. Slow head nods are usually taken as a sign of interest and willingness to listen, whereas fast head nods are interpreted as conveying impatience with the speaker. Likewise shaking the head slowly usually means 'I don't really agree' whereas shaking the head very quickly means 'I definitely disagree'! There is a range of other meanings that may be associated with various head positions in certain contexts; e.g.: head tilted slightly forward, eyes looking up through eyebrows (submissiveness); head tossed in the air (defiance); head tilted to one side (listening). Movements of the shoulders are clearly more restricted in terms of communication, though we can shrug our shoulders to indicate that we do not know what is being asked, or stiffen our shoulders to convey tension.
- **Legs and feet**. This region of the body is not typically used intentionally to communicate during interpersonal interaction. However, noticeable movements of the legs and feet are often interpreted by others as signs of unease, similar to self-directed gestures. Together, these have been referred to as 'social leakages' whereby the individual subconsciously displays evidence of tension or nervousness. These signals may be interpreted as a lack of confidence or as signs of deception, depending upon the context (Rozelle, Druckman and Baxter, 1997).

Facial expressions

One of the main functions of the face is to communicate emotional states, and facial expressions are therefore of vital importance during interaction between professionals and patients, in communicating affect. Ekman and Friesen (1982) identified a total of 46 'single action units', or separate facial movements, such as 'wink', 'lip corner puller', 'inner brow raiser' and 'nostril compressor'. Clearly, the variety of combinations of two or more of these facial action units allows for an enormous number of overall facial expressions. However, perhaps the most important of these in many instances is a combination of interest in the patient, coupled with a smile to indicate receptivity and friendliness. Likewise, practitioners may need to control their facial expressions by, for example, not showing disgust when changing an infected wound or interacting with a patient with halitosis.

Gaze

Eye contact is very important in our society. Since it is usually a pre-requisite for any interaction, gaze conveys a willingness to participate with another person. In Western society, the listener usually looks at the speaker about twice as much as the speaker looks at the listener (Argyle, 1988). However, the degree of eye contact engaged in depends upon the situation. Two young people in love may stare devotedly at one another, whereas the same degree of gaze between two males may be the prelude to physical aggression. Conversely, the absence of eye contact may convey embarrassment or lack of interest.

When dealing with patients, it is important to display appropriate levels of gaze, since too much or too little eye contact can be disconcerting. In the Larsen and Smith (1981) study mentioned earlier, it was found that greater use of eye contact by a doctor was associated with lower patient satisfaction during first-time visits. In this instance, the increased doctor gaze may have heightened the anxiety of patients when dealing with an unfamiliar physician. Interestingly, psychiatrists may put patients on a couch and sit in a chair behind them, to help reduce any possible embarrassment that patients may feel in discussing personal matters. In a review of eye contact in the health context, Davidhizor (1992) highlighted the importance of this domain in assessing patient needs, providing psychological support and evaluating patient reactions to the practitioner.

Appearance

This includes both the physical make-up of the individual, and the clothes, jewellery, etc. that they wear. As discussed in Chapter 3 this is an important dimension of communication, since we make judgements about the nature, character and disposition of individuals based upon their appearance. However, some aspects of appearance can be manipulated more easily than others. For example, dress and hair colour can be controlled, whereas height can be adjusted only slightly. It is important for health professionals to portray an appropriate image in terms of appearance so that they 'look the part' when interacting with patients.

Paralanguage

This refers to **how** something is said as opposed to **what** is said. Indeed, the manner in which a verbal message is spoken will directly affect the meaning of that message. Slight alterations in the tone, pitch, volume, speed or emphasis on certain words can change the overall meaning being conveyed. There are speech styles associated with different settings. In this way, sports commentators on TV, evangelical clergymen saying prayers in church and auctioneers selling goods, all have distinctive speech patterns. Health professionals, however, are required to display a range of speech styles. For example, the style associated with informing a patient of a terminal illness or death of a relative, will be markedly different from that associated with telling a young woman, who has been trying to have a baby for several years, that she is pregnant.

In one study of communication between nurses and the elderly, it was found that 'secondary baby talk' was a common feature of many interactions (Edwards and Noller, 1993). This involved high pitch and exaggerated intonation, coupled with patronizing terms such as 'good girl' and 'poor dear'. However, it was also found that while this secondary baby talk was rated as less respectful by nurses and psychology students who observed it, the elderly reacted less negatively to this form of communication. The reasons for this are not clear. It could be for example that the elderly have been conditioned to accept this, or that they actually enjoy being looked after in a manner resembling a form of 'second childhood'. Edwards and Noller argue that health professionals face the challenge 'of modifying communication to the elderly while at the same time conveying respect and nurturance' (p. 221). Thus, sensitivity and flexibility are required in terms of appropriate use of paralanguage and terminology.

Summary

These nine features of non-verbal communication are important dimensions of most interactive episodes. Although these aspects have been separated for the purposes of analysis, it will be obvious that they are in fact interrelated. Not only should these non-verbal features complement one another when communicating with others, they should also be consistent with the verbal message. Furthermore, the differences in meaning attached to non-verbal behaviours across cultures need to be borne in mind. Thus, a smile may be used to show deference or mask anger rather than to convey agreement or pleasure, while 'the verbal and non-verbal expression of pain or symptoms may be downplayed by patients of some cultures' (Lee *et al.*, 1992, p. 253).

4.3 REINFORCEMENT

From a very early stage of development the importance of social rewards, in the form of verbal and non-verbal reinforcement, can be observed. The smile of the infant is an important reinforcer for the mother, and likewise the smiles, caresses and soothing vocalizations of the mother are crucial to the mother–child bonding process. Furthermore, the social reinforcers of the mother are linked to the satisfaction of basic biological needs in the child, and therefore attain a significant associative role very early in life. Thus, when the child is being fed, changed or kept warm, it is also receiving concurrent social reinforcement.

This association between social and material rewards is a common one (Dickson, Saunders and Stringer, 1993). The child who wins a race or passes an examination will usually receive some form of material reward, but will also receive praise and attention from peers and from significant others. This therefore strengthens the link between social and material reinforcers. As Skinner (1953, p. 78) noted, 'The attention of people is reinforcing because it is a necessary condition for other reinforcements from them.' Over time, social reinforcement in itself acquires value for the individual even in the absence of more tangible rewards. As a result, the use of praise, encouragement, etc., can be implemented to influence the behaviour of others. Dickson, Saunders and Stringer (1993, p. 3), in their comprehensive review of this topic, asserted: 'Social rewards are of the utmost importance in interpersonal transactions and their effects wide-ranging.'

Although the term reinforcement was introduced by Pavlov (1927), it is the more recent work of Skinner (1969, 1976) that has influenced interest in this concept as a social skill. As Skinner (1971, p. 199) iterated, reinforcement is based, 'on the simple principle that whenever something reinforces a particular activity of an organism, it increases the chances that the organism will repeat that behaviour'. It is obvious that this latter Skinnerian application of the concept of reinforcement has direct implications for human behaviour. Thus a young male who is interested in a young female will give her concerted attention in the form of eye contact, smiles, nods and verbal rewards, in order to encourage her to continue talking to him. Similarly, if we tell a joke at work and our colleagues reward us by laughing, we are more likely to tell another joke than if they frown or declare that they are not amused. In this way, behaviour is shaped by the positive or negative consequences that ensue.

4.3.1 Functions of reinforcement

The use of social reinforcement serves a range of purposes.

- **Encouraging the involvement of the other person**. In order to obtain maximum participation during interaction, it is necessary to reinforce other people when they are communicating with us. Without such reinforcement, their level of participation will decrease markedly. Indeed, one of the problems with many psychiatric patients is that they give little or no reinforcement to others. As a result, they receive fewer communications, which in turn increases their social isolation (Hargie and McCartan, 1986).

- **Demonstrating interest**. We pay greater attention to, and reinforce more, people who are of interest to us. For this reason, if people do not reinforce us, we in turn feel that they are not really interested in us. Thus, Kasteler *et al.* (1976) found that patients who felt their doctors were not interested in them were more likely to change to another doctor. Similarly, Nelson *et al.* (1975) illustrated how schizophrenics were more likely to comply with treatment if they perceived their physicians as being interested in them. Conveying interest is therefore an important function of reinforcement.
- **Developing and maintaining relationships**. At the initial stage of relationship development people reciprocate high levels of reinforcement. Once a relationship has been established, reinforcement levels may subside. However, if reinforcement ceases, the relationship is likely to terminate. In health contexts the amount of reinforcement given will depend upon the setting. A patient who only occasionally sees the doctor, pharmacist or health visitor will expect more concerted attention than a patient in hospital will expect from a nurse on the ward.
- **Providing reassurance**. Although in certain instances reassurance can be employed to decrease behaviour, as when the professional reduces the anxiety of patients who may be mistakenly concerned about their well-being by reassuring them that they are quite healthy, it also can have a reinforcing potential. The very fact that the professional has taken the time to reassure the patient will probably encourage the patient to return to that person again. This will be especially true if the practitioner affirms the wisdom of the patient in seeking professional advice. Patients are often worried about their condition, the prognosis and the ability of medical staff to help them overcome their difficulties. Often, such worries are based upon mistaken beliefs or misinformation and their fears can genuinely be allayed by the practitioner. Leigh and Reiser (1980, p. 294) defined reassurance as consisting 'of a general optimistic and hopeful attitude and specific statements based on data and/or experience designed to allay exaggerated or unfounded fears of the patient'. Such reassurance should obviously be genuine, since false reassurance may well be counterproductive. DiMatteo and DiNicola (1982) emphasized the importance of a reassuring, reinforcing 'bedside manner' for practitioners, especially during ward rounds. They highlighted how patients, after such rounds, often reported feeling anxious, upset, depersonalized and even dehumanized, with resulting adverse changes in their physical condition.
- **Conveying warmth and friendliness**. Individuals who are perceived as being warm, friendly and approachable display much higher levels of verbal and non-verbal reinforcement than those who are perceived as cold or aloof. Several studies have shown that patient satisfaction and compliance with treatment are positively related to perceptions of practitioners as being warm and friendly (Dickson, Saunders and Stringer, 1993). Thus, it is important to employ appropriate reinforcers to demonstrate a warm, friendly approach when dealing with patients.

- **Helping to control the topic of conversation**. By selectively reinforcing particular aspects of the other person's communication it is possible to increase the incidence of these elements. This phenomenon is known as 'the Greenspoon effect', following a study carried out by Greenspoon (1955) in which he demonstrated that, by using the reinforcer 'mm-hmm' on each occasion during interviews that the interviewee used a plural noun, the total number of plural nouns used by interviewees could be gradually increased. Following this study, a range of similar investigations were conducted, confirming that the responses of interviewees could be subtly manipulated, through the selective use of reinforcement, to encourage them to discuss at greater length areas targeted by the interviewer.

White and Sanders (1986) carried out a series of interviews with patients suffering from chronic pain. Through the selective use of praise and attention they were able to influence the amount of **well talk** as opposed to **pain talk** of these patients. They also discovered that the reduction in pain talk was correlated with reductions in ratings of severity of pain intensity made by these patients. Quite often, of course, professionals subconsciously use selective reinforcement to encourage patients to discuss certain matters, but not others. Indeed, a review of recordings of interviews by Carl Rogers, the proponent of non-directive counselling, found that in fact he differentially (and presumably unintentionally) rewarded certain categories of client utterance (Truax, 1966). It is therefore clear that reinforcement can be applied in such a manner as to control the topic of conversation.

4.3.2 Behavioural components of reinforcement

There is a wide range of verbal and non-verbal behaviours that can be employed in order to reinforce others. Non-verbally, most of the behaviours described in the previous section can be used as reinforcers. Verbal reinforcers can be divided into five main types.

- **Acknowledgment/confirmation**. These are words or phrases that are employed in order to acknowledge or confirm the response of another person. Examples include 'Thank you', 'OK', 'I see', 'You are correct', 'Yes'. These are not very strong reinforcers but they are often expected as part of basic courtesy and if not given can leave the person feeling aggrieved. Thus, if we open a door for someone who walks through without saying 'Thank you', we tend to feel somewhat annoyed!
- **Compliments**. It is rewarding to be told that some aspect of our personal appearance is worthy of positive comment. This can be particularly true in the health field where statements such as 'You are looking well'; 'You haven't changed a bit'; 'Your hair is lovely' can be very rewarding, especially where a patient is feeling dejected or lacking in self-esteem.
- **Supportive comments**. Phrases such as 'That must have been very painful'; 'You have every right to feel like that'; 'I agree entirely' can be employed to

convey to others that they are speaking to someone who will offer encouragement, support and concern. This is very important when discussing personal and emotional matters. For instance, a doctor may say to a patient coping with an unexpected bereavement: 'This has been enormously difficult for you. I understand how painful it must be.'

- **Evaluative comments**. Here, rewards are given for some effort another person has made. Thus a nurse may say to a young boy who has valiantly withstood crying when receiving an injection, 'Well done! You're a very brave little man!' Similarly, a physiotherapist may say to a patient making a few tentative steps following a stroke, 'Great effort! You're really coming on remarkably well.' Such forms of encouragement are invaluable in many health contexts.
- **Response development**. This involves paying careful attention to what someone is saying and ensuring that their responses are built upon where appropriate. In this sense, developing and extending the topic of conversation raised by a patient is a potent form of reinforcement. In an investigation of topic initiation in consultations between elderly patients and doctors, Adelman *et al.* (1992) found that some two-thirds of topics were raised by the latter. They also found that doctors paid significantly more attention to topics they had raised than to patient-initiated topics. There may, however, be gender differences in the manner in which topics are selected. In a study of doctor–patient encounters, Ainsworth-Vaughan (1992) discovered that female physicians were more likely than their male counterparts to employ reciprocal topic shifts, where overt agreement is secured from both sides before moving from one topic to another. In her study, the ratio of reciprocal to unilateral topic shifts was 1.4:1 for males and 5:1 for females. Ainsworth-Vaughan argued that this differential may be because females are more likely to view the consultation as an activity in which power is shared, whereas males tend to prefer to be more dominant.

These are the main verbal and non-verbal components of the skill of reinforcement. The importance of this skill was highlighted in a review by Cairns (1986), who iterated that 'the way one person responds and reinforces another is a significant aspect of the communication between the people that leads to attraction, friendships or even more intimate relationships' (p. 136). Health professionals should therefore be aware of the potency and beneficial effects of the appropriate use of reinforcement. There is evidence to suggest that this skill should be incorporated into CST programmes, since studies of doctor–patient (Verby, Holden and Davis, 1979) and nurse–patient (MacLeod Clark, 1982) interactions have indicated a dearth of practitioner reinforcement. Furthermore, studies of speech-therapist–patient (Saunders and Caves, 1986), pharmacist–patient (Hargie, Morrow and Woodman, 1993) and physiotherapist–patient (Adams *et al.*, 1994) interactions have found 'positive reinforcement' to be one of the most important skills as evaluated by the practitioners themselves.

Exercise 4.1 can be employed by the trainer to encourage trainees to focus upon the skill of reinforcement, and generate a wide range of behaviours which can be employed as rewards during social interaction.

Exercise 4.1 Reinforcement

Aim

To sensitize trainees to the range of verbal and non-verbal reinforcers that can be used during interpersonal encounters.

Instructions

This exercise is not suitable for very large groups of trainees. It involves subdividing the class into dyads or triads and asking each subgroup simply to list, on a sheet of paper, as many examples of verbal and non-verbal reinforcers as they can within each of the reinforcement categories described earlier. Thus trainees should note as many examples as possible of situations where touch, proximity, orientation, etc. could be employed and should then itemize as many examples of acknowledgments, compliments, etc. as they can generate. Each subgroup should be given a specific order for listing examples (e.g. Group 1 could begin by examining 'Touch'; Group 2 'Proximity' and so on) so that a wide variety of examples will be generated. The subgroups should then be given a set time limit for completing the task.

Discussion

Using the blackboard or the overhead projector, the trainer should take each reinforcement category in turn and obtain from the groups as many examples as possible. This procedure is followed until all of the categories have been covered. During this feedback session the trainer should raise, for various examples, issues such as:

- the differential use of reinforcement with different age groups;
- gender differences in the use of reinforcers;
- cultural factors.

4.4 REFLECTING

Reference has already been made to the multidimensional nature of communication (Chapter 1). People can communicate at either a factual or a feeling level. When responding to others, we can decide to focus specifically on either one of these levels, or can take both into account. One technique that can be used to respond to patients is that of reflecting, whereby the practitioner rewords and feeds back to the patient the main elements of the latter's previous communication.

Where the emphasis is solely upon reflecting back the factual component, this is termed 'paraphrasing' (or 'reflection of content'); where it is solely upon feelings it is known as 'reflection of feeling'; and where both facts and feelings are involved this is referred to as 'reflection'. This last type of reflection has also been termed 'reflecting meaning' (Mader and Mader, 1993). As highlighted by Lang and van der Molen (1990), paraphrasing is concerned with showing an attempt to understand **what the client is saying**, while reflection of feeling involves trying to demonstrate an understanding of **how the person now feels** or **has felt**. These distinctions were neatly exemplified by Crute (1986) in relation to a health-visitor–client interaction:

> **Client**: 'I just don't understand my mother-in-law. One minute she's very kind and good to me, and the next she's treating me terribly.'
> **Health Visitor**: 'So, she's very inconsistent with you (Paraphrase). You feel confused (Reflection of feeling).'

Here, taken as a whole, the health visitor's response is an overall reflection, although either the paraphrase or the reflection of feeling could have been employed in isolation, had a decision been made to focus primarily on facts or emotions respectively.

However, there is some conceptual confusion concerning the actual meaning of the term 'reflection' (Dickson, 1997). For example, Hein (1973), in her discussion of nurse–patient communication, defined reflection as simply echoing the actual words used by the patient and used the term 'restatement' to refer to the process of reformulating the patient's verbalizations in the nurse's own words. Myerscough (1989) concurred with this view of reflection as the simple repetition of a word or phrase used by the patient. French (1994), on the other hand, conceived of paraphrasing as involving the activity of putting the patient's statements, thoughts and feelings into one's own words. This meaning was echoed by Buckman (1992), who made a distinction between paraphrasing, which he termed 'reiterative', since this was 'repeating what the patient has told you but in your own words, not hers or his', and reflection, which involved going beyond this by showing 'you have heard and have interpreted what the patient said' (p. 43). However, in this chapter the distinctions mentioned earlier will be used, and reflection will be regarded as involving the following steps:

1. recalling and restating the speaker's message correctly;
2. identifying the main factual and/or feeling aspects being expressed;
3. translating these factual and/or feeling components into one's own words;
4. reflecting the essence of these facts and/or feelings, without adding one's own interpretation;

5. checking the accuracy of the reflection by monitoring the reaction of the other person.

The use of reflection as an interviewing skill originated with the development by Rogers (1951) of client-centred, non-directive counselling. Here the emphasis is upon allowing the client to lead the interaction and dictate the topics to be discussed. The counsellor is viewed as a facilitator, encouraging clients to talk through and sort out their own problems and, as a result, the use of more directive techniques, such as questioning, are eschewed. Although reflection as a skill was identified within the field of client-centred therapy, this skill is also frequently employed in a wide range of interview settings (Millar, Crute and Hargie, 1992). Indeed, it is commonly regarded as a skill that can be most gainfully employed when accompanied by other interviewing skills, including certain types of question (see Chapter 5). As Hein (1973) put it, in the health context, reflection 'in particular needs to be used in conjunction with other skills. . . . Used exclusively, it can generate antagonism and frustration from our patients' (p. 46).

4.4.1 Functions of reflecting

The main functions of the skill of reflecting can be summarized as follows.

- **To demonstrate interest in and involvement with the patient**. Reflection is in fact a form of response development which, as discussed in the previous section, is in turn a potent form of reinforcement. It helps the speaker 'to express thoughts gradually more clearly and fully. It assures him of understanding. And it makes a public possession of a private meaning. The result is to encourage participation' (Dillon, 1990, p. 186). It is, however, quite difficult to listen, assimilate what is being said and then immediately reflect this back using different terminology. The ability to do so is clear evidence of careful listening and this is therefore appreciated by clients. This ability often takes time to develop and trainers may need to devote concerted time and effort to ensure that trainees acquire an effective grasp of this skill.
- **To use a patient-centred approach**. In their analysis of doctor–patient consultations, Byrne and Long (1976) identified a continuum of interactive styles ranging from doctor-centred at one end to patient-centred at the other. At the latter end, one of the techniques employed was that of reflecting. Byrne and Long underlined the value of a patient-centred approach but found it was seldom used by doctors. Livesey (1986) attributed this finding to the probable fear by doctors of losing control of the consultation and of being involved in protracted interactions with patients. However, these fears are groundless since control can be subtly maintained within a patient-centred approach and very few consultations will involve complex problems requiring lengthy interviews. Furthermore, in discussing doctor–patient interactions, Shorter (1985) identified two main conditions that were necessary for successful consultations: (1) the doctor showed an active interest in the

patient; and (2) patients were given the opportunity to present in a leisurely, unhurried manner.

Bensing and Dronkers (1992, p. 288) found that a patient-centred approach was characterized by 'doctors who show their attentiveness by paraphrasing the patient, reflecting or legitimizing his or her feelings and showing agreement or partnership'.

- **To check for accuracy of understanding**. Reflection is a useful skill for ensuring that both the practitioner and patient fully understand the latter's communications. In this sense, it allows the practitioner to periodically seek feedback, since the patient will indicate verbally and/or non-verbally following a reflection whether it has been accurate. This can also be valuable from the patient's point of view. When talking through a complex problem that has not been fully sorted out internally, the use of practitioner reflections can facilitate the coalescence of thoughts, ideas and feelings in a new and meaningful *Gestalt*, thereby providing insights and a deeper, more accurate understanding.
- **To highlight certain facets of the patient's communication**. By reflecting back particular parts of the message received, the practitioner is, in effect, encouraging the patient to discuss these more fully and is thereby using a form of selective reinforcement. As already mentioned, such selection may involve an exclusive focus upon either facts or feelings. Within these two domains, of course, there may be further selectivity. One of the most commonly cited advantages of reflection is that it allows, and indeed encourages, the exploration of feelings, in that the use of reflection of feeling conveys to the patient that it is acceptable to have such feelings and that the practitioner is willing to discuss them (Bensing and Dronkers, 1992).
- **To show respect for patients and their concerns**. The willingness to allow patients to freely express themselves, coupled with the use of practitioner reflections to demonstrate concerted listening, is an indicator that patients are valued and worthy of attention. This, in turn, facilitates the process of relationship development.
- **To demonstrate empathy**. In his analysis of the dimension of empathy in doctor–patient interactions, Authier (1986) highlighted the central role of reflections in communicating an awareness and understanding of the patient's perspective. As defined by Rogers (1975, p. 3), empathy involves 'pointing sensitively to the "felt meaning" which the client is experiencing in this particular moment, in order to help him focus on that meaning and to carry it further'. It is therefore clear that the skill of reflection will be a core technique in conveying an empathic approach.

4.4.2 Guidelines for the use of reflections

There are several points that need to be borne in mind when using this skill.

- **Avoid interpretations**. Reflections involve rephrasing what the patient has said, not going beyond this to analyse or interpret the message received. As Hein (1973) asserted, when using reflections 'No new information is being sought at these times. Validity, clarity and understanding of the old (i.e. previous) information are the major aims of this skill' (p. 46).

- **Be accurate**. While the occasional inaccurate reflection will not adversely affect a relationship, consistent inaccuracy will indicate a total lack of understanding. In particular, it is important to gauge the correct level of emotion to reflect back. When using reflection of feeling, Cohen-Cole (1991) recommended staying on the side of caution by using feeling words at a moderate level. Trainees can be sensitized to different emotional labels by having them distinguish three levels of emotion, namely low, medium and high. This can be achieved by giving them a few examples as follows:

Low	*Medium*	*High*
Annoyed	Angry	Furious
Pleased	Delighted	Ecstatic
Like	Love	Adore

Trainees can then be asked, either individually or in groups to identify as many of these emotional continua as possible, and their responses written on the blackboard.

- **Non-verbal considerations**. As well as verbally reflecting, the practitioner should non-verbally reflect the patient's communication. This may involve adopting a similar facial expression, posture, body movements or paralanguage. At times it may be necessary to reflect feelings based purely upon non-verbal signals, and in such cases it is wise to allow an opportunity for the patient to correct possible misinterpretations by using prefaces such as 'It seems to me that. . .'; 'You appear to be. . .'; 'I get the impression that. . .'.
- **Do not use stereotyped responses**. One of the common errors made by inexperienced interviewers is to begin every reflection with 'You feel. . . '. Other errors include either under- or overusing this skill and using questions in the mistaken belief that they are reflections. This latter misconception can partly be overcome by developing the ability of trainees to clearly identify appropriate reflections. One method whereby this can be achieved is for the trainer to display on an overhead projection transparency a number of patient statements and, for each statement, to instruct trainees to write down a relevant paraphrase and reflection of feeling. The trainer can then ask individual trainees to call out their responses.
- **Be concise and specific**. A reflection should be a brief reformulation of the essence of what the patient has said. Where feelings are involved, there should be a feeling 'label' in the reflection. Thus, general statements such as 'Boy, have you got a problem!' are not reflections.

These are the main points that should be considered when using the skill of reflection. This is a very useful skill for practitioners to acquire since Dickson (1997), in his review of research in this field, has shown how interviewers who employ reflections are perceived positively by both interviewees and external observers. It should also be realized that this can be a difficult skill for trainees to master. As Mader and Mader (1993, p. 284) emphasized: ‘Paraphrasing the content of a message is not always easy, but describing how someone feels is even more difficult’. This means that time and practice will be essential for trainees to become proficient in the use of this skill.

4.5 LISTENING

In terms of responding skills, the ability to demonstrate effective listening is of prime importance. In fact, many of the behaviours associated with all of the skills in this chapter, and in Chapter 5, can be employed as indicators of listening. Given this widespread range of listening behaviours it is hardly surprising that Pietrofesa *et al.* (1978, p. 243), in their discussion of counselling, concluded that ‘if we had to pin-point a crucial helping skill, it would be the ability to listen’. Furthermore, Porritt (1984, p. 80), in her analysis of nurse–patient communication, asserted: ‘Most life events, including admission to hospital, do not require highly skilled counselling but do require skilled listening.’ In his review of research into doctor–patient communication, Buckman (1992) summarized the main benefits of effective listening as: improved patient satisfaction; increased perceived competence of the physician; and enhanced compliance with the treatment plan. It is therefore vital that health professionals have a sound knowledge of, and capacity for, effective listening skills. Indeed, in their analysis of this field, Wolvin and Coakley (1993, p. xii) argued that ‘listening pedagogy ought to be central to communication education at all levels’.

Although several books have been written specifically on this topic (e.g. Borisoff and Purdy, 1991; Wolvin and Coakley, 1993; Burley-Allen, 1995), and indeed most texts on communication for health professionals include at least a chapter devoted to this skill, there is no one agreed definition. Ridge (1993), in reviewing definitions of listening, highlighted the fact that some theorists regard this as involving solely the reception of auditory information, while others view listening as encompassing the assimilation of both verbal and non-verbal messages. It is this latter perspective which will be adopted here, and in this sense listening can be defined as the process whereby one person pays careful attention to, and attempts to understand, the verbal and non-verbal signals being emitted by another.

This definition emphasizes the active nature of listening. It is possible to listen to someone (especially to their verbal messages) without showing that you are paying attention, in other words to listen **passively** (Hargie, Saunders and Dickson, 1994). However, in professional contexts it is necessary both to listen carefully and to indicate this verbally and non-verbally. Thus, the use of reinforcement, reflections, self-disclosure, probing questions and so on are potent indicators of **active listening**. Active listening is also required to ensure that maximum verbal and non-verbal information is received from patients. As discussed in Chapter 3, concerted effort is essential during interpersonal interaction to ensure that the selective nature of the perceptual process does not result in vital social information being lost.

4.5.1 The listening process

When we listen to others, a range of mental processes operates. Wolvin and Coakley (1993), used the acronym HURIER, to highlight the six core processes of **h**earing, **u**nderstanding, **r**emembering, **i**nterpreting, **e**valuating and **r**esponding. As we listen we attempt to make sense of, retain and judge what the speaker is saying, we plan what we are going to say in response, and we covertly rehearse (often subconsciously) our response. While these processes are an inherent part of interpersonal interaction, they should not interfere with the act of listening *per se*. In other words, we should not be concentrating so much on what we intend to say that we stop paying attention to what the speaker is saying.

In relation to the actual reception of verbal messages, three factors should be borne in mind.

- **Reductionism**. We can only cope with a limited amount of information and so if we are presented with too much detail it is necessary to reduce this in order to retain it. Care must be taken to ensure only less important elements are lost.
- **Rationalization**. This refers to the process whereby we attempt to make incoming data fit more easily with our own experience. To facilitate such assimilation we may rationalize it in three ways. Firstly, we may attribute different causes to those presented (e.g. the practitioner may regard the pain expressed by a 'hypochondriacal' patient as imaginary). Secondly, transformation of language may occur. There is an apocryphal story about the message 'Send reinforcements, we're going to advance' being sent by troops at the battlefront along the line, and eventually arriving at headquarters as 'Send three-and-fourpence, we're going to a dance'! Such acoustic confusions (Gregg, 1986) are not uncommon in reality, but can be potentially dangerous in the health sphere where products with similar-sounding names can easily be confused. For example, in one case in Belgium a patient died after being given the diuretic Lasix® instead of the anti-ulcer drug Losec®. Thirdly, there can be the addition of material, a classic example being gossip enlargement! As mentioned under the skill of reflection, care needs to be taken not to 'read too much into' what a patient is saying.
- **Change in the order of events**. Where the information received contains a chronological order or a set sequence, this can be mixed up. Thus, 'Take 2 tablets 4 times daily' may become 'Take 4 tablets 2 times daily'.

4.5.2 Obstacles to effective listening

In order to employ effective listening skills, it is necessary to be aware of a number of obstacles that can interfere with the listening process. These include the following.

Speech-thought rates

Research has shown that 'listeners pay attention to, and comprehend better, messages that are delivered at rates 25% or 50% faster than the normal conversational rate' (Buller and Street, 1992 p. 128). The average rate of speech is between 125 and 175 words per minute whereas the average 'thought rate', at which we assimilate information, is between 400 and 800 words per minute, and this differential means that we usually have spare thought time when listening to others. A faster rate of speech decreases this differential and encourages listeners to pay more attention to the message. However, in certain situations, it will not be appropriate to speak at a fast rate – for example when breaking bad news it is important to do so at a rate that takes cognisance of the emotional state of the recipient. When explaining complex information also, it will be necessary to proceed at the patient's pace.

When listening, it is important to use available spare thought capacity positively. As summarized by Brownell (1993, p. 246): 'Effective listeners use spare listening time efficiently; they consider the ideas presented in terms of their personal interests and needs, apply the information to concrete situations, formulate relevant questions, and otherwise participate in the communication event.' For example, the Royal College of General Practitioners Working Party (1972) recommended the following covert questions for doctors:

> What must I tell this patient? How much of what I learned about him should he know? What words shall I use to convey this information? How much of what I propose to tell him will he understand? How will he react? How much of my advice will he take? What degree of pressure am I entitled to apply?
>
> *Royal College of General Practitioners Working Party, 1972, p.17*

Without careful concentration it is probable that spare thought time will be filled with other mental processes unrelated to listening (such as daydreaming). Attention and memory can be facilitated by imposing organization on the material to be remembered. Four techniques have been identified for improving the reception, storage and recall of information (Morrow and Hargie, 1988a).

- **Categorization**. The organization of information being given by the patient, using categories such as presenting symptoms, current/previous treatments and medication dosage.
- **Sequencing**. The ordering of this information into a pre-set chronological order, such as symptoms ⇨ severity ⇨ duration ⇨ timing of ⇨ previous action taken, etc.

- **Mnemonics**. The most common of these is the use of acronyms – such as PAIL for the four types of skin cut: puncture, abrasion, incision, laceration. In addition, rhymes can be usefully employed to remember patients' details (e.g. Mrs Diane Adair, round glasses, red hair).
- **Visualization**. This involves painting a mental picture of what the patient is saying.

Distractions

Listening ability is impaired if the environment contains too many intrusive distractions that divert attention away from the speaker. This would include other people talking in the room or ward, telephone ringing, and so on.

Inattentiveness

Listening is hard work and requires constant concentration. As a result, listeners who are tired or have something preying on their mind are less likely to listen in an efficient manner.

Mental set

The initial frame of mind of the listener, including preconceptions of the speaker, can influence how the latter's message is received and interpreted. Judgements about the speaker are often made on the basis of age, sex, dress, appearance, status, etc. Similarly, patients are often evaluated on the basis of ascribed stereotypes (hypochondriac, troublesome patient). In this way, more attention is paid to who is speaking rather than on what is being said. Good listeners need to ensure objectivity during social encounters.

Individual bias

Listening can be impaired when an individual distorts the message being received. Thus the practitioner who is in a hurry may choose not to 'hear' a message because it would entail an extended interaction with a patient. On the other hand, seriously ill patients, or their relatives, may choose to ignore unpleasant facts being detailed by the professional because they are too threatening or disturbing. Another example of individual bias occurs where individuals do not listen simply because they wish to speak, and get their own message across, regardless of what others have said.

The speaker

Quite often the cause of ineffective listening lies with the speaker. If the speaker has a severe speech disfluency, speaks for long periods at an extremely fast or slow rate, has a marked foreign or regional accent, or is being deliberately vague and evasive, it will be very difficult for the listener to cope.

Blocking

Hargie, Saunders and Dickson (1994) identified a range of blocking tactics that a listener who does not wish to pursue a certain line of communication may employ. These blocking techniques, which include referring the person elsewhere, responding selectively to only part of the message or changing the topic completely, are used to divert or terminate the conversation. It should however be realized that in certain instances blocking tactics may be used positively: for example, a pharmacist suspecting a serious illness would be expected to refer a patient to see a doctor immediately.

4.5.3 Active listening

During interpersonal encounters, the practitioner must make the effort not only to listen to others but also to clearly demonstrate this, both verbally and non-verbally. This is not as simple as it may sound, since listening requires a great deal of effort and concentration to sort out the relevance of various points and to consider their possible relationships. In addition, listening can be a time-consuming activity which, in some health professions, may be regarded as a form of inactivity. For example, Hein (1973, p. 171) illustrated how, in nursing practice, listening often was 'supplanted by more immediate and visually apparent tasks or priorities. Listening skilfully during a nursing task is often a good utilization of time, but as a solitary activity (except perhaps with psychiatric patients) it is often considered unessential'. While this approach to patient care is changing, there still remains a residual attitude that listening is somehow an easy option and synonymous with 'doing nothing'.

Yet, the skilled use of listening when interacting with patients is useful in order to achieve a number of functions, including:

- to focus specifically upon the verbal and non-verbal messages being communicated by patients;
- to gain a full, accurate understanding of the patient's situation;
- to communicate interest, concern and sympathetic attention;
- to encourage full, open and honest patient communication;
- to develop a more non-directive, patient-centred style of interaction.

Listening, therefore, is a core skill for health professionals. In reviewing studies that have examined doctor–patient interactions, DiMatteo and DiNicola (1982) found that in almost every instance the doctor talked significantly more than the patient, yet most physicians believed that they spent much more time listening to their patients than talking to them. In a study, already mentioned, of doctor and patient perceptions of actual consultations, it was shown that doctors reported that they listened to the worries of and gave support to 58% of patients, whereas only 30% of patients reported that the doctor had done so (Martin *et al.*, 1991). Likewise, in a survey of members of the public, over 94% of respondents expressed the desire for community pharmacists to spend more time listening fully to their concerns (Hargie, Morrow and Woodman, 1992).

These findings underline the need for more concerted training in listening skills. As Armstrong (1991, p. 262) pointed out, 'patients report as what they most value: a doctor who listens', although he also noted that 'though it would seem that listening is a medical skill more valued than previously, this does not necessarily mean that doctors have yet learnt always to hear what patients are saying'. Davis and Fallowfield (1991, p. 336), in their review of this area, concluded: 'There is currently very limited emphasis placed upon the development of good listening skills in medical education. Active listening is very hard work initially and demands considerable attention and practice but the advantages in terms of eliciting information and developing a good therapeutic relationship with a patient are worth the investment of time'.

Wolff *et al.* (1983) suggested 10 main points that should be borne in mind to facilitate effective listening.

- Do not stereotype the speaker.
- Avoid distractions.
- Arrange a conducive environment (adequate ventilation, lighting, seating, etc.).
- Be psychologically prepared to listen.
- Keep an open, analytical mind, searching for the central thrust of the speaker's message.
- Identify supporting arguments and facts.
- Do not dwell on one or two aspects at the expense of others.
- Delay judgement or refutation until you have heard the entire message.
- Do not formulate your next question while the speaker is relating information.
- Be objective.

4.6 SELF-DISCLOSURE

In order to make accurate diagnoses about patients' illnesses, it is necessary to encourage them to openly and honestly disclose personal details about their condition and their situation. As Smith and Bass put it:

> Patients and new employees in a health-care setting must often be encouraged and helped to recognize some of the situations in which extra self-disclosure is necessary. Physicians and other health professionals often need to know personal or intimate details about a patient to make a diagnosis and either to prescribe or to carry out treatment. The patient's willingness to disclose himself may be crucial.
>
> *Smith and Bass, 1982, p. 157*

Self-disclosure, in this sense, can be defined as the act of verbally and/or non-verbally communicating to others some dimension of personal information. Thus, self-disclosure can be non-verbal, in that it is possible, for example, either to hide feelings such as happiness, sadness, anger, etc. or to express them through the use of facial expressions, gestures and so on. Most texts on self-disclosure, however, tend to emphasize the verbal component of this skill, since this aspect is less prone to misinterpretation, whereas we can be mistaken in our judgements about the non-verbal behaviour of others.

A knowledge and skilled use of self-disclosure is important for health professionals for two main reasons. Firstly, they should be aware of the factors that will encourage patients to fully present and openly express their needs. Secondly, practitioners need to be sensitive to situations in which it is apt for them to self-disclose to patients. The use of self-disclosure by professionals can be divided into two main categories (Hargie and Morrow, 1991): one's own personal experiences, or one's personal reaction to the patient's experiences (although Danish, D'Angelli and Brock (1976) argued that technically the former is a self-disclosing statement whereas the latter is a self-involving statement). Both of these types of self-disclosure can be appropriate, depending upon the circumstances. The first type can be used to reassure patients that they are not alone in their situation, and can demonstrate shared experiences. However, it should not be taken to extremes or to what Yager and Beck (1985) termed the 'we could have been twins' response! The second type keeps the focus of attention firmly upon patients and indicates a willingness to become involved in their experiences.

4.6.1 Elements of self-disclosure

There are three main elements of self-disclosure that need to be considered when evaluating the effectiveness of this skill in professional contexts.

- **Informativeness**. This relates to the amount (total number) of disclosures made by the individual and to their depth (or intimacy). There is a relationship between psychological adjustment and self-disclosure, in that people who are not well-adjusted tend to be either extremely high or low disclosers. For example, clinically depressed patients will be very reticent about imparting personal information, whereas neurotic patients are generally quite verbose in providing details of their personal affairs. The depth of self-disclosure increases as a relationship develops. During initial social encounters with strangers, disclosures tend to be fairly superficial, but they gradually become more intimate as a relationship grows. This underlines the importance of practitioners developing a good relationship with patients.
- **Appropriateness**. Self-disclosures are most frequently used between people of equal status, followed by disclosures from low-status to high-status individuals. The least frequent usage is from high- to low-status, so that too

much self-disclosure from professionals to patients would not be deemed appropriate (Derlega *et al.*, 1993).

- **Accessibility**. Certain individuals will be more inhibited than others when presenting personal information. This may be due to personality differences (e.g. extroverts will disclose more than introverts), upbringing (i.e. the child may be taught not to reveal too much of his/her business to others) or culture (some cultures encourage more disclosure than others). With embarrassing, intimate problems, practitioners may find more difficulty in accessing complete disclosure. Often patients will present a problem that is not in fact the primary problem, and health professionals need to ensure, therefore, that they encourage patients to disclose fully, thereby getting to the heart of their true concerns.

4.6.2 Influencing factors

Self-disclosure will be influenced by a range of factors pertaining to the speaker, the listener, the overall relationship, and the situation itself (for a fuller review see Hargie, Saunders and Dickson, 1994).

The speaker

Research findings indicate that, generally, self-disclosure increases with age, although the most problematic stage seems to be that of mid-adolescence, when disclosure tends to be lowest. Overall, females disclose more easily and at a greater depth than males. Interestingly, firstborn children seem to disclose less than their siblings, a finding attributed to the possibility that with later-born children parents will have developed more experience of child-rearing, coupled with the fact that younger children are usually able to seek support from their older and therefore higher-status brothers and sisters. As mentioned earlier, personality differences affect disclosure, as does cultural background (so that for example Americans tend to disclose more than comparable groups from Europe or the Middle East).

The listener

As a general rule, people tend to disclose more to members of the opposite sex. However with intimate problems, patients may prefer to deal with a practitioner of the same sex. Disclosure also increases if we perceive the listener as attractive, either in respect of physical appearance or in terms of holding similar values, beliefs, attitudes, etc. (Hargie, Dickson and Hargie, 1995). We also disclose more to people who are friendly, accepting and empathic. Not surprisingly, therefore, doctors who adopt a more open, patient-centred approach have been shown to encourage greater disclosure from patients, especially about psychosocial matters (Verhaak, 1988). Conversely, it has been shown that, when dealing with elderly patients, physicians often respond in ways that actively discourage disclosure, one hypothesized reason for this being that 'some physicians may fear that by showing any interest in an elderly patient's presentation of self they will open a Pandora's box of concerns and issues' (Greene *et al.*, 1994, p. 231).

The relationship

Trust is a crucial factor in encouraging self-disclosure from patients, who will confide more in practitioners in whom they have confidence. Reciprocation of self-disclosures at a similar level is the norm in most situations although, as already pointed out, in the professional context the patient will do almost all of the disclosing. As Greene *et al.* (1994) highlighted, the norms of initial medical interviews allow doctors to ask questions that would not be acceptable in other settings, such as 'How many sexual partners do you have and what gender are they?' or 'Do you take drugs?'.

Furthermore, the nature of the encounter means that patients would not expect to ask the doctor such questions. Indeed, Fisher and Groce (1990), in an analysis of 43 medical interviews, found that 'it was a rare occurrence in our data for doctors to disclose even the most obvious about themselves'. Likewise, while the community pharmacists participating in a study by Hargie, Morrow and Woodman (1993) identified 'disclosing personal information' as an important pharmacist skill, few examples of such disclosure emerged in recordings of some 350 consultations with patients. However, there is a considerable body of evidence to indicate that therapist self-disclosures encourage client self-disclosures (Stricker and Fisher, 1990).

In the health context, Weiner (1980) has emphasized that appropriate practitioner self-disclosure is beneficial in fostering a positive relationship with patients. For example, one doctor in the Fisher and Groce study did disclose 'I'm a little overweight myself, but gee, I like to drink beer and eat steak,' and a pharmacist in the Hargie, Morrow and Woodman (1993) investigation said to a patient receiving antibiotics for a dental problem, 'I must admit, I've suffered in the past from several abscesses. They've been very painful.' The use of such brief disclosures can help the practitioner to present a 'human' face, while not of course taking the focus away from the patient as the centre of concern.

On some occasions patients may seek advice from a professional with whom they are not acquainted. This has been likened to what is known as the 'stranger-on-the-train' phenomenon – more recently referred to as 'in-flight intimacy' – wherein two people who meet on a long train or plane journey and realize they are unlikely ever to meet again will disclose quite intimate personal information (DeVito, 1993). One advantage of so doing is that there is not the likely embarrassment of interacting with that individual again, having initially disclosed a great deal of very personal information.

The situation

Patients will disclose more where there is greater privacy. Thus, a doctor's surgery will be more conducive to self-disclosure than a public hospital ward or a pharmacy shop floor. Indeed in relation to the latter, research has shown that members of the public would value a private consulting area (Hargie, Morrow and Woodman, 1992). In their report, the Audit Commission (1993) was critical of the fact that 'surgical and gynaecological clinics in a number of hospitals are held in cubicles with nothing more than a curtain to separate patients having intimate examinations and private discussions' (p. 29). Such an environment is clearly not conducive to self-disclosure.

Greater levels of disclosure also occur in 'warm' environments with potted plants, carpets, curtains and effective use of colour and lighting. Furthermore, where people find themselves in a crisis situation, such as prior to surgery or following bereavement, they are also more liable to divulge their personal feelings. Finally, people who are isolated or 'cut off' from the rest of society, for example patients in a hospital ward, tend to engage in more self-disclosure.

4.6.3 Functions of self-disclosure

Given the above aspects, it will be clear that self-disclosure serves a number of important functions in the health setting. These include:

- to open conversations (e.g. 'Hello. My name is Mary Hilton. I'm a pharmacist here at the hospital and I would like to talk to you about the medicines you are currently taking. . .');
- to encourage reciprocation – as Archer (1979, p. 47) pointed out, 'the most frequently demonstrated determinant of disclosure is disclosure itself';
- to provide reassurance – sometimes a patient may feel foolish having to discuss a particular problem; here, a reassuring disclosure from the professional can be of great benefit. As Cohen-Cole (1991) illustrated, a disclosure such as 'I can understand why you would be worried about this' can be used to legitimize or validate a patient's feelings;
- to share common experiences – this is useful to demonstrate to patients that you are 'on the same wavelength' and can empathize with them;
- to express concern for others;
- to facilitate self-expression – it can frequently be therapeutic for patients just to be allowed to talk things through with a caring professional. There is truth in the adage that 'a problem shared is a problem halved'. Indeed, it has also been shown that getting people to disclose in writing their feelings about severe traumatic events has positive health benefits (Greenberg and Stone, 1992);
- to develop relationships – Wilmot (1995) has clearly demonstrated the paramount importance of self-disclosure in the development and maintenance of relationships. How and what we disclose will influence the types of relation-

ship we develop, and likewise once we have established a relationship we expect to give and receive higher levels of disclosure.

An awareness of the skill of self-disclosure is therefore crucial for health professionals. DiMatteo and DiNicola, in reviewing the importance of practitioner self-disclosure, concluded that:

> If it is appropriate in timing, dosage and content, self-disclosure can enhance the therapeutic relationship and hence patient cooperation . . . a limited amount of practitioner self-disclosure has been found to promote clients' perceptions that the therapist is genuine . . . to increase clients' self-disclosure . . . strengthen interpersonal attraction and social influence . . . (and during first visits) increases the chances of clients returning for a second session.
>
> *DiMatteo and DiNicola, 1982, p. 107*

Practitioners can also increase the level of self-disclosure from patients by establishing a relationship of trust, confidence, acceptance and empathy by:

- ensuring an attractive, professional, appearance;
- providing a warm private environment in which intimate matters can be discussed freely;
- dealing with patients in a relaxed, unhurried style.

Exercise 4.2 can be used to introduce trainees to the concept of self-disclosure within the context of a practitioner–patient interaction.

Exercise 4.2 Self-disclosure

Aim

To sensitize trainees to some of the important elements of self-disclosure.

Materials

Blank acetates and felt-tip pens.

Instructions

Divide the total class into small groups each comprising three or four trainees. Each subgroup should then generate a number of low-, medium- and high-level self-disclosure statements, some of which in each category should be health-related. Examples can be given as follows:

Low level: 'I have a headache'; 'My name is Philip'.
Medium level: 'I have trouble passing water'; 'I'm separated from my husband'.

High level: 'I have AIDS'; 'I've tried to commit suicide twice'.

Having generated a range of such disclosing statements and listed these on the acetate the groups should then evaluate some of the difficulties faced by patients disclosing each health statement, of either a medium or high level, to the practitioner. Some examples can be given to stimulate trainees (e.g. The patient may find it embarrassing having to disclose 'I have trouble passing water' to a practitioner of the opposite sex). However, the onus should be put upon trainees to generate specific difficulties for each statement and to then suggest methods for dealing with these difficulties.

Discussion

Each subgroup in turn (or a spokesperson) comes to the front of the class and presents the acetate detailing the disclosing statements. They then relate the difficulties they have identified and their suggested methods for coping with these difficulties. At this stage, other groups should be asked for their comments, and a general open class discussion should ensue concerning the problems presented by each self-disclosure.

4.7 OVERVIEW

This chapter has examined five skills central to effective practitioner–patient interactions. These skills – non-verbal communication, reinforcement, reflecting, listening and self-disclosure – are essentially responsive in nature. They are particularly useful in encouraging patients to participate fully in consultations. Together with the skills provided in the following chapter, these are the core communication skills used by health professionals. As such, they can appropriately form the basis of CST programmes. The intention of this chapter has been to provide a brief overview of the central facets of each skill and the trainer is recommended to pursue further some of the references employed throughout the chapter.

Initiating skills

5

5.1 INTRODUCTION

This chapter extends the analysis of communication skills covered in Chapter 4 by focusing upon those areas where the practitioner initiates the interaction or plays a leading role in it. The initiating skills included here are questioning, explaining, opening interactions, closing interactions and assertiveness. Again, it is the purpose of this chapter to provide a summative overview of each skill, which should act as a useful *aide-memoire* for the trainer to consult. While the skills are discussed in relation to health situations, the reader is strongly advised to pursue some or all of the references used.

5.2 QUESTIONING

The ability to use questions effectively is a core skill for most health professionals. Before appropriate advice or information can be given, the practitioner must obtain all relevant information from the patient. As Morrow and Hargie (1988a) pointed out, the acronym FUN (**f**irst **u**ncover **n**eeds) is useful for trainees to remember, in that it is only when the needs of patients have been fully established that the interaction can progress satisfactorily. The most direct method of assessing needs is to ask questions, and therefore a knowledge of the nature, functions and types of question is of particular importance in facilitating accurate diagnosis.

However, given that the skill of questioning has a high face validity, there is a danger that practitioners will rely too heavily upon this skill, and indeed even misuse it, at the expense of effective communication with patients. Fisher and Groce (1990, p. 230), in their examination of doctor–patient interaction, found that 'it is doctors who ask most of the questions and patients who respond most of the time'. White (1988) characterized many doctor–patient consultations as being represented by the expression 'stop telling me about your problems and answer my questions'! The ideal patient is often seen as a passive object, answering questions precisely as required – in a brief, factual manner and only discussing the medical problem (Mishler, 1984). In his review of research in this area, Dillon (1986, p. 114) concluded that 'the doctor is observed to speak almost nothing but questions, to ask numerous, response-constraining questions (yes/no, multiple choice), at a staccato pace with incursions into patient turns, and with an even briefer pause between the patient's answer and the doctor's next question – as little as one-tenth of a second'. Indeed, Hargie, Saunders and Dickson (1994) argue that health professionals frequently use questions to manipulate patients and maintain control of the interaction. It is not surprising, therefore, to learn that high levels of question-asking by health professionals may be related to a decrease in patient satisfaction (Thompson, 1994).

In most social situations it is the person with high status and power who asks the questions. Thus, questions are asked by lawyers in the courtroom, by teachers in the classroom, by detectives in interrogation rooms and so on. In all of these settings clients do little questioning and in fact are often discouraged from it. West (1983) reported similar outcomes in a study of 21 doctor–patient interactions where it was found that doctors posed over 90% of the total number of questions asked. It was further discovered that, when patients did ask questions, many of these were marked by speech disturbances indicating that they felt uncomfortable requesting information from the doctor. Likewise, in their analysis of doctor–patient interactions, Stimson and Webb (1975) found that patient requests were posed in the impersonal form such as, 'What can be done?' rather than in the personal form of 'What can you do?', again indicating a reluctance to ask direct questions of the doctor.

In another study, Skipper (1992) video-recorded all patient assessments in a hospital swallowing clinic over a 4-month period. Her results showed that patients asked 12% of the total number of questions and also indicated an age difference in questioning behaviour with 'older patients expressing a reluctance to ask questions' (p. 586). In the community pharmacy context, however, Morrow *et al.* (1993) discovered that patients asked some 38% of the total number of questions, indicating a greater readiness to request information from pharmacists than from doctors. Interestingly, some patient questions were requests for clarification of what the doctor had told them. This pattern of patient questioning was confirmed by Dillon (1990, p. 56) in his review of this area, when he concluded that 'Patients sense that they are **not to ask** questions of the doctor; and they know they can ask their questions more easily of other medical personnel – nurses, technicians, pharmacists.' He further urged these latter professionals to continue to encourage, and answer, patient questions. However, we would also recommend that doctors and consultants be trained to do likewise.

These findings are somewhat disconcerting, given that there would seem to be distinct positive advantages that can accrue from encouraging patient questions. Roter (1977), for example, found that an experimental group of patients who were encouraged by a health counsellor to formulate questions they would like to ask prior to consultation with their doctor, asked more questions and subsequently demonstrated higher appointment-keeping ratios than a control group who were given no such counselling. Later results also demonstrated that the earlier in the consultation the first question was asked by the patient, the more questions they asked overall, the shorter the time the consultation lasted and the higher the appointment-keeping ratio (DiMatteo and DiNicola, 1982).

Parrott, Greene and Parker (1992) illustrated that the volume of questions asked by patients could be increased, since when paediatricians addressed concerns raised by the parents of patients, more questions were then asked by these parents. As Hargie, Saunders and Dickson (1994, p. 95) put it 'patient questions can be encouraged (and of course discouraged!) by the approach of the doctor'. The Audit Commission (1993), in their report on eight hospitals in England, found that patients did not have much opportunity to ask questions, and recommended that patients should be invited to prepare for their next consultation by making a list of questions they would like answered. Clearly, health professionals need to ask questions of their patients. Equally, however, they should also expect and encourage patients to ask questions of them. By so doing, they can develop a style of interacting that allows patients to negotiate their own needs and become active participants in the health-care process.

5.2.1 Definition and functions

A question can be defined simply as a request for information, whether factual or otherwise. Such requests can be non-verbal and may take the form of raised eyebrows, a quizzical facial expression or the use of a high pitched vocalization ('hmmm?'). However, most requests for information are verbal, and it is this aspect that will be focused upon. Questions serve a number of important purposes for the practitioner, including:

- to obtain precise information from patients;
- to open interactions (e.g. 'How are you today?')
- to diagnose particular difficulties that patients may be experiencing;
- to focus attention upon a specific area;
- to assess patient condition, and knowledge and understanding thereof;
- to maintain control of the interaction;
- to encourage maximum participation from patients;
- to demonstrate an interest in the patient;
- to help create enlightenment (e.g. 'Did you know that. . .?');
- to facilitate the discussion of attitudes and feelings.

5.2.2 Types of question

A number of different types of question have been identified. Rudyard Kipling recognized the main categories in the lines:

I keep six honest serving men
(They taught me all I knew);
Their names are what and why and when
And how and where and who.

The main categories of question are closed, open, leading and probing.

Closed questions

These are questions worded to encourage the respondent to answer in a limited fashion. In this way, they limit the options available to patients; in other words they close down the available scope for the response. There are three types of closed question.

- **The identification question**. Here the patient is expected to identify a piece of information and present this as the response, e.g. 'Where exactly is the pain now?'; 'When did you first notice the swelling?'; 'What type of contraceptive do you use?'
- **The selection question**. This form of closed question requires the patient to select one from two or more alternatives, and as a result is sometimes referred to as 'forced-choice'. Examples include 'Would you prefer aspirin or paracetamol?'; 'Is it worse at night or in the morning?'; 'Is the pain at the front or the back of your knee?'
- **The yes/no question**. In this instance the patient is simply expected to respond either 'yes' or no'. For example: 'Does it keep you awake at night?'; 'Have you been physically sick?'; 'Do you have any difficulty passing water?'

Closed questions are particularly useful in obtaining limited pieces of factual information. They are also easy for patients to answer, and can therefore assist patients who are unused to talking at length. As Hein (1973, p. 34) put it: 'Often patients with a limited vocabulary, minimal education, or lack of culturally enriching experiences are more comfortable in responding to closed questions.' However, when overused, closed questions can be counterproductive, in that they have been shown to be a powerful influence for controlling and blocking the development of conversation (Hargie, Saunders and Dickson, 1994). They can also be frustrating for the more articulate patient who is capable of elaboration without constant questioning.

Open questions

This type of question allows the patient much more scope in determining the response – the answer is left open to patients who can therefore more easily negotiate their own needs. Open questions are broad in nature and require more than a one- or two-word answer. However, there are degrees of openness in that some open questions allow more scope than others. Morrow and Hargie (1985) gave the following example to illustrate how a questioning sequence can gradually become more restricted:

> How has your new medication affected you?
> What types of problems has it caused?
> What sort of pain have you had?
> What is the pain like now?

All of these questions are open, but of course the sequence could continue, ending in a closed question such as 'Is it painful now?'

This process of questioning has been referred to as a 'funnel sequence' (Hargie, Saunders and Dickson, 1994), 'narrowing' (Enelow and Swisher, 1986) or the 'open-to-closed cone' (Cohen-Cole, 1991).

Open questions tend to produce longer responses than closed questions, and indeed it may be a fear of patients answering at length, or giving irrelevant information, that causes practitioners to rely heavily on the closed type of question. Both types of question can, of course, be useful, and Fisher (1992, p. 268) highlighted how practitioners 'can benefit from a combination of both open-ended and closed-ended questions during patient consultations'. Where time is limited, and an urgent diagnosis is required, closed questions are often appropriate, whereas if patients are being encouraged to express feelings or attitudes open questions are more apt. However, studies have shown that health professionals often rely almost entirely upon closed questions, indicating a need for training in the use of open questioning skills (Hargie, Morrow and Woodman, 1993; Dillon, 1997).

Leading questions

These are questions which, by the way they are worded, lead the patient to give a response that the professional expects to receive. There are four types of leading question.

- **Conversational**. Here the question anticipates the response that the patient would probably have given. The conversational lead is used to stimulate the flow of conversation, e.g. 'Isn't this lovely weather we're having?' When they are used appropriately such questions have been shown to facilitate the development of rapport (Hargie, Saunders and Dickson, 1994).
- **Simple**. These are straightforward leads that clearly exert pressure upon the patient to acquiesce with the practitioner's viewpoint. MacLeod Clark (1984), in her study of nurse–patient interactions, provided some examples of simple leads employed by nurses, including: 'There, that didn't hurt, did it?'; 'You're all right, aren't you?'
- **Subtle**. In this instance the question may not be immediately recognized as leading, since subtle leads use a particular wording style in order to influence

patients in a particular direction (for this reason they are also known as directional questions). For example, Loftus (1975) found that when people were asked 'Do you get headaches frequently, and if so how often?', the average response was 2.2 headaches per week. However, when the word 'occasionally' was substituted for 'frequently' the average figure given was 0.7 headaches per week. A range of similar studies have confirmed how subtle changes in question wording can influence the responses obtained (Hargie, Saunders and Dickson, 1994).

- **Implication**. This form of leading question either requires the patient to respond as expected or accept a negative implication. Examples would include: 'Presumably you weren't stupid enough to drink alcohol when you were taking these tablets?'; 'As a responsible parent, wouldn't you agree that it's a good idea to give your child a vitamin supplement?'

The latter three types of leading question need to be used with caution since they may 'put an individual in a defensive position . . . there is a rather clear suggestion of manipulation . . . (and) . . . an increased probability that inaccurate information will be given' (Fritz *et al.*, 1984, p. 97).

Probing questions

These are follow-up questions, which can be employed to encourage the patient to develop a particular theme. Probes can be open, closed or leading.

The main types of probing question are as follows.

- **Clarification**. 'What exactly do you mean?' 'Could you describe it?'
- **Justification**. 'What makes you think that?' 'Why do you say that?'
- **Exemplification**. 'What type of pain is it?' 'When has this happened in the past?'
- **Extension**. 'Go on.' 'Then what happened?'
- **Accuracy**. 'You definitely took one tablet every day?' 'It is only sore at night?'
- **Echo**. This involves simply repeating in an inquisitive fashion the last few words uttered by the patient, e.g. **Patient**: 'It has been very painful for the past three days.' **Practitioner**: 'Three days?'
- **Non-verbal**. The practitioner can indicate a desire for further information by raising or lowering the eyebrows, or uttering vocalizations such as 'Oh?' These, and other forms of non-verbal behaviour, can be used as probes.

5.2.3 Related factors

There are other facets of questions which need to be considered and to which we now turn.

Prompting

When the patient either does not answer or gives an answer that is clearly unsatisfactory the practitioner can prompt, to encourage a more meaningful response, by:

- restating the question or rephrasing it in parallel language;
- rewording the question using simpler language;
- reviewing material previously covered to remind the patient of the context in which the question is being asked.

Pace

The use of pauses is important. The professional can pause after asking a question and after receiving a response. There is evidence to suggest that by pausing for at least 3 seconds at either juncture the amount of talk-time of the respondent will increase. As Dillon (1990, p. 199) pointed out: 'Against all appearances, silence is a positive practitioner behaviour; and seemingly against all expectations, people respond positively to it.' It also ensures that the interaction does not become like an interrogation, with continual rapid-fire questioning.

Multiple questions

This involves asking two or more questions simultaneously. Walton and MacLeod Clark (1986) found that patients reported being unable to formulate a reply when asked more than a single question. Despite this, they note that nurses frequently ask multiple questions, and give the following example: 'Come on, take your trousers off. How do you like your pillows? Do you want the back rest out or not?' Such questions only serve to confuse the patient and decrease the probability of receiving accurate information. They should, therefore, generally be avoided.

Structuring

Where a number of questions are to be asked of a patient it may be important to give advance information concerning the reason why answers to these questions are required. This process of 'accounting' allows the patient to get mentally prepared for what is to follow and become more amenable to responding (providing the reasons given are accepted as valid). Another facet of structuring involves combining together all questions relating to one specific topic before progressing to a different area. This is important, since it allows the patient to follow the rationale for the questions. However, Dillon (1990, p. 60) illustrated how in many doctor–patient consultations, 'The **sequence** of questions is disconnected, one question following another without apparent reason or relation', such that the patient is constrained simply to provide answers, not knowing what to expect next.

Affective questions

Numerous studies of interaction in health contexts have indicated that it tends to be essentially task-centred focusing upon physical symptoms. MacLeod Clark (1982) found that only 1.3% of all nurse–patient communication was concerned with emotional or psychosocial matters. Similar findings have been reported in studies of doctor–patient interaction. Indeed, Maguire (1981) suggested that the dearth of questions relating to the affective domain is the main reason for the poor rate of detection of psychosocial problems in patients. Thus, the use of affective questions, which specifically relate to the emotions, attitudes and feelings of the respondent, should be an important aspect of focus during CST.

Morrow and Hargie (1988b) have identified the skill of questioning as forming a continuum from facilitative at one end to restrictive at the other. The facilitative style allows patients to be centrally involved in the consultation, whereas the restrictive style largely ignores the needs of the patient. In the former, the scope of the questions tends to be open, their content includes psychosocial dimensions, there is a low level of bias in terms of fewer leading questions, the pace is appropriate to the patient, the questions are less direct, they are at a deeper level, and the professional encourages patient questions and is accepting of responses.

There is evidence to suggest that practitioners may become fixed in their style of interacting soon after qualifying (Maguire, Fairbairn and Fletcher, 1986). It is therefore crucial for trainees to develop an effective style of questioning prior to qualifying, and this should be an important task for trainers during CST. Exercise 5.1 can be employed by trainers to illustrate the disadvantages of closed, as opposed to open questions.

Exercise 5.1 Questioning

Aim

To highlight some of the differential effects of open, as opposed to closed, questions.

Instructions

This is a short, easily executed exercise. Inform the class that you are about to play the role of a patient presenting an illness. What they are required to do is to ask only closed questions in an attempt to ascertain exactly what the illness is. Ask someone in the class to count the total number of questions employed. As 'patient' you should only answer the questions as they are asked, and should not volunteer any information beyond this. The illness can be of various types, although we have found that even a simple one such as pruritus can produce a large number of closed diagnostic questions. Repeat the exercise a second time, using a different illness, but on this occasion allow class members to ask open questions.

Discussion

Evaluate the differences between the two types of questioning strategies in terms of (1) total time taken, (2) effort on the part of the practitioner and (3) patient satisfaction. This exercise neatly illustrates same of the advantages of using open questions during patient consultations.

5.3 EXPLAINING

All health professionals have to give explanations to patients, and it is therefore important to address this aspect of practice during CST. There is firm evidence that patients value, and benefit from, the effective communication of information by practitioners (Hamilton, Rouse and Rouse, 1994). Conversely, 'Patients who are not able to understand and remember the diagnosis and treatment are likely to be dissatisfied with the entire medical encounter' (Jackson, 1992, p. 199). However, 'the most common reason for dissatisfaction of patients is that they cannot get sufficient information or explanation from their doctors about either the drugs they receive or the diseases for which they are intended' (International Medical Benefit/Risk Foundation, 1993, p. 8). Yet the benefits for the patient of receiving and comprehending a full account of his/her condition are well-documented, such that 'many research studies point to the critical role of information in permitting patients to adapt to the stress of illness, in reducing anxiety and in promoting recovery' (Brearley, 1990, p. 43). In her study of prescribed medication-taking, Parrott (1994) found that effective explanation resulted in better informed patients who would be more likely to collect their prescriptions and take medication in the correct manner. In his review of the area, Kreps (1993) demonstrated how patients who were well informed by their practitioners were more satisfied with the medical care they received; were less likely to discontinue treatment; experienced less stress prior to difficult medical examinations and procedures; and seemed to actually benefit more from treatment.

Despite these findings, information-giving to patients would not seem to be one of the strengths of many health professionals. For example, Fisher, Corrigan and Henman (1991), in their examination of 40 community pharmacies, demonstrated how the time spent by pharmacists in talking to patients about their medicines was, on average, equivalent to only 3.5 minutes per hour. In another study, Bensing (1991) found that doctors overestimated, by a factor of nine, the time they actually spent giving information to patients and underestimated the patient's desire for information.

In relation to information-seeking by patients, a distinction can be made between 'monitors' – patients who actively search for and request information about their condition – and 'blunters' who deliberately avoid such information particularly if it may have negative implications (Miller, Brody and Summerton, 1988). Thus, patients who complain most about lack of information or explanation may paradoxically be better informed than those who do not complain (Armstrong, 1991). In their study of information-giving in community pharmacies, Blenkinsopp, Robinson and Panton (1994) classified patients as either 'active' or 'passive' depending upon the extent to which they introduced new topics into the consultation. Information given was measured in terms of a 'unit' which was defined as 'a phrase which, standing alone, could be considered meaningful (and so could be remembered)' (p. 88). Not surprisingly, active patients received more units of information than passive ones (15.9 and 8.5 respectively), but in a follow-up 1 day after their visit it was found that both groups had forgotten some two-thirds of the information they had received.

Other research has indicated that patients in general forget some 50% of the information they are given by practitioners (Jackson, 1992). Furthermore, Norton and Mann (1994) found that when patients were prescribed a new medication, of those who did have the possible side effects explained (and one in three patients was either not told of any or did not know if he/she had been told), 45% did not list the main side effect in a postconsultation questionnaire, indicating that 'patients may not be aware of significant symptoms, even though they have been explained by the doctor' (p. 11). One consequence, as highlighted in a report by the International Medical Benefit/Risk Foundation (1993, p. 14), is that 'at least 50% of patients in Europe, Japan and North America fail to take their medicines properly'.

These findings were supported by the Audit Commission (1993), who compared 12 consultant surgeons on eight criteria relating to how they dealt with women referred with breast lumps. Their findings illustrated a wide variation between surgeons and a low overall score on most criteria. The actual results were as follows, with numbers of surgeons scoring on the criterion presented in brackets.

- Patient dressed on meeting the surgeon (2).
- Patient dressed for discussion of the prognosis (4).
- Patient invited to bring a companion (6).
- Consultant working with a breast nurse (7).
- Nurse included in the discussion of treatment (3).
- More than one chance to discuss the treatment (6).
- Discussion of radiotherapy before a decision taken on surgery (2).
- Written information used (1).

One surgeon did not score on any of the criteria, three scored on only one, while the best score was one surgeon who used seven out of the eight criteria. Not surprisingly, patients expressed dissatisfaction with their treatment. One woman interviewed by the Commission, who had been diagnosed as having a breast lump, commented: 'I didn't even know it was malignant. Perhaps they leave it to your imagination.'

In noting the consistently reported failure of doctors to provide adequate explanations to patients, Livesey (1986) reached the somewhat depressing view that, since this is so widespread, it may be intentional. Maguire, Fairbairn and Fletcher (1986), however, attributed the failure to lack of training and asserted that 'some young doctors do discover for themselves how best to give patients information and advice, but most remain extremely incompetent. This is presumably because they get no training as students in this important aspect of clinical practice. This deficiency should be corrected, and competence tested before qualification to practise' (p. 1576).

The importance of effective information-giving to patients has been emphasized in recent studies of various health professions. The trainer, during CST, should therefore attempt to ensure that trainees develop an awareness of and expertise in a range of techniques central to the effective use of the skill of explaining.

5.3.1 Definition

In everyday usage the verb 'to explain' has two meanings. One of these emphasizes the **intention** of the explainer ('I explained it to him but he was too stupid to understand') while the other highlights **success** ('I explained it to him and he was able to do it'). In professional contexts it is the latter usage that is recommended and, in this sense, to explain is to give understanding to another person. Thus, if the recipient does not comprehend the message, it has not been fully explained. However, there are two levels of explanation:

- **Level 1**. At this simple level, explaining involves giving information of a descriptive or prescriptive nature and involves telling, describing or instructing. For example: 'I am giving you a prescription for Paracodol which you should take instead of the soluble aspirin you are taking at the minute. I'm also giving you Fybogel to keep your bowels active.'
- **Level 2**. At this more complex level an explanation provides understanding in the mind of the listener by going beyond simple description to reveal causes, make links, give reasons, demonstrate relationships, etc. For example: 'You should stop taking soluble aspirin, since this will upset your ulcer and cause you pain. I will give you soluble Paracodol, which you can take for your headaches. These will do the same job as the aspirin but will not affect your ulcer. However, they can cause constipation, so to keep your bowels active I am also giving you Fybogel, a natural fibre medication.'

5.3.2 Types of explanation

Explanations can be divided into three main categories.

Verbal

This type of explanation usually occurs where no aids are available and the practitioner has to rely solely upon verbal skills. In cases where it is vital that patients understand what they have been told, the consultation can be audio-taped and a copy of the tape given to the patient to take away. While it seems self-evident that at the very least patients should be given verbal information about their medications, Wiederholt, Clarridge and Svarstad (1992) ascertained that the percentage of patients receiving no such information about new prescriptions ranged between 17% and 30% for doctors and between 30% and 87% for pharmacists. Such a state of affairs clearly needs to be rectified. Indeed, as well as presenting information orally, practitioners should give careful consideration to the provision of written information to patients, since 'there is ample evidence that written information reinforces oral messages and that patients who receive it understand more about their condition and retain information that helps them manage their own care' (Audit Commission, 1993, p. 31). However, while the importance of written information has been clearly documented (O'Connell and Johnson, 1992; Hammond and Lambert, 1994), studies have shown that only 26% of patients were provided with it when obtaining prescription medications from pharmacists (Morris *et al.*, 1987).

Illustration

Here audiovisual aids are employed to facilitate explanation. Such aids have been shown to improve the retention of information by the listener, as well as resulting in the person using them being perceived as more professional, better prepared, more persuasive and more interesting (O'Hair and Friedrich, 1992). Aids are particularly useful where the information being conveyed is difficult to relate in purely verbal terms. Illustrations can also help to underline the most important elements in an explanation. Many products (suppositories, inhalers, etc.) are accompanied by patient package inserts with illustrative diagrams and these can be employed by the professional to 'talk through' an explanation with a patient. Alternatively, where such commercially produced aids are not available, to help explain certain types of problem for patients it is often useful for the practitioner to draw a simple diagram which can be executed very quickly. The advantage of illustrations is evidenced by the maxim 'One picture is worth 1000 words.'

Demonstration

Where the information being imparted relates to a practical activity, the use of a demonstration by the practitioner can be of particular benefit, since it has been said that 'One demonstration is worth 1000 pictures'. An important part of any demonstration should be allowing the recipient to attempt the procedure as soon as possible. This is underlined by the old Chinese proverb: 'I hear and I forget. I see and I remember. I do and I understand.'

5.3.3 Functions of explanations

Depending upon the context, the skill of explanation serves a number of purposes, some of these being situation-specific. For example, in their investigation of community-pharmacist–patient consultations, Hargie, Morrow and Woodman (1993) identified the seven main explaining subdivisions as instructing, directing, informing, reassuring, reasoning, reiterating and emphasizing. They also found that on occasions, and only with non-prescription related consultations, the pharmacist used the skill of 'suggesting/advising', which was defined as 'the offer of personal/professional opinion as to a particular course of action, while simultaneously allowing the final decision to lie with the individual' (p. 84). Thus, they would proffer advice prefaced by remarks such as: 'You'd be wiser getting . . .'; 'I think I would go to the doctor . . .'; 'I would advise you to . . .'.

In general terms, the main functions of explaining are to:

- provide information;
- simplify complexities;
- correct mistaken beliefs;
- give advice;
- aid patient compliance;
- highlight the important elements of any procedure;
- offer reassurance and reduce uncertainty;
- justify one's actions and recommendations;
- increase patient satisfaction;
- ensure patient understanding.

5.3.4 Features of explanation

Several reviews of the central features of the skill of explanation have been carried out (e.g. Ley, 1988; Hargie, Saunders and Dickson, 1994; Brown, 1997) and there is general agreement about the nature of the component elements.

Planning

In some instances, the practitioner will have more opportunity to plan an explanation than in others. When planning, consideration should be given to three aspects:

- the identification of the key elements in the problem to be explained;

- the relationship between these elements and how they can best be linked during explanation;
- the ability level, background knowledge, and possible reactions, of the recipient of the explanation.

Presentation

This is the crux of any explanation. How the explanation is presented will determine how successful it is. Success in explaining can be achieved through a number of techniques.

- **Speaking fluently**. Messages are more easily understood when delivered in a clear, fluent style, with the use of short sentences and an avoidance of 'ums', 'ers', etc.
- **Structuring**. Explanations should follow a logical sequence, moving from the known to the unknown and from the simple to the more complex. In order to do this it is necessary to ascertain at the outset what the patient already knows or believes. Structuring also involves informing patients in advance of what is to be said, so that they can 'tune in' to the explanation. This includes the use of 'signposts', which are periodic statements indicating where the explanation is going. For example 'I am going to show you how to use this inhaler. . .' 'I want to move on now to talk about your diet. . .'.
- **Reducing vagueness**. As Kitching (1986), in his discussion of pharmacist–patient interaction, illustrated, the ambiguity of terms such as 'plenty', 'a lot' and other similar expressions can cause confusion for patients and should therefore be avoided. In other words, the practitioner should use specific, rather than vague, expressions.
- **Pausing**. By using pauses appropriately, the professional can move at a moderate pace and thereby ensure that he/she does not cover too much material too quickly. Research evidence also illustrates the importance of speaker pauses of a minimum of 3 seconds duration in facilitating the understanding and recall of information by listeners (Hargie, Saunders and Dickson, 1994).
- **Using appropriate language**. Health professionals, like all groups of professionals, have a specialized terminology which can facilitate communication within the profession. However, the use of such 'jargon' should be avoided when dealing with patients, or if technical terms are used they should be explained concisely. For example, Jackson (1992) found that an explanation to undergraduates about mononucleosis led to greater satisfaction, recall and comprehension when non-technical as opposed to technical language was employed. Another pitfall to avoid is the use of middle-class (elaborated code) language with working-class (restricted code) patients. Indeed Waitzkin (1985), in a study of doctor–patient consultations found that fewer explanations were given to lower-social-class or less educated patients. In this study it was also found that more information was given to patients who

had an unfavourable rather than favourable prognosis, and that more explanation was given to patients whom the doctor had known for a longer period of time.

A balance needs to be maintained, however, since another danger is that of 'talking down' to patients. This is confirmed by Jackson (1992, p. 198) who noted that 'one of the most frequent patient complaints involves a feeling of being patronized by doctors'. It should be realized, for example, that at the age of 2 years the average child has a vocabulary of over 400 words, at six years 2500 words, and by the age of 14 years this reaches 50 000 words (Kopp and Krakow, 1982). Thus, even young children, and in particular adolescents, are quite capable of understanding appropriate explanations from practitioners.

- **Providing emphasis**. Important parts of a message can be emphasized verbally and/or non-verbally. Verbal emphasis can be achieved by repetition of the important points, by using verbal cues ('This is very important. . .' 'What you must never forget is. . .'); and by verbal foci ('first . . . second . . .'; 'major'; 'crucial'; etc.). Emphasis can also be achieved non-verbally by, for example, raising or lowering the volume of the voice; and by hand gestures, facial expressions, sudden body movements, etc. Morrow and Hargie (1994) recommended the use of action-oriented phrases to emphasize what the patient should **do**. They give the following example from a community pharmacist who has just sold a sunscreen lotion to a client going on a continental holiday.

  > Avoid hot sun between the hours of 11.00 am and 2.00 pm. Re-apply the lotion every two or three hours or after swimming. Pay special attention to sensitive areas like the nose, ears, top of head. Remember the sun's rays can penetrate glass, cloud, water and even fine fabrics so wear the sunscreen at all times
  >
  > *Morrow and Hargie, 1994, p. 313*

- **Using examples**. These are effective during explanation since they help to relate new or unfamiliar concepts to situations that are familiar (Brosius and Bathelt, 1994). Indeed, Livesey (1986) outlined how the use of simple analogies, which may technically be inexact, can facilitate understanding, giving the following suggestions: 'the heart is a simple pump with one-way valves, atheromatous arteries may be likened to furred up water pipes, and brown fat stores are radiators which burn up calories and radiate heat' (p. 92).
- **Being expressive**. The manner in which an explanation is delivered can influence its effectiveness. In particular, the demonstration of enthusiasm, concern, friendliness and humour by verbal and non-verbal means can make an explanation more appealing and interesting for the listener.
- **Summarizing**. It is often useful to briefly recap the main points covered, especially if an explanation has been quite lengthy. This helps listeners to assimilate and retain the information presented.

Hargie and Morrow (1995) have discussed how, while the focus of CST programmes in health has been primarily on one-to-one communication, much less attention has been devoted to presentational skills in small- or large-group settings. Yet practitioners are often faced with the task of speaking to groups, and Hargie and Morrow illustrated how a CST course can be designed to cater for this dimension. They demonstrated how many of the above features of explanation also apply in such contexts (opening the talk, structuring, clarity of expression, using examples, summarizing). They also highlighted other dimensions of explanation in public presentations, including stimulus variation, which refers to the process of **change** in presentations, to arouse and maintain the interest and attention of the audience.

Variations in presentations can be achieved by three main methods. Firstly, presenters should introduce changes in verbal and non-verbal behaviour, since expressiveness, enthusiasm and humour are three of the main characteristics of effective presenters. Secondly, there is a need to vary the sensory focus of listeners (e.g. from listening to looking). The use of audiovisual aids can help to stimulate such changes in sensory focus. Thirdly, audience participation should be encouraged where possible. Another aspect of presentations covered by Hargie and Morrow is that of responding to audience questions, in that presenters should attempt to anticipate possible questions and prepare related answers. Questions can also be adapted to suit the message the presenter wishes to give (e.g. 'To answer that question you first need to look at. . .'), and should be geared to the whole audience and not just the questioner.

5.3.5 Feedback

The definition of explaining given earlier emphasized the importance of its success, and in order to evaluate whether an explanation has been successful it is necessary to obtain feedback from the listeners. This can be achieved by the following methods.

- attending to the non-verbal expressions of listeners to identify signs of confusion, puzzlement or bewilderment;
- asking listeners if they understand – the danger here, of course, is that many patients are likely to respond in the affirmative regardless of whether they understand or not;
- asking specific questions designed to test comprehension – to overcome the likelihood of any embarrassment, the practitioner can take the blame for any possible failure by using expressions like: 'I don't know whether I explained that very well, can I just check. . .'; 'This is quite difficult and I may have gone too quickly. . .';
- asking listeners if they have any questions;
- asking listeners to summarize the explanation, or complete a procedure if a practical task is involved.

The Audit Commission (1993) highlighted the problems of explaining and interpreting feedback with non-English-speaking patients. If an interpreter is needed, there can be distortions in translation, especially where the interpreter is a family member (often a sibling) who may be embarrassed to use certain terms or discuss difficult issues with a close relative. One Indian woman interviewed in the report by the Audit Commission said 'I don't always tell the doctor everything, because I have to tell my daughter what it is. I feel it is very embarrassing' (p. 54). This suggests the need for professional interpreters where possible, and underlines the need for care and sensitivity on the part of practitioners during foreign language consultations.

It is clear that the skill of explaining is central to effective communication in health contexts. Armstrong (1991) argued that patients require answers to three basic questions: 'Why me?', 'Why now?' and 'Why this particular illness?', while Morrow and Hargie (1988a) identified four questions to which patients need answers regarding their medication: 'What is this medicine for?', 'How do I take it?', 'Are there any side effects?', 'How long do I need to take it for?' There is also the remaining question of 'What is going to happen to me?' Practitioners will have to explain to patients the nature of an illness and its aetiology, the treatment being prescribed and its effects, the prognosis and, often, what other professionals have said to them!

The following statement was agreed as part of a consensus statement published by an international conference on doctor–patient communication: 'Explaining and understanding patient concerns, even when they cannot be resolved, results in a significant fall in anxiety. . . . The level of psychological distress in patients with serious illness is less when they perceive themselves to have received adequate information' (Simpson *et al.*, 1991, p. 1386). Concerted training in explaining skills is therefore an essential component of CST.

Exercise 5.2 can be utilized in the classroom to demonstrate to trainees some of the processes and difficulties involved in giving explanations.

Exercise 5.2 Explaining

Aim

To highlight some of the techniques, processes and difficulties in explaining effectively, and to relate these to the health context.

Instructions

This is a short, easily executed exercise. Give each group an index card bearing the name of an abstract concept which they will have to explain to the rest of the class. The rules are: (1) they must not mention the name of the concept; (2) they are not allowed to use the 'blank' technique, e.g. 'The Beatles had a song called "All You Need is **Blank**" for the concept 'love';

(3) they cannot use the 'sounds like' method e.g 'Sounds like fate' for the concept 'hate'. Concepts which can be employed here include 'aesthetic'; 'dogma'; 'pragmatic' and 'hostile'. Allow each group 3 minutes to prepare the explanation and then take each group in turn and ask them to present the given concept, while the rest of the class members try to guess what it is. If the class cannot guess the concept after it is fully explained, then they are allowed to ask questions of the explainers. Allow no more than 4 minutes for the total explanation of each concept, after which time it should be revealed if not guessed.

Discussion

When all the groups have presented their concepts, hold an open discussion on the techniques employed to facilitate explanation. For example, explainers will usually use examples relevant to the listeners, try to paint mental pictures, use synonyms and antonyms, emphasize and repeat key areas. Why were some explainers more successful than others? How did explainers and class feel when the explanation was unsuccessful? What were the main difficulties encountered? In the light of the difficulties presented by this task, the implications of the exercise for giving explanations to patients should then be discussed.

5.4 OPENING AND CLOSING

Two important parts of any interaction are the opening and closing stages. It has long been known that the first (primacy effect) and last (recency effect) events in any sequence tend to be best remembered. The primacy and recency effects are also prevalent during social encounters. For this reason, elaborate greeting and parting rituals have been developed to help smooth the interpersonal process. Lamb (1988, p. 103) postulated that 'greetings and partings are moments of tension. You are on display. Your status or your expectations about a relationship may be brought into question. You may make a fool of yourself.' It also follows that, if people are more likely to remember what we do when we meet them or just before we leave them, we should devote time and effort to these interactive phases. Indeed, it is interesting to note that even very young children are taught by their parents to be aware of the importance of 'hellos' and 'goodbyes'! In health contexts, the practitioner should therefore take cognisance of the impact which can be made at the beginning and end of encounters with patients.

5.4.1 Opening skills

During the first few minutes of an interaction people make judgements which can then influence how they perceive one another and how they interpret each other's behaviour. As Riggio (1992, p. 11) pointed out: 'Initial impressions can influence the length, tone, and quality of first social encounters. Indeed, impressions formed from brief exposure to visual and auditory non-verbal cues . . . [and] . . . verbal statements, may determine whether an interaction takes place at all.' Such judgements, when made by patients, can be based upon factors such as the physical appearance, dress and grooming of the practitioner, initial verbal and non-verbal greeting behaviour or the room layout. This is especially true when the professional is meeting the patient for the first time: there is truth in the maxim 'You don't get a second chance to make a first impression.' In his analysis of how to break bad news, Buckman (1992, p. 39) noted that a good opening 'only takes twenty or thirty seconds and it saves many moments of dissatisfaction (on both sides) later'. Once a conducive relationship has been developed with a patient, the practitioner may be excused the occasional hurried introduction, but during initial encounters this will not be acceptable and a more relaxed, attentive and receptive style will be appreciated.

The significance of the opening segment of patient interviews has been emphasized in most texts on communication in the health professions. Heath (1986, p. 25) identified the following sequence at the beginning of doctor–patient consultations: 'Greetings are exchanged, identities checked, the patient establishes an appropriate spatial and physical orientation, and the doctor sorts out equipment and documentation, not infrequently reading the medical card.' However, Livesey (1986) illustrated how, with many doctors, little effort is devoted to this process of 'meeting, greeting and seating'. He speculated that this is because for the physician the next patient is just one of many to be interviewed. On the other hand, for the patient the consultation may be a 'one-off', special and perhaps even anxiety-provoking. In recognizing this point, Shuy (1983) commented that 'the medical interview can be cold and frightening to a patient. If the goal of the physician is to make the patient comfortable, a bit of personal but interested and relevant chitchat, whatever the cost in precious time, is advisable. The patients are familiar with normal conversational openings that stress such chitchat. The medical interview would do well to try to move closer to a conversational framework' (p. 200).

There is evidence, however, that practitioners could improve their greeting skills considerably. Davis and Fallowfield (1991, p. 7) found one of the main deficiencies of health professionals to be the 'failure to greet the patient appropriately, to introduce themselves, and to explain their own actions'. This was evidenced by Maguire, Fairbairn and Fletcher (1986, p. 1575) who, in a study of the consultation skills of young doctors, reported that 'few doctors explained the purpose of the interview or the time available. They had questioned the value of this mode of beginning as students and still rejected it.'

In discussing the vital role of such skills during nurse–patient interactions, French (1994) proposed that the nurse should complete some or all of the following tasks at the beginning of an encounter with a patient.

- Tell the patient what is going to happen.

- Give reasons why any information being sought is necessary.
- Ascertain if the patient has any concerns, and answer any questions fully.
- Explain what the patient will be expected to do.
- Check the accuracy of any information previously collected, where appropriate.
- Gain the attention and co-operation of the patient.

Buckman (1992) and Hargie, Saunders and Dickson (1994) provide reviews of a range of techniques that can be employed to good effect at the beginning of interactions. These include the following.

- **Arranging an appropriate environment**. This encompasses the reception area and waiting room. If these are bleak, cold and uninviting this can have an initial off-putting effect upon patients. Likewise, the practitioner's office should be arranged in a cooperative fashion (see Chapter 4). Where possible, 'creature comforts' should also be provided, including a soft chair, a cup of tea or coffee and reasonable heating and lighting.
- **Appropriate greeting behaviour**. This may involve meeting the patient at the door and shaking hands. In noting the importance of the handshake, Buckman (1992, p. 36) highlighted how this 'reduces tension at the start of the interview. It is, of course, a personal touch (literally), and requires a certain commitment to intimacy on the part of both participants. It is therefore a way of telling the patient that you are (at least partly) a human being.' Other forms of greeting include smiling, engaging in eye contact, the use of non-task comments (e.g. about the weather) and offering a seat.
- **Motivating the patient**. By appearing interested, concerned and attentive at the outset, the practitioner helps to motivate the patient to participate fully in the consultation. As Livesey (1986) pointed out, if a doctor is still making notes about a previous patient, does not look up from the notes and merely grunts a welcome, this can certainly be demotivating for patients! Indeed, there is evidence that individuals who display higher levels of non-verbal emotionally expressive behaviours are more attention-getting in interpersonal encounters (Riggio, 1992).
- **Checking details**. This can involve introducing oneself, checking the patient's name, stating one's function (this is especially important in the hospital, where the patient may be meeting a host of different health professionals) and ascertaining the expectations of the patient. Buller and Street (1992, p. 120) underscored the fact that patients are active agents in the communication process 'who help shape the exchange based on their goals and expectations for the medical consultation'. By establishing the patient's goals at the outset and matching these against the realities of the situation, patient satisfaction and empowerment can be enhanced. Indeed, Bensing (1991, p. 13), in her study of doctor–patient communication, emphasized the importance of clarifying the reasons for the patient coming for a consulta-

tion, pointing out that 'there is growing evidence that not meeting patient's expectations is one of the most important reasons for patient dissatisfaction'. For this reason Cohen-Cole (1991), in his analysis of the medical interview, asserted that effective interviews begin with an explicit statement or acknowledgement of goals. Any previous information that may have been gathered should also be reviewed, the objectives of the interaction outlined and the patient informed as to what exactly is about to happen.

5.4.2 Closing skills

As well as paying attention to how interactions are opened, professionals need to arrange a smooth, effective closure. However, this can often be more difficult, since the nature and content of a closing sequence is dependent to a large degree upon what has taken place during the interaction. Furthermore, the practitioner cannot simply decide to terminate the interaction without the agreement of the patient, since to do so would be likely to cause resentment, pique or anger. Rather, as Heath (1986, p. 150) observed in relation to doctor–patient communication: 'bringing the consultation to an end is a progressive, step-by-step process in and through which doctor and patient cooperate and coordinate their actions'. On occasions this process can be difficult, particularly where what Byrne and Long (1976) referred to as the 'by the way. . .' syndrome occurs, whereby a patient introduces a new, often important, problem just as the interaction is about to end. This has also been termed the 'door handle phenomenon' (Lang and van der Molen, 1990). The professional is then faced with the difficult decision of whether to discuss this problem or arrange another consultation with the patient in the immediate future.

Livesey (1986), however, argued that in doctor–patient consultations physicians often terminate their interviews before the patient expects it, and that the usual manner in which this is achieved is by handing over a prescription. Livesey believed that this state of affairs is due both to the pressure under which a doctor may be working and to the mistaken belief that what patients really want are prescriptions. He suggested that by encouraging patients to participate early on in the consultation, the 'by the way. . .' phenomenon can be circumvented and a smooth closure effected. In discussing the techniques associated with closing interactions in a skilled fashion, Hargie, Saunders and Dickson (1994) identified the following central methods.

- **The use of closure indicators and markers**. In order to convey to the patient that the time is approaching when the interaction will terminate, a variety of verbal and non-verbal behaviours can be employed as closure indicators. These include breaking eye contact, looking at a watch, writing a prescription, organizing papers together, orienting towards an exit, and utterances like: 'Well we've covered just about everything. . .'; 'Right, I'll call in again on Friday at the same time. . .'. These behaviours are useful, since the patient needs some warning that the practitioner is about to draw the proceedings to a close. When the interaction is finally terminating, this is underlined by the use of final closure markers such as standing up, shaking hands, tearing a prescription from the pad and handing it to the patient, and making utterances such as 'Come back and see me if the pain persists'; 'Take this form to the receptionist'; 'Goodbye'.

- **Summarizing**. At the end of an interaction it is often useful for the practitioner to provide a summary, reminding the patient of the main points covered. As Hein (1973, p. 49) remarked, summaries are 'a capsule review of the content and feelings discussed during an interview . . . (they) . . . allow time not only for review, but also for patients to begin adjusting to the end of the interview. Just as summaries give evidence of progress, they also give evidence of the areas needing development.' In their detailed analysis of social closure, Albert and Kessler (1976) described the summary as a 'historicing act', in that it refers to the interaction as something that has already happened, and in this way signals that the encounter is at an end.
- **Obtaining feedback**. In the Maguire, Fairbairn and Fletcher (1986) study of the consultation skills of young doctors mentioned previously, one of the identified weaknesses of this group of physicians was their failure to check that the information they had obtained from patients was accurate and reflected key problems. One of the important closure skills is, therefore, ensuring that both parties are in agreement about what has been discussed and what decisions have been taken. This is sometimes referred to as a procedure of 'checking out'. It can be accomplished by the use of appropriate questions by the practitioner and by inviting the patient to make comments or ask questions about anything that has been discussed.
- **Making future links**. This refers to the 'what happens next' element. It may involve a simple statement, such as, 'OK, Mrs Rodgers, I'll call back tomorrow' or 'Take these tablets for a week and it should clear up. If not, come back and see me.' However, a patient at the preoperative stage of surgery, for example, may require much more detailed discussion and analysis about the procedures involved and their likely effects.
- **Motivating the patient**. On occasions, it is useful for the practitioner to motivate and encourage the patient at the end of a consultation. For example, a physiotherapist may end a session by underlining for a patient the importance of following a set exercise routine, or a doctor may stress the continued benefits of not smoking to a patient who has recently given up cigarette smoking.
- **Reinforcing the patient**. The process of relationship development and maintenance can be enhanced by providing the patient with appropriate rewards at the end of an interaction. These may be task-related, as when a dentist says to a young child 'You were very brave', or a health visitor says to a mother coping with her first baby 'You are doing really well'. On the other hand they may be non-task-related reinforcers, such as 'I really enjoyed talking to

you'; 'Thanks for the tea. Your home-made cake was delicious.' By employing such reinforcers the practitioner can give patients a sense of achievement, as well as facilitating the development of rapport with future encounters in mind.

- **Using non-task statements**. Once the substantive business has been conducted, it is often appropriate for the professional to make some comment unrelated to the actual task itself. Such comments are often about the weather, although they may relate to holidays, traffic problems, topical events, etc. By taking the time to engage in such dialogue the practitioner is thereby highlighting the social, as opposed to the purely task, dimension of his/her relationship with the patient.

Opening and closing skills are clearly crucial to the effective delivery of health care by all practitioners. In her review of these skills, Saunders (1986, p. 175) stated that 'while most people can recall the difficult openings and closings they have experienced, few can clearly and systematically analyse how the difficulties have been overcome, if indeed they have'. For this reason it is vital, during CST, for trainees to be sensitized to the importance of these two phases of any interaction and to recognize the variety of strategies that can be implemented to ensure that opening and closing skills are effectively executed.

5.5 ASSERTIVENESS

The ability to assert oneself skilfully is crucial to effective interpersonal functioning in many situations. It has been clearly documented that 'assertion is a **skill**, not a "trait" that someone "has" or "lacks"' (Rakos, 1986, p. 408). However, within the health professions it would seem that certain groups find this skill quite difficult to implement. Morrow and Hargie (1987a), for example, found that pharmacists rated assertion skills as the most important yet most difficult to put into practice, especially when dealing with other professionals and with ancillary health-care workers. The importance of assertiveness in this context was further confirmed in a later study by the same authors into effective skills in community pharmacy (Hargie, Morrow and Woodman, 1993), and a programme of training has been shown to be of value for practising pharmacists (Batty *et al.*, 1993). Likewise, McCartan and Hargie (1990) have reviewed the difficulties faced by nurses in being assertive, given that their work role involves being kind, considerate, often humble and non-confrontational. Busby and Gilchrist (1992), in a study of interaction during medical ward rounds, found that nurses were indeed unassertive, especially with more senior staff members in general and medical staff in particular, and expressed a desire to become more involved and assertive.

Thus, assertion is clearly a skill that should be included as part of CST. Another reason for sensitizing health professionals to this skill is that they will be dealing with many patient groups who find difficulty in asserting themselves and who will therefore need help and support in overcoming such difficulties. For example, physically disabled adults confined to wheelchairs have been found to experience discomfort in social situations that necessitate refusing help, managing patronizing remarks or giving directives (Glueckauf and Quittner, 1992). The skilled health professional should recognize such situations and be able to take steps to alleviate the problems faced by such patients.

Numerous definitions of assertiveness have been proposed, and all of these emphasize the core components as standing up for personal rights, respecting the rights of others and expressing thoughts and feelings openly and honestly. However, to fully understand the meaning of this skill, it is necessary to distinguish between four main styles of responding – non-assertive, assertive, aggressive and indirectly aggressive.

- **Non-assertive style**. Here the individual hesitates, speaks softly, avoids eye contact, denies true feelings, does not express opinions, avoids contentious issues, is subservient, appeases others, accepts blame needlessly, is self-effacing and apologetic, fidgets frequently and generally lacks confidence.
- **Assertive style**. In this approach the person responds immediately, speaks in a firm yet conversational tone, expresses true feelings, maintains eye contact, gives opinions, addresses contentious issues, is self-respecting, protects the rights of both parties, seeks equality with others and generally conveys confidence.
- **Aggressive style**. This style involves interrupting others, speaking loudly and abusively, glaring at others, vehemently expressing opinions, fuelling contentious issues, seeking superiority over others, not being concerned with the rights of others, being self-opinionated and generally being overbearing and intimidating.
- **Indirectly-aggressive style**. This style involves a range of behaviours such as sulking, huffing and pouting, using emotional blackmail (for example, crying in order to make someone feel guilty) and employing Machiavellian tactics to subtly manipulate others. It may also involve deflected aggression, such as banging doors or drawers.

In discussing these four styles, Hargie, Saunders and Dickson (1994) give the following example of each style being used in response to someone smoking in a designated no-smoking zone.

- Not mentioning your discomfort, and hoping that someone else will confront the smoker (Non-assertive).
- 'Excuse me, but do you realize that this is a "no smoking" area? Cigarette smoke affects me quite badly, so I'd be grateful if you would not smoke here' (Assertive).
- 'Hey, you, there's no smoking allowed in this area. Either put out or get out!' (Aggressive).

- Coughing loudly and vigorously waving a hand towards the smoker, as if to fan the smoke away (Indirectly aggressive).

Of these four styles, assertion has been found to be the most effective in most situations (Rakos, 1991). People who are either directly or indirectly aggressive may initially get their own way, but they will be disliked, whereas non-assertive individuals are often viewed as weak, incompetent and easily manipulated. Assertive people, on the other hand, tend to be respected and are seen as competent, strong, fair and confident. One interesting research finding, however, is that while people tend to **respect** assertive individuals, they often do not **like** to have to deal with assertive responses. This highlights the importance of employing assertiveness in a sensitive, skilful manner.

The skilled use of assertiveness can serve a number of functions namely to:

- maintain and protect personal rights;
- recognize the rights of others;
- make reasonable requests;
- withstand unreasonable requests from others;
- handle unreasonable refusals;
- avoid unnecessary conflict;
- confidently and openly communicate one's own position.

5.5.1 Types of assertion

A distinction can be made between three main types of assertion.

- **Direct assertion** involves a short, straightforward statement in support of one's personal rights.
- Using **indirect assertion** the person does not actually confront the issue but rather indirectly states a point of view.
- **Complex-direct assertion** includes the use of an embellishment to 'soften' the assertion. The main types of embellishment include:
  - an explanation for being assertive;
  - showing empathy towards the other person;
  - the use of praise;
  - giving an apology for any negative consequences;
  - suggesting a compromise.

One of the authors received a telephone call from a colleague at another institution inviting him to present a paper at a conference, but for various reasons he did not wish to accept this invitation. Using this scenario, the three types of assertion can be exemplified in the following responses:

- **Direct**: 'No, I can't undertake such a commitment at this time.'
- **Indirect**: 'Phew . . . I've got so much on my plate at the minute: I have a deadline to meet on two books and I know I have another commitment around that time. . . .'

- **Complex-direct**:
  - 'I couldn't undertake this commitment, since I am behind with the deadline for a forthcoming book, and I already have another speaking engagement in June' (Explanation).
  - 'I know you have a lot on your plate organizing the Conference, but. . .' (Empathy).
  - 'It's really nice of you to ask me and you know if I could do it for you I would. . .' (Praise).
  - 'I'm sorry to give you more problems in organizing speakers, but. . .' (Apology).
  - 'I can't undertake this, but I have a colleague whom I think could. . .' (Compromise).

Generally, the use of complex-direct assertion is recommended since this will be more favourably received by the target. Direct assertion can seem like aggression, while indirect assertion can lead to further pressure to relent. Furthermore, a number of the above embellishments can, of course, be used in combination to protect the relationship with the other person.

5.5.2 Assertion techniques

There are several techniques associated with the use of assertion.

Escalating assertion

The initial assertion employed should be at the level of the minimal effective response. In other words, the person should use only the minimum amount of assertiveness that could be successful at the outset, but gradually escalate the degree of assertion as required to ensure a successful outcome.

Confrontive assertion

This is required when someone's words and actions do not concur and the individual is forced to confront the person with this discrepancy. For example, a ward sister may say to a nurse: 'You said you would bed-bath Mrs Johnson before 3.30. It is now 3.45 and you still have not done so. Would you please do so immediately!'

Progressive assertion

Rose and Tryon (1979) identified three stages of assertion. These can be exemplified in relation to a situation where someone is being continually interrupted:

- Description of the behaviour – 'Excuse me, that is the third time you have interrupted me.'

- Description, plus indication of non-compliance – 'Excuse me, that is the third time you have interrupted me. I find it very disconcerting.'
- Description, non-compliance, plus request for behaviour change – 'Excuse me, that is the third time you have interrupted me. I find it very disconcerting. Would you please let me finish what I was going to say.'

Rose and Tryon found that ratings of assertiveness increased as individuals progressed from simply using the first stage through to employing all three stages.

I-language assertion

The use of self-reference pronouns ('I', 'me', etc.) can help to underline the fact that a response is intended to be assertive, whereas the use of 'you-language' statements tends to be associated with aggression. Compare, for example, the statements (a) 'I am upset because I feel that I am doing more than my fair share of the work.' and (b) 'You are annoying me in the way that you never do your full share of the work.' While statement (a) is less accusatory than (b), care must be taken when using I-language to avoid giving an impression of selfishness and lack of care for the other person. For this reason, Hargie, Saunders and Dickson (1994) recommended the use of 'we-language', which 'helps to convey the impression of partnership in, and joint responsibility for, any problems to be discussed' (p. 275). Continuing with the above example, a we-language response would be (c) 'It would be useful to talk about how we are both contributing to the overall workload, so that we can work out what we both feel would be an equitable distribution.'

Process factors

The way in which assertive behaviour is executed is also important. For example, this may involve arranging or altering the environment to make the situation more conducive to assertiveness. Thus, a community pharmacist may invite a dissatisfied patient to discuss a grievance in a private area away from the main shop floor. Likewise, a doctor may select a central seating position at a case conference, thereby increasing his/her ability to influence the proceedings.

Other process skills include: seeking the opinion of a third person who is known to hold a similar view on any particular issue; asking for more time to consider a request; and using rewards (praise, encouragement, etc.) to reduce any negative feelings engendered by assertiveness and also to help maintain and protect the relationship. Finally, the non-verbal behaviour of the asserter is very important and should include medium levels of eye contact, direct body orientation, upright posture, smooth use of gestures when speaking yet inconspicuous gestures when listening and the use of smiles, which serve to emphasize that a response is intended to be assertive and not aggressive (Wilson and Gallois, 1993).

5.5.3 Covert aspects

There are three main covert elements involved in assertiveness.

- **Knowledge**. In order to be assertive it is necessary to know what one's rights actually are as well as knowing how to protect them. Where we are unsure about our exact rights, we often consult the opinions of others to ascertain whether these have been infringed (e.g. 'Has he the right to ask me to do that?'). There is evidence to show that those who are aware of the exact parameters of their job role are better able to assert themselves in the work setting (Rabin and Zelner, 1992). As summarized by Porritt (1984, p. 105): 'If you have not thought about your rights as a health professional and the rights of others now is the time. Once you hold beliefs about your rights and their accompanying responsibilities you will find it easier to act in a way which expects those rights to be upheld and also accepts the responsibility attached to any action you take.'
- **Perceptions**. People may be unassertive owing to mistaken perceptions, such as perceiving unreasonable requests to be reasonable or perceiving a tyrant as being a strong boss. Such individuals need to learn to be more accurate in judging the behaviour of others or they may be viewed as 'easy touches' who can easily be manipulated.
- **Beliefs**. Some people are submissive as a result of mistaken beliefs, such as believing that they must always do what their superiors tell them. Again, a learning process is necessary here in order to educate the individual to develop a more realistic set of positive beliefs. Indeed, training non-assertive individuals to change their negative beliefs to more positive ones has been shown to result in significant gains in assertiveness (Rakos, 1991).

5.5.4 Influencing factors

A range of factors influence the degree, nature and effectiveness of assertion. The gender of both parties is important, since it is often easier to be assertive with someone of the same sex. In the health context, it is difficult to be assertive with seriously or terminally ill patients and their relatives, with physically or mentally handicapped people and with the elderly. It is also more difficult to be assertive with close friends and with people of higher power and status. Similarly, practitioners will often find it more difficult to be assertive in the patient's home as opposed to the health clinic. The importance of setting was highlighted by Kilkus (1993), who discovered that nurses working in less traditional contexts (schools, public health contexts, etc.) were more assertive than those working in hospitals, nursing homes or clinics, as measured by responses on the Rathus Assertiveness Schedule. He also found that nurses who had received assertion training reported higher levels of assertiveness than those who had not been so trained.

The status of the professional is another important factor, in that it is easier to be assertive from a position of power and authority. Thus, Gerry (1989) found that the assertion level of nurses was related to their place in the hierarchy. In her study of hospital nurses, she found that nursing sisters were more assertive than staff nurses who, in turn, were more assertive than enrolled nurses. Interestingly, however, Gerry also found that these work trends did not influence everyday life contexts outside the work setting, since here it was the enrolled nurses who had fewer problems with assertive situations.

There are also cultural differences, in that some (especially Western) cultures value this skill whereas other (notably Eastern) societies may emphasize non-assertive responses such as humility, indirectness, 'fitting in' and tolerance (Thomlinson, 1991). This has been shown to have important ramifications for the professional who works in a multiracial society (Kreps and Kunimoto, 1994). For example, Rasinski (1993), in her review of cultural factors that impinge upon practitioner–patient communication, illustrated how in certain Arabic and Semitic cultures the doctor is treated with the utmost respect and trust, such that 'for a physician to ask the patient or the family for a decision regarding the patient's future care would raise in their minds the thought that the physician was not competent or confident of the diagnosis or treatment' (p. 171). In other words, even within a society where the general trend is for patients to be viewed as partners in care, certain subcultures will expect the practitioner to be the sole decision-maker. This means that health professionals need to be sensitive to the cultural nuances of those with whom they interact. As discussed by Hargie (1997b), skilled individuals require high levels of such cultural expertise.

All of the above factors are important in that they contribute to the fact that some professionals will find it relatively easy to be assertive in many situations, whereas others will find it difficult to be assertive in any (Slater, 1990). However, the skill of assertiveness is important for every health professional. Briggs (1986, p. 24), describing a 2-day course on assertion skills for nurses, pointed out, 'Assertion training is about improving personal, and thereby professional, effectiveness. It is concerned with the building of self-confidence and esteem, and the ability to translate this into improving communications and relationships.'

Exercise 5.3 provides details of an exercise which can be employed by the trainer to encourage trainees to develop their awareness of assertiveness, and distinguish this approach from other response styles.

Exercise 5.3 Assertiveness

Aim

To encourage trainees to identify, and discriminate between, assertive, nonassertive, and aggressive styles of responding.

Materials

Blank acetate sheets and felt-tip pens. Two (or more) prepared acetates or hand-outs depicting a situation where assertive skills are required. One of these situations should relate to the professional situation, whereas the other can be of a more generic 'life' situation. For example (1) 'You are a nurse on ward duty. A consultant is dealing with a female patient whom you know to be sensitive and shy. He is being markedly abrupt and rude with her and you can see she is visibly upset and close to tears.' (2) 'You have loaned £50 to a close friend who promised to pay it back the following week. Four weeks have now passed and there has been no mention of the money at all. You do not need the money urgently, but are worried about never receiving it if you do not raise the issue.'

Instructions

Having presented the scenarios divide the class into small groups. Provide each group with blank acetates and felt-tip pens. Each group is then requested to generate and list on the acetate, an assertive, a non-assertive and an aggressive response to each of the given statements, and to discuss the possible outcomes of each type of response.

Discussion

Each subgroup in turn, or a spokesperson, comes to the front of the class and presents the acetate detailing the three types of response. They also discuss the anticipated outcomes of each response. At this stage, a general class discussion should be encouraged, concerning the identification of response styles and the implications of employing each style in different contexts.

5.6 OVERVIEW

The focus of this chapter has been upon the skills of questioning, explaining, opening interactions, closing interactions and assertiveness. We have termed these 'initiating skills', since they are used primarily in contexts in which the practitioner takes the lead during interaction with patients and other professionals. When taken in conjunction with the skills reviewed in Chapter 4, this provides a coverage of core interpersonal skills relevant to health situations. The purpose of this chapter has been to provide a summative overview of each skill, and the trainer is advised to pursue some of the references given throughout the chapter for further information on the skills. In the following chapter we examine higher-order interactional strategies, which build upon the skills covered in this chapter and in Chapter 4.

6 Interactional strategies

6.1 INTRODUCTION

This chapter builds upon the preceding two chapters. It examines four interactional strategies, each of which is dependent upon the effective implementation of a number of the interpersonal skills covered in Chapters 4 and 5. A strategy in this sense can be regarded as a planned course of action featuring elements of various social skills which are combined and implemented in order to achieve a particular goal. Strategies are therefore situation-specific. For example, in a context where a patient is worried or distressed and needs to talk through a problem, the practitioner might usefully employ a counselling strategy. Counselling is the first strategy analysed in this chapter, the other three being influencing, interviewing and working in groups. These four strategies will be reviewed in terms of their applications to the work of health professionals.

6.2 COUNSELLING

The importance of counselling as a legitimate strategy for health professionals is increasingly being recognized (Morrow and Hargie, 1992). Unfortunately, the term 'patient counselling' is often used to mean simply all forms of practitioner–patient interchange, or, more specifically, situations in which the practitioner gives advice. Indeed, the term 'counselling' frequently has this latter meaning in everyday usage (e.g. investment counsellors, legal counsel). However, in relation to professional interaction, counselling should be regarded as a therapeutic process that involves: 'helping someone to explore a problem, clarify conflicting issues and discover alternative ways of dealing with it, so that they can decide what to do about it; that is, helping people to help themselves' (Hopson, 1981, p. 267).

As this definition illustrates, counselling is definitely not simply about giving advice. Rather, it involves developing a relationship with patients that will facilitate their full expression of feelings, emotions and thoughts, in order to enable them to make personal decisions. In other words, patients are encouraged to mobilize their own expertise and employ their own resources in searching for a solution to their own particular problems. The counsellor does not take the role of an expert who already has the answers, but instead devotes time and effort to actually finding out exactly how the patient feels, and to attempting to understand fully the patient's situation. In this sense, counselling, as a strategy, is altruistic since the emphasis is upon patient 'self-empowerment' through exploring and negotiating personal needs with no overt, directive guidance from the practitioner.

The development of counselling as a widely researched and well established therapeutic activity has resulted in the establishment of a range of full-time and part-time counsellors in various settings (for example, full-time student counsellors in colleges or part-time counsellors in organizations such as the Samaritans, Relate, etc.). Within the health domain, however, most professionals use counselling as a subrole, so that the practitioner may employ this strategy as an alternative form of intervention when dealing with patients (Morrow and Hargie, 1989).

There are a number of different forms of 'helping' that the practitioner can use, including:

- counselling;
- giving advice (e.g. advising a patient to stop smoking);
- giving information (e.g. informing a patient that smoking increases the risk of coronary heart disease);
- taking direct action (e.g. dressing a wound);
- teaching (e.g. showing a recently diagnosed diabetic how to use a hypodermic syringe);
- offering sympathy (e.g. following a bereavement);
- giving reassurance (e.g. where a patient is mistakenly worried about something);
- systems change (e.g. a GP may change an appointment system to ensure easier access, especially for patients in distress).

All of these are valid and valuable helping strategies and one or more of them may be effective, depending upon the context. However, they all serve different purposes. Hopson (1981) identified the main functions of counselling as helping patients to:

- enter into a relationship where they feel accepted and understood and are therefore prepared to talk openly about their problems;
- achieve an increased understanding of their situation;
- discuss alternative courses of action;
- make a decision about what to do;
- develop specific action plans;
- do, with support, what has to be done;

- where necessary, adjust to a situation that is unlikely to change.

It should be realized, however, that there is a range of theoretical perspectives on counselling, each with its own conceptual underpinning linked to practical implications for dealing with the counsellee (for a useful review of these see Ivey, Ivey and Simek-Dowling, 1987). In this chapter it is not possible to review these differing perspectives: we will present some general information central to the overall process of counselling *per se,* together with a sequential analysis of the stages involved in this strategy.

In addition to being aware of the nature of counselling, an important factor for the practitioner is knowing **when** to implement it. Counselling is associated with one of three 'c's' – making a **c**hoice, making a **c**hange, or sorting out **c**onfusion. Typical situations in which patients or their relatives might be in need of this form of help would include following a loss of some kind (such as bereavement or amputation of a limb) or when receiving bad news (such as terminal illness or the need for major surgery). As Lang and van der Molen (1990) iterated, counselling is generally indicated when emotional factors are causing problems for the individual. Criticisms of the lack of attention to this psychosocial domain appear regularly in the popular press. The following newspaper quote is not atypical of such feature articles: 'What health professionals often have trouble accepting is that a person's well-being involves the whole of the person – his or her psychological, social, economic, historical and cultural situation, as well as the actual medical symptom that may have brought them to the clinic in the first place' (*The Independent on Sunday*, 14 November 1994).

It has already been recognized in this book that practitioners are often reluctant to deal with the emotional and psychosocial dimensions of patients' problems. Indeed, Evans, Stanley and Burrows (1992, p. 156) argued that over a period of time physicians' 'ability to attend to patients' emotional needs may even decline, leading in subsequent medical practice to inattention to psychosocial correlates to illness and neglect of patients' concerns'. One possible reason for this may be the lack of training given in how to handle such problems. As Kelly, Moran and Myatt (1994, p. 137) pointed out, there is a 'great need for the teaching of communication skills and the importance of psychosocial factors in the assessment of medical presentations, both at under graduate and post graduate levels'. This holds for the encoding as well as decoding of emotions, since research has shown that the physician's ability to encode emotional information accurately is related to increased patient satisfaction, greater physician popularity and fewer patient cancellations (Tickle-Degnen and Rosenthal, 1992). In noting the many studies that have charted poor communication by health professionals, and in particular the failure to address psychosocial aspects of patient care, Davis and Fallowfield (1991, p. 19) argued that 'many of the deficiencies in communication would be removed if all professionals had basic counselling skills'.

Another reason for health professionals becoming skilled in counselling techniques is that we are 'moving out of an era in which **curing** is dominant into an era in which **caring** must take precedence' (Watson, 1988, p. 175). Indeed, cure only occurs in about 10% of patients seen by doctors, given the decreased mortality rate from former life-threatening conditions (Montgomery, 1993). The prevalence of chronic conditions means that health professionals will need counselling skills to deal with the other 90% who cannot be cured. Furthermore: 'As many as 30% of patients present in general practice with problems which are primarily emotional in origin' (Rowland, Irving and Maynard, 1989, p. 118).

6.2.1 Counselling stages

There are four main phases involved in the counselling process: attending, exploring, understanding and action. In order to gain a fuller understanding of the overall process, it is useful to examine each of these stages separately.

Attending

At this stage the practitioner needs to pay careful attention to the patient by demonstrating an active listening style (see Chapter 4). In particular, the manner in which the interaction is opened will have an important bearing upon how the patient responds (Chapter 5). If the professional conveys the impression of having the time, disposition and energy to devote to the consultation, then the patient is more likely to enter into a counselling relationship. Since patients frequently open the discussion with a 'presenting' problem, and will often only reveal their real problems when encouraged to do so, it is important to be aware of verbal and non-verbal signals which patients may emit to indicate a desire for a deeper level of discussion. In this regard, Bensing (1991, p. 17) highlighted the importance of not just 'listening to what is said, but also to what the patient is unable to say (his anxiety, uncertainty, the problem-behind-the-problem)'. Furthermore, the portrayal of warmth, which involves communicating a liking for the other person and an indication of being willing to engage fully in interaction, is crucial to the establishment of a good rapport conducive to a helping encounter. The use of verbal and non-verbal reinforcers (see Chapter 4) would seem to be central to the communication of warmth.

Exploring

Following the initial relationship-development phase, the next step is to attempt to gain a full and accurate understanding of the patient's situation. This necessitates allowing the patient to talk freely, with as little direction as possible from the practitioner. One way this can be achieved is through the use of reflections (see Chapter 4), which to a large extent permit the patient to control the flow of the discussion (Bensing and Dronkers, 1992). Where questions are used, these should be open rather than closed (see Chapter 5), thereby again placing minimum restrictions upon the respondent. A third skill which is important at the exploration stage is the use of spaced reviews. By employing this type of intermittent summary, the practitioner can ensure that both parties are in agreement about the information presented before moving on to explore further issues.

Understanding

Before progressing to the final stage, it is imperative to ensure optimum awareness by both parties of issues, thoughts and feelings raised during the exploratory phase. The practitioner will need to demonstrate empathy, by attempting to take the perspective of, and making a concerted effort to see the world through the eyes of, the patient. Empathy has been described as 'feeling with', whereas sympathy is 'feeling for', the other person (Bruneau, 1993). In his review of research in this field, Authier (1986) itemized the behavioural components of empathy as:

- good eye contact;
- close seating distance;
- a forward lean;
- the use of touch when appropriate;
- concerned facial expressions;
- the use of reflections of feeling;
- self-disclosure;
- confrontation.

The last technique necessitates tactfully yet firmly drawing attention to conflicting or contradictory aspects of the patient's communications.

Self-disclosure is also important. This can either be about experiences that the practitioner has had, or has dealt with, which are similar to those being described by the patient, or it can involve commenting upon how the practitioner feels about the patient's situation. The patient also needs to feel accepted and the practitioner therefore must demonstrate positive regard, which involves being non-judgemental and treating the patient with respect. In addition, the practitioner should be genuine and without facades and should not be simply playing a role. Rather, for effective counselling, congruence should exist between how the counsellor feels about, and in turn responds to, the counsellee (Patterson, 1986). In other words, honesty, sincerity and altruism are essential attributes for the counselling practitioner.

Geldard (1993) highlighted two techniques that can be useful at the understanding stage. The first is that of **reframing**, where the practitioner metaphorically puts a new frame round the picture being presented by the patient, so that it can be viewed in a different way. This is particularly important where patients are seeing the world from a position such as depression, anxiety or low self-esteem. For example, a woman who is ill describes how her husband is annoying her by always fussing around, never giving her a minute's peace and continually interfering. The practitioner could reframe this by saying 'This is obviously annoying for you, having him under your feet all the time. Yet I also get the impression that you must be really important to your husband and that he is very keen to take care of you.' However, such reframing must not deny the patient's view of the world and therefore needs to be presented in a sensitive and tentative fashion.

The second technique is that of **normalizing** the patient's emotional state, by giving an assurance that it is not abnormal. This is useful in response to questions such as 'Am I going crazy?'; 'How could I feel like this?'; 'Is it only me?' For example, those who have been recently bereaved may experience a mix of feelings, including anger, depression, guilt and despair. It can be made clear to the patient that this is part of a normal grief reaction, without diminishing the personal pain involved. Learning that one's emotions are experienced by others in similar circumstances can serve to reduce the patient's anxiety. At the same time, the need for the patient to work through these emotions should be given cognizance.

Action

By this stage, the patient should have fully explored and achieved a full understanding of the problem and be ready to take action to alleviate it. The patient needs to be the decision-maker, knowing what needs to be achieved and the steps which have to be taken, with the practitioner acting in a supportive role. The patient should also be aware of those factors that will either facilitate (**benefits**) or hinder (**barriers**) goal achievement. Success in goal achievement usually occurs where the benefits clearly outweigh the barriers. Action may also include educating the patient to goal achievement, and teaching can therefore be a final part of the counselling process. For example, a female who has had a mastectomy will need to be taught how to use appropriate cosmetic aids. However, such teaching should never preclude, or be a substitute for, counselling. A final aspect of the action stage may necessitate referring the patient elsewhere for specialist advice and guidance.

6.2.2 Effective counselling

While a considerable volume of research has been conducted in this field, there is no easy answer as to what exactly constitutes effective counselling. This is because success in this sphere is dependent upon a range of factors, such as the type of patient, the nature of the problem and the time available. In relation to the latter dimension, counselling may be a long process involving a series of interactions between practitioner and client, or might be satisfactorily concluded in a single encounter. One difficulty faced by many practitioners, of course, is the lack of time available to enter into a therapeutic helping relationship on a long-term basis.

However, there is evidence to indicate that many patients only require one interview in order to relieve emotional distress, and that the result of encouraging patients to ventilate their feelings and emotions is a decreased dependence upon medical services (Davis and Fallowfield, 1991). It is now widely accepted that in the past there was an overemphasis upon drug treatments for emotional problems. More recently, the need for other 'non-medical' approaches, such as counselling, is increasingly being recognized. These alternative approaches need not always overall be more time-consuming. As Bernstein and Bernstein (1980, p. 188) pointed out: 'The time required for counseling is unlikely to be more than that taken up by repeated medical visits. The few patients who require long-term counseling could be referred to more appropriate sources.'

Indeed, it is also recognized that some health professionals will have more time available for counselling than others. For example, Macmillan nurses in oncology care are able to devote more time to patients than would doctors. Likewise, those working in a hospice setting will regard counselling as being central to their communication repertoire with patients and their relatives. In hospitals, resident social workers can also undertake intensive counselling with patients. Another approach is for the practitioner to arrange for a specialized professional to be available if required, and indeed several GP practices in the UK now have a counsellor attachment.

This has been facilitated by the fact that it is possible for GPs to recoup between 70% and 100% reimbursement from government for the costs of hiring such counsellors. Harris (1994), in noting this trend, has presented a vitriolic argument against employing such counsellors. He portrays counselling as a very time consuming, nebulous activity, akin to magic or religion, and in many ways alien to the traditional stiff-upper-lip stoicism of the British. In concluding he asserted that:

> Counselling is a religion like any other. Left alone to take its chance in the mainstream of religious competition it will almost certainly founder. But installed in the doctor's surgery, paid for out of state funds and regulated by state laws it takes on a far more sinister aspect. The right to be unhappy, to dissent, will be denied us not by political officers and state torturers, but by benign therapists – mental hygenists – with our 'best' interests at heart. The interests of the state will then conform with the interests of happiness; a world in which the individual will no longer have a place!
>
> *Harris, 1994, p. 35*

While counselling if misused, like any form of helping strategy, is not without dangers, such extremist views are very much in the minority.

In one survey of 100 patients, Thomas (1993) found that 85% of respondents indicated they would prefer to see a counsellor in the surgery, while 56% said they would be more likely to do so if the doctor first explained the benefits. Thomas argued that seeing an 'in-house' counsellor probably does not attract the same stigma as a psychiatric referral. Rowland, Irving and Maynard (1989) also supported counsellor attachment schemes, arguing that this form of specialized help requires concerted training, which may be outwith the time and role of the doctor. An alternative perspective, however, is presented by Gray (1988), who purported that health professionals need to have counselling skills and be able to use them since, if counsellors are available, 'there may be a temptation for doctors and nurses to opt out of the care of a major group of their patients and this must be avoided at all costs' (p. 51). Health professionals will need to use counselling skills in their interactions with patients, but should also be able to recognize when to refer patients for more specialized and extensive counselling. Another dimension here, of course, is that health professionals themselves have been shown to benefit from counselling, especially where their work involves dealing with severe physical and emotional trauma (Garrud, 1990).

Counselling would therefore appear to be a crucial strategy for health professionals. In their review of research in this field, Davis and Fallowfield (1991, p. 314) concluded that 'counselling and communication can improve professional satisfaction, patient satisfaction, diagnostic accuracy, and treatment adherence. They have obvious benefits to the psychosocial care of patients, are associated with improvements in the patient's understanding and retention of information about their illness and treatment, have significant effects upon the physical outcome of disease, and have demonstrable preventive effects.' Programmes of CST have been shown to develop the ability of general practitioners to use counselling techniques effectively (Evans, Stanley and Burrows, 1992).

In concluding this section it is useful to highlight the main factors that would seem to contribute to successful counselling. As summarized by Authier (1986), this occurs where the practitioner is able to participate completely in the patient's communication, fully understands how the patient feels and successfully communicates this understanding, follows the patient's line of thought and treats the patient as an equal co-worker on a common problem.

6.3 INFLUENCING AND PERSUADING

An important dimension of the role of every health practitioner is to, at one time or another, persuade patients to pursue a recommended course of action. This may occur when initially explaining, following diagnosis, what action the patient will be expected to take, or if resistance is shown and objections raised to the treatment, it may be necessary to employ persuasion techniques to overcome such objections (Hargie and Morrow, 1987a). In this section, we will be concerned with this type of direct interpersonal influence as a social strategy, rather than with, for example, wider mass media campaigns often using a form of propaganda aimed at securing changes in health behaviour.

In discussing this distinction, Mulholland (1994) illustrated how propaganda uses strong – often covert – tactics, hardly allows for resistance to influence attempts, exerts even greater pressure in the face of opposition, and has as its goal the imposition of its own wishes on others. By contrast, interpersonal influence involves less pressure, follows a cooperative rather than a coercive path, and may involve the acceptance of partial success or even failure to persuade.

Although the terms 'influence' and 'persuasion' are often used interchangeably, there are differences in these two processes, in that persuasion implies both success and intentionality (Hargie, Saunders and Dickson, 1994). Thus, it does not really make sense to say 'I persuaded them to do it but they didn't' – here what is implied is that an **attempt** was made to persuade. Also, when we make persuasion attempts we are aware of so doing, whereas we can influence others without doing so consciously. For example a patient who sees a health professional smoking may conclude that it must not be that harmful and so be influenced to continue to smoke. In this case, the professional's influence would be unintentional.

Raven and Haley (1982, p. 427) defined social influence as 'a change in the cognitions, attitudes, or behaviour of a person (target) which is attributable to the actions of another person (influencing agent)'. Influence that leads to positive attitude change is termed 'private acceptance', while influence that changes behaviour in the intended direction (regardless of internal attitudes) is termed 'public compliance' (Turner, 1991). The former type of influence is necessary to ensure lasting change in behaviour. In attempting to influence others we can use a range of what Miller *et al.* (1987) termed 'compliance-gaining message strategies'. A knowledge of the range of influencing tactics that can be used to increase patient compliance is clearly of importance for health professionals, given the wealth of research evidence to indicate that patients frequently do not follow advice about medication or changes in life-style. This type of social influence and persuasion is an emergent area of study, which in recent years has witnessed 'a veritable explosion of research and theory' (Zimbardo and Leippe, 1991, p. xvii). Numerous books have been devoted to this topic (e.g. Reardon, 1991; Perloff, 1993; Bettinghaus and Cody, 1994) and there has been a proliferation of research articles published during the past decade. This interest is hardly surprising, given the pervasive nature of the process in health and other contexts.

Burgoon, Birk and Hall (1991) identified the following seven attributes of influencing, which characterize the health-care setting.

- In most cases targets (patients) enter into the transaction voluntarily and are free to decide whether or not to comply with the suggestions and directives of the agent (health professional).
- Patients enter into a contract (often economic) in which they agree to receive compliance-gaining directives.
- Compliance is almost always for the benefit of the target and is rarely seen as

being of benefit to the agent. (Although not recognized by Burgoon, Birk and Hall, there are of course benefits to the professional, including job satisfaction and a decrease in return visits.)

- There are recognized and significant differences in the perceived normative status of agent and target.
- Well-defined expectations provide agents with the freedom to employ many influencing tactics.
- There is no standard reaction by the agent to non-compliance by the target.
- The effects of non-compliance for the target range through death, serious illness, discomfort to perhaps nothing at all.

Given these parameters, we will now examine the core influencing tactics available to health professionals.

6.3.1 Influencing tactics

A number of tactics have been identified and the remainder of this section is devoted to an overview of those methods that have been shown to be effective in influencing others.

Power

There are six types of social power which can be exerted by practitioners.

- **Expert power**. Most health professionals are regarded as 'experts' by the lay population, in that they possess expertise or knowledge that others do not have. However, in terms of interprofessional communication, there is also a hierarchy of expert power within the health-care team. Expert power is underlined by three main factors. Firstly, the use of **titles** such as doctor, nurse, etc. sets the professional apart from others. Jackson (1994), in a study of patients suffering from back-pain, found that the use of a 'credibility enhancing cue' in an educational booklet given to patients resulted in significant increases in adherence to recommended exercise and confidence in medical advice, when compared to a group of patients given the booklet with no such cue. In this study, the cue was that it was a statement at the beginning of the booklet that it had been written by a physician with expertise in this field. Secondly, the **clothing** worn by many practitioners clearly indicates that they have a specialized function. Thirdly, **trappings** can convey expertise, in the form of diplomas on the wall, large tomes on a bookshelf, stethoscope round the neck, and so on. Raven and Rubin (1983) illustrated how, in many instances, in order to maintain respect as an expert one not only has to display an impressive front, but must also carefully withhold information and keep the source of one's knowledge a mystery. The use of this latter technique has obvious dangers for health professionals in terms of patient understanding of instructions (see Chapter 5).

- **Information power**. Here, the content of the message is the basis of the power. Thus, a dentist might persuade a mother to give her children fluoride drops by showing her the positive results of research studies comparing this course of action with a control group who received no fluoride drops. Another form of this type of power occurs when someone has access to information that another person either wishes to discover or does not want to be revealed. Bribery and blackmail respectively may be the result!
- **Legitimate power**. In this instance, power emanates from the position occupied by the individual, so that a ward sister will have power over nurses, but if she retires this is obviously relinquished. The authority is vested in the role or position, not in the person. Interestingly, patients have legitimate power over practitioners, so that a doctor will be expected to help a distressed patient.
- **Referent power**. We can be influenced by others because we want to be accepted by them and be part of their group. One good example of this is dress, hair-style, etc. among teenagers, where there is often enormous peer pressure to conform to the current fashions. Likewise, television advertisers use famous people to sell products. Recently, this has been termed the 'wannabe' phenomenon, based upon thousands of teenage girls who wanted to be like the pop star Madonna. Practitioners can use referent power to influence patients by, for example, stating that the medication they are recommending has been very effective when used by many other 'caring mothers' (or other appropriate reference group). The process of demonstrating the acceptability of a medication or recommended course of action by referring to others has been termed 'social proof' and has been shown to be a highly successful technique (Cialdini, 1988).
- **Reward power**. This stems from the ability of the person to reward others if they comply with requests. Parents have reward power over their children ('If you're good I will give you some chocolate'). Likewise, a nurse may comply with the sister's commands in order to receive a positive evaluation and increase the chances of promotion.
- **Coercive power**. This is the converse of reward power, since it refers to the person's capacity to administer punishments. Policemen clearly have this form of power, and we are therefore likely to obey their requests. Well publicized extreme cases have been described where coercive power has been used to control the behaviour of the senile elderly in sheltered accommodation (being given cold baths, tied to a chair, etc.). Such abuses are clearly at odds with codes of professional conduct. Practitioners may wield power more constructively to the extent that patients are concerned about receiving positive social reinforcement from them or are dependent on them for other rewards.

Fear

Dillard (1995) illustrated how fear appeals have been very common in health campaigns concerned with, *inter alia*, dental care, smoking, breast self-examination, sexually transmitted disease, nuclear radiation, and drug and alcohol abuse. He further highlighted how fear or threat messages can be effective in influencing attitudes and behaviour. Boster and Mongeau (1984) itemized the four stages involved in using fear as an influencing technique:

- You are vulnerable to this particular threat.
- If you are vulnerable, then you should take action to reduce this vulnerability.
- To reduce this vulnerability, you must accept certain recommendations.
- This is what you must do.

In reviewing research into the effectiveness of fear-arousing messages, Sutton (1982, p. 323) concluded that 'increases in fear are consistently associated with increases in acceptance (intentions and behaviour)'. However, in their overview of the area Heath and Bryant (1992, p. 134) found that 'some studies concluded that high amounts of fear produce attitude change, but other studies found low amounts to be more effective'. Dillard (1995, p. 304) summarized current research in this area by concluding that 'fear is reliably and substantially related to acceptance of the message. . . . However, it is not a simple effect, but one that is apparently qualified by interactions with age and anxiety.' In some instances an intense fear component may inhibit attention and increase distraction, which in turn will reduce comprehension or result in the message being ignored.

It would seem that the success of the fear tactic is dependent upon three critical elements:

- the magnitude and severity of the negative outcome as perceived by the target;
- its probability of occurring if no action is taken to avoid it;
- the likely availability and effectiveness of the recommended course of action (Rogers, 1984).

The greater the extent to which these three factors are present, the more effective the fear message is likely to be. Equally, if any one of them is missing, then the message loses its efficacy.

Roser and Thompson (1995) highlighted the distinction between threat appraisal and response-efficacy on the one hand – which refers to the acceptance by the individual of the severity of the threat and the effectiveness of the proposed response in reducing it; and coping appraisal and self-efficacy on the other – the individual's perception of personal ability to carry out the response successfully. Thus, a patient may recognize the importance of giving up smoking to reduce the risk of another coronary, but may believe that to stop smoking is something that would be personally not achievable or sustainable. Leventhal (1970) noted that where such a situation arises, patients may either feel hopelessness ('I'm probably going to get cancer anyway, so I might as well smoke and enjoy myself') or defensiveness ('This couldn't possibly happen to me'). Leventhal differentiated between fear control and danger control. The former is concerned with the reduction of internal states and feelings of fear, whereas the latter involves coping with the environment and overtly responding in such a way as to reduce the danger that is present. To continue with the smoking example, the most effective danger control technique would be to stop smoking. However, individuals who respond primarily in terms of fear control can simply avoid negative messages about smoking, rationalize their behaviour (e.g. 'I know a man who smoked 60 cigarettes a day who lived to a ripe old age') or, as Fishbein (1982) demonstrated, smokers may convince themselves that while others may suffer as a result of smoking (general beliefs), they personally will not be adversely affected (personal beliefs). It is therefore important to ensure that patients are clearly shown, and capable of carrying out, danger control responses to overcome any threat inherent in fear-arousing messages.

Moral appeals

Many people are susceptible to exhortations that they have a duty to carry out a particular course of action and that if they do not fulfil their moral obligations they will feel guilty. Marwell and Schmitt (1967a, b) identified the potency of **self-feeling** in either a positive ('You will feel better if you comply') or negative ('You will feel very bad about yourself if you do not comply') mode. They also illustrated the importance of **altercasting** in influencing others, either used positively ('A person with good qualities would comply') or negatively ('Only a person with bad qualities would not comply'). Another technique recognized by Marwell and Schmitt was that of **altruism,** where an appeal is made to the 'better side' of an individual (e.g. 'We are all depending upon you, please don't let us down'). An appeal to morals is one of the techniques employed to persuade individuals to use condoms for the protection of self and others. Interestingly, moral appeals are also used by insurance companies to sell life policies, with a high degree of success!

The relationship

We are more likely to be influenced by people we like, are friendly with, or for whom we have high regard (Yoder, Hugenberg and Wallace, 1993). For this reason, it is important for health professionals to develop and foster a positive relationship with patients. Most of the skills covered in Chapters 4 and 5 can be employed to build a conducive relationship. In particular, the skill of reinforcement can be very potent. Dickson, Saunders and Stringer (1993) reviewed research that illustrates how praise and compliments are effective techniques to employ when persuading others. It would seem that the receipt of praise leads to liking for the sender, which in turn can facilitate the process of influencing (flattery, it appears, may indeed get you everywhere!). Furthermore, where the practitioner has similar attitudes and values to the patient, or has a common interest or hobby, this can also facilitate the relationship. Many salespeople are, in fact, trained to use this latter 'we have something in common' approach. When interacting with customers they are taught to search for clues as to the interests of the customer (e.g. golf) and use this accordingly.

Similarity of language (accent, terminology, etc.) has also been shown to aid compliance and is part of communication accommodation, wherein an attempt is made to converge towards the vocal, verbal and non-verbal responses of the other person in order to enhance the relationship (Buller and Aune, 1992). For example, it has been shown that accommodation of language intensity enhances message credibility (Aune and Kikuchi, 1993). An example of high language intensity would be the use of terms such as 'absolutely', 'excellent', 'wonderful' as opposed to their low-intensity equivalents of 'perhaps', 'fair', 'acceptable'. Using the patient's name is another useful strategy which, when not overused, can lead to positive evaluations of the practitioner (Kleinke, 1986). Attractiveness, in terms of physical appearance and dress, is also important as we are more likely to be influenced by attractive individuals. Another important dimension in the establishment and maintenance of relationships is the use of humour, since 'Studies of persuasion have revealed that humorous people are perceived as more likable, and this in turn enables them to have greater influence' (Marsh, 1988, p. 113).

Reciprocation

One way to influence other people is to use the 'trade-off' method, whereby an exchange of favours is arranged. This may take the form of **pre-giving** where the target person is 'buttered-up' by being given rewards before any requests for compliance are made. This tactic is used by many sales companies when they give away free samples of their goods in the knowledge that this will increase their overall sales. Such a procedure increases the pressure on others to reciprocate, since they tend to feel in debt to the giver. An alternative approach is to make a **promise** ('You do this for me now, I will do that for you later'). Practitioners can employ the reciprocation tactic by pointing out to patients the efforts they have made on their behalf, before requesting compliance with a recommended course of action.

Logical argument

Raven and Rubin (1983) identified a number of features of arguments and the way they are delivered that tend to increase their persuasive appeal. The message conveyed should be fully comprehensible with clear conclusions being drawn and the important aspects repeated to underline them. The advantages of the recommended course of action and disadvantages of the alternatives should be firmly stated, both at the beginning (primacy effect) and at the end (recency effect) of consultations. In terms of delivery, a reasonably fast rate of delivery (around 200 words per minute), an open posture and a 'powerful' authoritative speech style (few hesitations or expressed doubts, coupled with the use of **intensifiers** such as 'definitely', absolutely', etc.) increase the influencing power of an argument.

Scale of the request

Two separate approaches have been identified in terms of the scale of the initial request. The first is the 'foot-in-the-door' (FID) tactic, where a small response is required at the outset and, if agreed to, future requests gradually increase in size. This technique has been found to be fairly successful, although if the costs of later requests are very high it may not be effective (Hargie, Saunders and Dickson, 1994). A doctor might use this technique by asking a patient to stop smoking for a day and gradually increasing the time span. Similarly, a physiotherapist will often ask patients to try to progressively bend a joint a little further. The second method is the 'door-in-the-face' (DIF), or reciprocation of concessions, tactic wherein a very large request is made in the knowledge that it is very likely to be refused. Then a much smaller request, which is equivalent to a concession, is made and is more likely to be successful, since the target will feel under some pressure to reciprocate the concession. Thus a doctor might ask a reluctant patient if she would be willing to go into hospital for a week to undergo some tests. This request could then be scaled down to a request to attend for only a morning as an out-patient. Research has shown FID and DIF techniques to be equally effective sequential influencing strategies (Seibold, Cantrill and Meyers, 1994).

Aversive stimulation

Here the agent subjects the target person to unpleasant experiences which will only be removed when the agent's request or demand has been complied with. An extreme example of this is the torture of a subject during interrogation, while an everyday example would be nagging by a spouse or child, aimed at wearing down the resistance of the target. Indeed, advertisers recognize the value of aversive stimulation when they target television adverts at children, whom they know will then continually request the product from their parents – a process they refer to as 'pest power'. A practitioner could obviously employ a variation of this technique with patients, but in a tactful fashion.

Scarcity value

Highlighting that an object or experience is in limited supply can influence people to seek it. Hence the appeal of 'limited editions' or 'once in a lifetime' opportunities. A parallel tactic is to indicate a time-limit on an offer (e.g. 'This sale ends on 19 January'). Thus, a patient might be encouraged to undergo an operation by being told that if he/she does not do so immediately it would be some considerable time before it could be arranged again.

Using influencing strategies

These are the main influencing strategies available to health professionals. It should, of course, be realized that 'many tactics can be employed at a time to achieve influence. And in many cases the use of multiple tactics can be more successful than using just one' (Mulholland, 1994, p. xvii). In using these tactics, it is useful to be aware of the following sequential stages involved in persuasion, as identified by McGuire (1981).

- Exposure to the message
- Attending to the message
- Becoming interested in it
- Understanding it
- Learning how to process and use it
- Yielding to it
- Memorizing it
- Retrieving it when required
- Using it when making decisions
- Executing these decisions
- Reinforcing these actions
- Consolidating the decision based upon the success of the actions.

The practitioner can use influencing tactics with patients at any of the above stages. It should of course also be realized that numerous factors may have an effect upon patient compliance, including the illness (e.g. life-threatening or a minor irritant), the nature of the treatment (e.g. injections, oral administration, side-effects etc.), patient motivation and mental state, age, gender, race, and so on. Much more research is needed in this field, however, before any firm conclusions can be reached with regard to optimum techniques that can be used to influence particular types of patients in specific contexts of practice. Ethical considerations surrounding their use must not be overlooked.

Exercise 6.1 can be employed to allow trainees to practise skills of influencing in a group context.

6.4 FACT-FINDING INTERVIEWING

The third strategy that we will examine in this chapter is that of the fact-finding interview. A range of different types of interview is carried out within health situations, and the nature and objectives of each type will vary depending upon the specific context. However, as Sheppe and Stevenson (1963) noted, all medical interviews have three general goals:

- to establish a good relationship with the patient;
- to elicit specific information;
- to observe behaviour.

An interview can be defined as 'a face-to-face dyadic interaction in which one individual plays the role of interviewer and the other takes on the role of interviewee, and both of these roles carry clear expectations concerning behavioural and attitudinal approach. The interview is requested by one of the participants for a specific purpose' (Millar, Crute and Hargie, 1992, p. 3). Of these characteristics, four key aspects were identified by Bernstein and Bernstein (1980) as being central to the medical interview.

- It is held more for the benefit of the patient than the practitioner.
- It has a specific purpose.
- It is a formal interaction.
- The interaction centres on the problems, needs or feelings of the patient.

All health professionals are involved in interviewing. For example, nurses conduct medical history interviews, hospital pharmacists interview patients to obtain drug histories and doctors carry out diagnostic interviews. The ability to interview effectively has long been recognized as a key dimension of health communication. Thus, Bermosk and Mordan (1964, p. 3) asserted that 'knowledge of interviewing and ability to interview are necessary for every nurse', while Enelow and Swisher (1986, p. 3) argued that 'a good doctor–patient relationship requires effective interviewing'. In this sense, interviewing is 'a very important, perhaps the most important part of the diagnostic process' (Bensing, 1991, p. 11). It is therefore essential to provide trainees with instruction in the methods and techniques of interviewing as part of CST.

6.4.1 Types of interview

There are a number of different types of interviewing formats (for a review of these see Richardson, Dohrenwend and Klein, 1965). In relation to doctor–patient interviews, Gill (1973) distinguished three main types. Firstly, there is the traditional short diagnostic medical interview focusing purely upon physical symptoms. Enelow and Swisher (1986) referred to this as 'directive-interrogative', noting that features of this type of interview include (1) early attempts by the patient to introduce personal concerns which are frustrated, (2) the patient then becomes a passive supplier of information to increasingly specific practitioner questions, (3) there is no deepening of the relationship, and (4) no picking up of important psychosocial cues. Secondly, there is the more personal, patient-centred type of interview, which is much longer and deals with feelings, relationships and psychosocial dimensions of the patient's well-being. Enelow and Swisher (1986) termed this 'open-ended', since the practitioner exerts 'the least amount of authority necessary to obtain the information he is seeking within the time allotted for the interview' (p. 18). Thirdly, there is the 'flash' type of interview, which involves having a free-flowing interaction, without the doctor having any preconceptions, during which there is the chance that a flash of insight will occur in terms of sudden mutual understanding by doctor and patient about what has caused some of the problems faced by the patient.

6.4.2 Interview structure

Carlson (1984) identified four degrees of interview structure applicable to health contexts.

- **Non-structured**. Here the practitioner merely has a general idea of the topics and subtopics that could possibly be discussed. No exact questions are prepared in advance and there is no predesigned order in which the interview is expected to progress. This format is quite close to the counselling strategy discussed earlier in the chapter.
- **Moderately structured**. In this type of interview, the major questions to be asked are decided upon before the interview is conducted. However, there is a degree of flexibility inherent in the interaction, in that while the questions to be asked have been worked out, these do not have to be posed in a set, preordained order. Rather, they can be raised in the context of a more natural conversational style of interaction.
- **Highly structured**. Using this approach, the precise wording of all questions is decided upon in advance of the interview, and usually these are posed in a predetermined sequential fashion. In most instances, they are written out and the practitioner reads them to the patient.
- **Highly structured standardized interviews**. In this instance not only is the exact wording and sequence of questions decided in advance, but the interviewee response options are also predetermined. Almost all of the questions are closed, to allow a tight control of the interview. This also facilitates coding of responses for subsequent data analysis, if the interview is part of a research investigation. The questioning schedule for the interview really takes the form of a questionnaire to be administered orally rather than simply completed individually by the patient. French (1994) noted that an interview, rather than a questionnaire, is often necessary for three reasons. Firstly, while most of the points to be covered can be standardized in a closed format, there is usually a need for some degree of probing at certain points to allow for expanded information. Secondly, the practitioner may have to code answers into particular boxed categories, especially where computer analysis is to be conducted. Thirdly, the interview can allow the practitioner to reassure and motivate the patient while at the same time clarifying any uncertainties regarding particular questions.

The interviewing structure employed depends upon the goals of the interaction. If there is certain specific factual information to be obtained then the interview can be highly structured, allowing the practitioner to direct and control the interaction. On the other hand, if the objective is to find out emotional as well as factual information and to gain as complete a picture as possible of the patient's situation then a less structured approach can be employed, thereby giving the patient a much higher degree of control over the content and direction of the consultation. The less structured approach also facilitates the establishment of rapport and the development of a conducive relationship.

6.4.3 Interview stages

Interviewing can be subdivided into five main stages.

The pre-interview stage

Before the interview takes place the practitioner should take steps to ensure it will be as successful as possible. Carlson (1984) suggested a number of questions that the practitioner should bear in mind at this stage: 'What is the general purpose of this interview?'; 'What are my specific goals?'; 'What are the ways in which I can best achieve these goals?'; and 'Out of all the ways I could achieve my goals, what is the best way for the patient as well as myself to achieve these goals?' The preparatory stage also involves thoroughly scrutinizing any referral data, organizing a suitable environment for the interaction by providing as much privacy as possible, minimizing any possible interruptions or distractions (e.g. by ensuring telephone calls are intercepted if the interview is taking place in an office setting), setting aside adequate time for the interview, and arranging suitable seating, ventilation and so on (Newell, 1994).

The opening stage

At this juncture all the skills of meeting, greeting and seating the patient are crucial (see 'Opening' in Chapter 5). It is essential for the practitioner to develop a good initial rapport with the patient to facilitate the exchange of information in the interview. The actual objectives of the interview should also be carefully itemized, the probable duration should be given and some idea of the main areas to be covered should be outlined. If the patient expresses concern or shows resistance at this stage there are a number of steps that can be taken. Klinzing and Klinzing (1985) recommended the following.

- The purpose of the interview can be reiterated.
- The benefits of cooperation should be underlined.
- The need to obtain the information requested should be stressed.
- The patient's fears should be fully identified and allayed.

Where none of these tactics work, the interview may have to be postponed and, where necessary, another practitioner asked to conduct it. The health professional must gain the confidence of the patient at the outset if the interview is to be successful.

The information collection stage

This is the main body of the interview, during which a number of skills need to be effectively employed. The appropriate use of questions is essential to ensure active patient participation, accuracy of information received and a logical flow of conversation (see Chapter 5). The maintenance of rapport can be achieved through the apposite use of reinforcement and active listening, while in patient-centred interviews the skill of reflecting may be employed to allow the patient to influence the direction of the interaction and play a more active role throughout. An awareness of non-verbal communication is also crucial in terms of interpreting the cues being emitted by, and sending appropriate messages to, the patient. Likewise, techniques for encouraging maximum patient self-disclosure should be implemented (see Chapter 4).

In many interviews it will be necessary for the practitioner to make notes. Where this is the case, the reasons for note-taking should be explained and the patient should be aware of what exactly is being written down. It would also seem that note-taking interchanged rather than concurrent with conversation is more effective in terms of remembering what has been said, while also facilitating a more natural interchange (Millar, Crute and Hargie, 1992). Gorden (1980, p. 356) emphasized the importance of providing **transitions** 'to provide specific material to act as a bridge from one topic to another'. This can serve to show the patient the relationship between the old and new topics, help to relate the new topic to the objectives of the interview and prepare the way for a smooth change in subject matter. Transitions are therefore lead-ins to questions, which give patients time to fully assimilate the question itself.

The closing stage

Drawing the interview to a satisfactory conclusion is an important skill for practitioners to master (Chapter 5). The patient should be prepared for the termination of the interview through the use of closure indicators (e.g. 'This is the final question. . .'), and closure markers of either a verbal (e.g. 'Well, that's it. . .') or non-verbal nature (e.g. gathering papers together, putting pen away, etc.) by the professional. Other components of the closing stage may include giving a summary of what has been covered, inviting and answering patient questions, providing rewarding statements ('You have been very helpful') and making future links in terms of informing the patient how the information gathered will be used.

The post-interview stage

After the interview the practitioner should check that all the information received has been recorded and correctly coded. At this final stage it may also be necessary to make further notes regarding the patient. As French (1994) pointed out, this is particularly true in the case of subjective judgements based upon the reactions of the patient throughout the interview. These activities should occur as soon as possible following the interview, since a prolonged time delay may result in inaccuracy or distortion in the recording of what actually took place. By carefully checking the details of the interview at this stage it is also possible to quickly identify any material which may have been inadvertently omitted, or not fully covered, and return to the patient to obtain it.

6.4.4 Interviewing in practice

Steps should be taken to ensure the accuracy of information provided by patients. This can be achieved by attempting to reduce those factors that may bias the responses given. There is clear evidence to indicate that interviewees often try to please interviewers by offering responses they believe are expected or socially desirable (Dillon, 1990). It is therefore important for practitioners not to lead patients, either directly or indirectly, to give certain types of responses. Thus, the questions asked should not be leading (Chapter 5) and the verbal and non-verbal reactions of the practitioner should be non-judgemental. Bias can be very difficult to eliminate, however, since it would seem that factors such as the age, sex, social class and race of the interviewer in comparison to the interviewee can have marked effects upon how the latter responds (Millar, Crute and Hargie, 1992). Nevertheless, all possible steps should be taken to maximize the objectivity of the interview. The language employed by the professional, for example, should be appropriate to the level of the patient. Bradburn and Sudman (1980) illustrated how respondents reported having drunk twice as many cans of beer and masturbated three times as often when familiar, rather than formal, forms of wording were used to describe these activities.

Interviewing is clearly an important strategy for health professionals. At the same time, this dimension of practice is perhaps one of the most difficult to master. Indeed, it has long been known that 'the diagnostic interview as practised by the physician is certainly one of the most complex and demanding of skilled interviewing techniques' (Kahn and Cannell, 1957, p. 258). Furthermore, in his review of this field, Newell (1994, p. 1) asserted that 'Although interviewing takes up a good deal of time in nursing and other health care professions, it is. . . by and large done poorly'. If practitioners are to become effective interviewers it would therefore seem that time and effort will need to be devoted to this strategy during training.

6.5 WORKING IN GROUPS

It has been recognized for some time that all health professionals need to work effectively in groups. Sampson and Marthas (1981, p. 14) highlighted the fact that, for most aspects of daily practice, 'health professionals find themselves among several others with different kinds of responsibility for managing the care of patients. A person's skill as a team member or organizer are vital to the effectiveness of practice.' Likewise, Singleton (1983, p. 78) emphasized that 'each hospital doctor is part of a team or group whose specific aim is to look after the patient. Much of the real skill of a good and successful doctor is his or her ability to be a useful team member.' More recently, Kreps and Kunimoto (1994) highlighted the importance of the small group as a ubiquitous work unit in health care, while Harding, Taylor and Nettleton (1994, p. 44) illustrated how 'successful provision of health services to the public requires communication, cooperation and collaboration between members of the primary health care team'. Indeed, the Audit Commission (1993), in underlining the possible dangers inherent in a system whereby staff working with the same patient belong to different clinical teams, recommended the setting up of interdisciplinary teams in hospitals. Lecca and McNeil (1985) have illustrated how such teams also operate in a wide variety of other settings including rehabilitation facilities, mental health centres, hospices, nursing homes and drug/alcohol treatment programmes. This means that a knowledge and understanding of group skills, processes and dynamics should form part of any CST programme.

Health professionals will engage in many different types of group and may have to employ differing skills in each group context – a process that is not always easy (Kreps, 1993). Group situations include a team carrying out surgery or other medical procedure, meeting a patient's family, interdisciplinary team meetings, participating in a management executive meeting, and teaching a small group of patients. In relation to the latter context, for example, Pugh (1995) has described a programme of group skills designed specifically for HIV-positive drug misusers. With regard to the management context, Garko (1992) highlighted how it is often the case that as doctors make the transition from clinician to manager they persist with ways of behaving akin to the clinical modality. That is, they function independently and autonomously from others and regard themselves as in ultimate authority, displaying a reluctance to engage in collaborative team management. This can be dysfunctional, since 'while clinical behaviours are critical for success in the practitioner role, they tend to create conflict, resistance, and tension in the managerial role' (Kurtz, 1988, p. 66). Thus, doctors and other health professionals will require training to effect a smooth transition from one role to another, including from practitioner to team manager.

6.5.1 Defining features of groups

The study of groups has been a major focus for research and analysis within the social sciences for many decades (Worchel, Wood and Simpson, 1993). The main reason for this is that groups are functional units for humans, in essence serving five main purposes:

- helping us to more readily achieve desired goals and fulfil specific needs;
- providing a source of identity;
- enabling us to engage with people we perceive to be similar to ourselves;
- offering a sense of belonging, worth and acceptance;
- affording a greater potential for influencing others (Hargie, 1994).

But what exactly is a group? While there is no one agreed definition of the term 'group', alternative conceptualizations tend to have a high degree of consensus. For example, Rubin (1984, pp. 16-17) defined a group as 'two or more people, existing in an arrangement that permits some degree of interaction, and sharing some sense of identity as members'. A similar, but extended, definition given by Johnson and Johnson (1987, p. 8) was 'two or more individuals in face-to-face interaction, each aware of his or her membership in the group, each aware of the others who belong to the group, and each aware of their positive interdependence as they strive to achieve mutual goals'. The defining features of a small group are therefore as follows.

- It involves at least two people who interact with and attempt to influence one another in face-to-face encounters. Usually, small groups comprise more than two but less than 20 members (Hargie, Saunders and Dickson, 1994).
- The members are interdependent.
- People define themselves, and are recognized by others, as part of the group.
- Common goals are pursued.
- Matters of mutual interest are dealt with through a system of interlocking roles.
- The group provides a source of rewards for the individual.

6.5.2 Advantages and disadvantages of groups

It has long been assumed that decisions made by groups are superior to those of the same number of individuals working alone. For example, Feldman (1985, p. 385), in his review of this area, asserted: 'Years of research have yielded a consistent pattern of findings showing that groups typically produce more, and produce better, solutions to problems than the same number of individuals working alone.' In a more recent review, however, Stroebe (1994, p. 4) contradicted this finding when he concluded that 'scientific evidence has consistently demonstrated that people produce many more ideas when they work alone rather than in groups'. He referred to what has been termed 'the illusion of group effectivity', which relates to the conviction in academic and business circles that group discussion is an effective technique for decision-making. He further argues that this is caused by the 'baseline fallacy', whereby more ideas are produced by a group than by any **one** individual member, but when individual totals are added this is higher than the group score. Brown (1988), however, pointed out that much research on groups has been conducted under artificial experimental conditions where people are brought together and asked to perform as a 'group'. He reviewed studies that indicate that when people are allowed to form an identity, or already have an established identity, they actually do work harder than the same number of individuals working alone. This would underscore the importance for health professionals of fostering each member's identity with any group for which they are responsible.

It may also be the case that people believe group decisions to be more effective because the group process itself is often enjoyable. Certainly, people report higher levels of satisfaction when working in groups than alone, and they also believe that the group has been more effective (Wilke and Meertens, 1994). This is important, since it means that members are more likely to be committed to what they see as a better decision – and one taken by a group of which they have been a part. If the idea came from one person working alone, then others are not likely to feel so committed to its implementation. Enjoyment and commitment are therefore two important advantages of groups. The sharing of ideas, feelings, fears or concerns is another positive feature of groups. In this way, people undergoing similar experiences (pregnant mothers, coronary patients, etc.) can be brought together to form a network of support for one another.

However, groups are not always effective, and it should be realized that there are merits and demerits attached to group work. As Harding, Taylor and Nettleton (1994) have shown, a range of factors can inhibit effective team work in the health context, including differences in the status, prestige and power of different health professionals. In general terms, 'groups can and do exert powerful influences on their members. These influences are often destructive, and must be understood and overcome in order to promote effective decision making' (Swap, 1984, p. 69).

Being watched by others can have a detrimental effect upon performance – a process known as 'social inhibition' or 'evaluation apprehension'. In particular, complex tasks or tasks that have not been fully mastered are more likely to suffer an impaired performance in the presence of observers. The negative effects of groups on the individual can include physiological reactions of increased heart rate, perspiration and feelings of nausea, together with impairments in intellectual performance and memory, as well as interactional problems such as prolonged silences, reduced ability to break such silences, less talk time, lack of eye contact and increased use of self-oriented gestures (Hargie and McCartan, 1986).

Interestingly, there are two sides to the group coin, since there is also what is termed the 'social facilitation' effect in groups which is 'the effect whereby a person will carry out a task with more zest . . . if there is even the mere presence of another person or group' (Blumberg, Davies and Kent, 1986, p. 273). In other words, groups can have a motivational effect upon the individual, increasing the level of arousal for performance. For example, athletes will tend to record their best performances in front of spectators in a stadium, rather than in practice sessions. In summary: 'Performing a task in the presence of others can under certain conditions create anxiety and apprehension and under different conditions inspire and energize' (Johnson and Johnson, 1987, p. 3). Health professionals therefore need to take steps to maximize the facilitating, while minimizing the inhibiting, effects of groups for which they have responsibility.

6.5.3 Factors affecting groupwork

Groups operate at three related levels: that of the **task** to be performed, the **procedures** required to perform this task effectively and the **interpersonal** relationships associated with operating as a team. A number of factors impinge upon the performance of groups at these levels, including the following.

Size

As the number of people in the group increases, so too does the number of potential relationships. For example, in a group of three there are six, increasing in a group of seven to 966 possible relationships (Napier and Gershenfeld, 1993). As a result, increases in group size tend to result in decreased individual satisfaction with the group, fewer people participate, a greater number of members will say nothing (this is known as 'the anonymity phenomenon'), the affectional ties of members decrease and one person is more likely to emerge as a dominant leader, since more directive control is required. In general it has been found that in discussion groups 'above the size of five, members complain that a group is too large' (Napier and Gershenfeld, 1993, p. 39).

Participation levels

Those who participate most tend to be extroverts, people with most information about the topic of discussion, those with high status, including designated leaders, or those located in a central physical position in the group (Tubbs, 1995). Often these factors are related, in that an extrovert is more likely to attempt to become leader and try to secure a central dominating position in the group. Another dimension of participation is that high contributors tend to direct their remarks to the entire group, whereas low contributors direct most of their comments to one other person. Not surprisingly, those who initiate most contributions also receive most from other members. One implication here is that if health professionals wish to be noticed in discussion groups, they should speak frequently and address their remarks to the entire group.

Physical layout

The shape of the group will affect participation levels. For example, members are more likely to participate in groups with circular or horseshoe-type layouts than where one person faces the rest of the members in traditional classroom-style rows.

Group structure

This refers to the interdependent relationship between roles and status. Roles allow for a division of labour and bring order to the group task as well as facilitating self-definition within the group. However, studies of interprofessional communication have shown that health professionals often hold conflicting views of what the roles of other professions in the health care team are, or should be (Skipper, 1992; Harding, Taylor and Nettleton, 1994). This obviously creates problems in team working and such conflict in role expectations has been shown to be detrimental to group functioning (Wilke and Meertens, 1994). Indeed, although Skipper (1992) found that all professions in her hospital study emphasized the need for a team approach, 'the understanding of what constituted a team varied considerably' (p. 574). As a result, she recommended that training in team work be implemented to ensure optimum functioning. Part of the problem is that the development of effective interdisciplinary teams necessitates a move away from an emphasis on individual professions towards a patient-focused approach (Diller, 1990). This raises the threat of possible loss of status by some professions. Status, in this sense, implies the consensual prestige of other members and allows those of higher status a greater opportunity to initiate ideas and activities, and influence and control other members (Brown, 1988). Groups where roles and status differentials are clearly delineated and accepted will function more smoothly.

Norms

People in groups like to know what is expected of them, and norms, which are 'rules of conduct established by the members of the group to maintain behavioral consistency' (Shaw, 1976, p. 250), serve to fulfil this function. Such rules, which are usually unspoken, serve to increase the regularity and predictability of behaviour, help to prevent conflicts and establish parameters for power and influence. It is particularly important for new members to learn what the group norms are, so that they can rapidly and painlessly become accepted by the rest of the group. At the same time, the dangers of 'groupthink', where the norms are that conformity is expected, that the leader's opinion should not be challenged and that dissent is frowned upon, need to be avoided (Wilke and Meertens, 1994). The result of groupthink is that minority opinions are not heard and so any decisions made are not fully evaluated, with possibly disastrous consequences. In groups it is useful to appoint at least one person to specifically formulate reasons to challenge each decision taken, so that the full implications are considered. To avoid groupthink, leaders should also be trained to actively seek dissenting views during meetings.

Communication networks

In a study of interdisciplinary team functioning, Butterill, O'Hanlon and Book (1992) illustrated how the group process can be facilitated or hindered by the organizational structure. In many organizations there is a formal hierarchical communication network, whereby A can only talk to C by going through B. The contrast is where people are allowed to communicate freely and easily with others at all levels. The former type of communication network is referred to as centralized and involves a great deal of leader control, while the latter is decentralized and relies more upon member cooperation. Research suggests that 'while more centrally organized groups tend to be more productive and efficient (especially when dealing with simple problems), members frequently manifest low morale and express little satisfaction with group activities' (Hargie, Saunders and Dickson, 1994, p. 303). One solution to this dilemma of increased productivity but decreased satisfaction in centralized networks is to introduce participative decision making (PDM) within the organization, wherein decisions are made by the relevant group members. PDM seems to work best when:

- it is important for the organization that all members accept the decision and facilitate its implementation;
- the decision is seen to be of relevance to all members;
- those in the group have sufficient expertise and information to contribute meaningfully (Wilke and Meertens, 1994).

However, PDM also requires that group leaders have skills in conflict resolution and mediation, and this usually requires training. Furthermore, subordinates may enter the process believing they will have a great deal of influence and rapidly become demotivated if their views fail to hold sway. It is also important that any decisions made as a result of PDM are implemented, otherwise the process will be regarded as a sham veneer of democracy. An extension of PDM is the use of self-managing teams (SMT), where groups of between 10 or 15 people are given total responsibility for their area of work within an organization. These SMTs then make all of the decisions, coordinate their tasks, and manage their own budgets. This gives increased responsibility and power to these small SMTs, and as a result there is high member identification and productivity (Barker and Tompkins, 1994).

The main problems facing interdisciplinary health teams have been summarized as falling into three categories (Cooley, 1994). The first is **disorganization**, where the group's procedures, objectives and decisions are unclear; secondly, **miscommunication**, where diverse professionals speak in their own 'jargonese', hold misconceptions about the roles of others and see things from their own particular perspectives; finally, **inadequate problem solving**, where decisions are taken in a haphazard fashion, discussion lacks structure and members do not all participate equally in the process. In order to overcome these problems, Cooley carried out a CST programme specifically designed to improve the group skills of 25 staff members (from a variety of disciplines including medicine, physiotherapy, social work, occupational therapy, psychology) in a rehabilitation clinic specializing in chronic pain treatment. The skills covered included listening, paraphrasing, probing, summarizing, giving examples, closing, consensus testing and problem solving. Results from the training were very positive in terms of increases in staff skills and receptivity to the programme.

6.5.4 Leadership

An important distinction needs to be made between the terms 'leader' and 'leadership'. In analysing this distinction, Gulley (1968, p. 171) regarded leadership as a process of 'influencing others within a particular situation and social context in a way that induces them to follow, to be modified, to be directed'. Similarly, and after reviewing various definitions, Bryman (1986, p. 2) defined leadership as: 'a social influence process in which a person steers members of the group towards a goal'. Bryman further viewed leadership as the display of the skills of controlling, directing and influencing other group members, through 'enhancing their voluntary compliance . . . [which] . . . relates to the leader's ability to motivate, an ingredient which is often taken as the *sine qua non* of leadership' (p. 3).

A leader is someone who has either been designated as such, or has clearly emerged as the person displaying most leadership during group discussion. Thus, a designated leader will be expected to display leadership skills. For example, the chief executive (CE) in a health organization would be the designated leader at senior management team meetings and be expected to initiate, direct, control and terminate the discussion. Indeed, other members will ascribe this role to the CE and will, in turn, play the role of subordinates. In contexts where there is no designated leader, one person will tend to 'emerge' as leader, and the longer the discussion time or larger the group the more likely it is that this will occur. For example, studies of juries have shown that leaders do emerge (and that these are usually people with power or status in the outside world), some people try to become leader but fail, some fit passively into the group structure, while others withdraw or become isolates (Napier and Gershenfeld, 1993). One thing is clear – leaders are expected by group members to have good leadership skills and if they do not, then dissatisfaction will increase and the group will not function smoothly. For this reason, in the current health environment, Schneider and Tucker (1992, p. 19) emphasized that 'doctors need to develop democratic leadership skills: listening, empathy, team decision making, and delegation of responsibility'.

In their analysis of leadership, Hargie, Saunders and Dickson (1994) identified six core skills. Most of these skills can be employed at various times by any group member, but all will be expected from the leader. The first four of these are concerned with the completion of the group task and the final two with the maintenance of group cohesiveness.

Initiating/focusing

This involves opening the discussion at the outset, making any necessary introductions and outlining what is to be discussed and why. It also includes introducing new topics at appropriate moments, as well as allocating time limits for discussion.

Clarifying/elaborating

The purpose here is to ensure that everyone understands points being made during discussion. This may involve paraphrasing or summarizing contributions – especially where these have been lengthy or convoluted, asking probing questions to encourage members to elaborate on points made or providing relevant information or examples to clarify specific issues. The leader should also ensure that members keep to the topic under discussion and disallow the pursuit of irrelevant issues.

Promoting contributions

Yank, Barber and Spradlin (1994), in their analysis of mental health treatment teams, highlight this as one of the important functions of the leader. The two extremes of the participation continuum range from those who attempt to hog the discussion at one end to those who say nothing at the other. Since low participators often have very valuable ideas it is important that these be heard, and since satisfaction levels will decrease if one or two vocal members do all of the talking, the leader must promote a balanced discussion. Whittington (1986, p. 300) aptly summarized her advice to group leaders in the phrase: 'Bring in non-participants and shut out monopolizers'. This action, of course, should be executed in a sensitive fashion, through the use of phrases such as 'I want now to hear what each person thinks of this. . .'; 'OK, Peter, you have expressed your views very clearly, but I am now going to open the discussion to bring in other points of view. . .'. It may be necessary to 'protect' more introverted members by allowing them time to express their views while keeping the more vociferous individuals silent. The leader should also ensure that the physical layout is conducive to participation by all members, stop members interrupting one another and intervene where more than one person is speaking.

Summarizing

In long discussions, transitional reviews are useful to remind the group what the key issues raised, or decisions taken, have been. At the end of discussion, the leader will then be expected to give a summary of the main points covered, decisions taken and what will happen next. In fact, the relationship between being group leader and summarizing is so strong that if another member attempts to give the final summary this will be seen as a personal challenge to the authority of the leader (Hargie, Saunders and Dickson, 1994).

Relieving tension

When group members become embroiled in heated arguments, it is necessary to defuse the hostility or tension which has built up. Here mediation is needed, with the leader emphasizing the strengths of the views of both sides, highlighting areas of agreement, underlining the need for compromise and focusing discussion upon substantive issues and away from personality clashes. Tension can also be relieved through the use of humour, which 'provides a smooth and acceptable means of changing the level or direction of a conversation. . . . It also helps to indicate to others that they are taking things too seriously and need to look at their problems from a more detached or balanced perspective' (Foot, 1986, p. 362). Indeed, in many groups one person, other than the leader, may play the role of joker or 'social leader' – a very useful function in maintaining group cohesiveness.

Supporting/encouraging

When group members make useful contributions, these should be rewarded and supported by the leader. This will, in turn, encourage them to make further meaningful inputs. The leader is a potent source of reward power for group members, who are more likely to value reinforcement from this source than from other members (Dickson, Saunders and Stringer, 1993).

6.5.5 Making groups effective

There are clear differences, on a number of key features, between effective and ineffective groups (Johnson and Johnson, 1987). In effective groups:

- goals are agreed and pursued by all members;
- communication is open and free-flowing;
- leadership is shared;
- ability and information determine influence and power;
- consensus is sought for important decisions;
- disagreement is seen as a positive indicator of commitment;
- cohesion is encouraged through high levels of inclusion, acceptance, affection, support and trust;

- members evaluate group performance and how it could be improved.

By contrast, in ineffective groups:

- goals are either not fully clarified or are imposed;
- communication is mainly one-way;
- members' feelings are ignored or suppressed;
- leadership is based upon status and position;
- participation levels are unequal;
- high-status members dominate and make the decisions;
- disagreements are regarded as unhelpful;
- members are controlled by force/threat;
- conformity is promoted;
- only the highest-authority members evaluate the group's effectiveness.

Groups can therefore be functional or dysfunctional work units. Health professionals therefore need to learn how to organize, participate in and lead effective group work. Exercise 6.1 can be employed to study many of the key features of group discussion.

Exercise 6.1 Group decision-making

Aim

To provide an arena for the study of influencing and negotiating skills in a group context. Although this exercise is written for community pharmacists, it can be applied, *mutatis mutandis*, to any health-professional group.

Materials

Duplicate copies of steps 1, 2 and 3 for all trainees.

Instructions

Distribute step 1 and have each trainee complete this individually. Allow 10 minutes for this part of the exercise. There should be no discussion during this step. Now distribute step 2 sheets to everyone, and then divide the class into sub-groups of no less than five and no more than eight members. Ideally each subgroup should then be located in a separate room with video-recording facilities, although the exercise can also be conducted in a large room in which sub-groups are dispersed. Each subgroup is then instructed to complete step 2 and given a time limit (this can be a minimum of 40 minutes or maximum of 1 hour). The discussions should either be video recorded or an observer should be attached to each group.

Discussion

At the end of step 2, bring the class together and compute the step 3 scores. The difference between the OR (own ranking) and GR (group ranking) scores is a measure of how much individuals have been influenced by the group to change their original decisions – the higher the difference in score the more they have been swayed. Good negotiators will tend to have lower difference scores. Once these scores have been computed, each subgroup should review the video recording of the discussion (or discuss this with the observer) in the light of the difference scores. Who had the lowest/highest scores? What influencing and negotiating skills and strategies did these individuals employ in the discussion? Did a leader emerge and if so how? Were the objectives of the group clarified at the outset? Was the group an example of PDM in action? How could the discussion have been improved? The practical should end with the entire class coming together to discuss the main themes emerging from the exercise.

Qualities of an effective community pharmacist

Step 1. Name:

Instructions

Below are listed 15 factors related to the effectiveness of a community pharmacist. Your task is to evaluate each, in terms of their importance. Place the number 1 by the most important factor, the number 2 by the second most important factor, and so on through to number 15, the least important factor. Think carefully about your reasons for these rankings, since you will have to present these reasons in the next step of this exercise, when you will have to come to a group consensus about the rankings. At this stage, however, you should complete the column marked 'OR' individually.

	OR
Physical appearance	
Flexibility when dealing with people	
Good powers of interpersonal communication	
Enthusiasm	
Physical fitness	
In-depth knowledge of products	
Ability to make decisions quickly	
Ability to be persuasive	
Social sensitivity	
Willingness to work long hours	
Personal motivation to be successful	

Ability to sustain relationships	
Creative thinker	
Good self-awareness	
Good organizer	

Qualities of an effective community pharmacist

Step 2. Name:
Instructions
Now that each individual in your group has rank-ordered the 15 individual factors your next step is to reach a group consensus about the ordering. This means that the prediction for each of the 15 individual factors **must** be agreed upon by each member before it becomes part of the group decision. Consensus is difficult to reach, so not every ranking will meet with everyone's complete approval. Try, as a group, to make each ranking one with which all group members can at least partially agree. Write each member's rankings in the columns under the numbers, and then as a group agree a Group Ranking (GR) for all factors with number 1 again being the most important factor, through to number 15, the least important factor.

	1	*2*	*3*	*4*	*5*	*6*	*7*	*8*	*GR*
Physical appearance									
Flexibility in dealing with people									
Good powers of interpersonal communication									
Enthusiasm									
Physical fitness									
In-depth knowledge of products									
Ability to make decisions quickly									
Ability to be persuasive									
Social sensitivity									
Willingness to work long hours									
Personal motivation to be successful									
Ability to sustain relationships									
Creative thinker									
Good self-awareness									
Good organizer									

Qualities of an effective community pharmacist

Step 3. Name:
Instructions
In order to ascertain the difference between your own ranking (OR) and the group ranking (GR), enter your ranks for each of these below. To get the Change Score for each item simply subtract the lower score from the higher score in each case. Then sum all the Change Scores to get the Total Change Score.

	OR	*GR*	*Change*
Physical appearance			
Flexibility in dealing with people			
Good powers of interpersonal communication			
Enthusiasm			
Physical fitness			
In-depth knowledge of products			
Ability to make decisions quickly			
Ability to be persuasive			
Social sensitivity			
Willingness to work long hours			
Personal motivation to be successful			
Ability to sustain relationships			
Creative thinker			
Good self-awareness			
Good organizer			

Total Change Score:

6.6 OVERVIEW

This chapter has been concerned with four dyadic and small-group strategies central to the role of health professionals – counselling, influencing, interviewing and working in groups. As with the skills covered in Chapters 4 and 5, the purpose of this chapter has been to offer a summative analysis of each strategy, and the trainer is recommended to pursue some of the references used for further information on these areas. When taken together, these three chapters provide an overview of the central skills and strategies employed by practitioners in various contexts of practice. A knowledge of the material covered in these chapters will facilitate an understanding of the overall process of CST as detailed in the remaining chapters.

PART THREE

The Process of Communication Skills Training

In Part Three we turn our attention from matters of content *per se* to systematically examine the CST process. As presented in Figure I.1, the three main stages in the instructional sequence which are essential to the effective implementation of programmes of this type are **preparation**, **training** and **evaluation**.

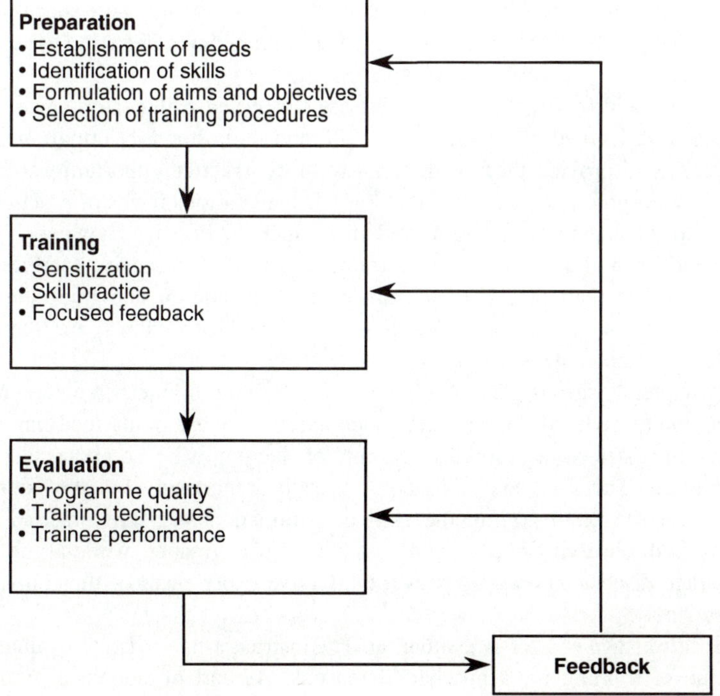

Figure I.1 A sequential analysis of CST.

At the initial preparatory stage it is necessary to identify those communication skills deemed most suitable to meet the needs of the particular group of trainees. With groups undergoing basic-level training, these will probably be the core skills outlined in the previous section. When CST forms part of continuing education and is designed to provide instruction of a more specialized nature (e.g. communicating with the elderly), then more refined skills may be required. In either case, it is important for the instructor to be familiar with the general approaches and specific techniques that can be used to uncover the essential skill content prior to commencing CST. These issues of skill identification are dealt with in Chapter 7.

The second major stage of CST is the implementation of the training programme. Here there are four main steps involved. It will be recalled from Chapter 1 that, in terms of communication competence, a distinction can be made between knowledge of communication ('knowing that'), ability to use it ('knowing how') and actually doing it (performance). This distinction is reflected in these four training steps. The first, **skill analysis**, involves introducing trainees to each of the skills, in turn, through the use of lectures, guided reading, etc., thereby providing background knowledge regarding components of skills and their effects during various contexts of practice. In other words, it is concerned largely with ensuring that trainees 'know that'. The second step, **skill discrimination**, has to do with illustrating the skills in operation through the use of model videotapes or other forms of demonstration, and is necessary to provide trainees with knowledge about 'how' to use the skill successfully. The overall process of skill analysis and discrimination is referred to as 'sensitization' and is fully described in Chapter 8.

The third and fourth steps of training are concerned with performance. Once trainees have learned to identify each skill, and understood its importance, the next step is to provide them with some form of **practice** opportunity to allow them to attempt to operationalize that knowledge. Various forms of practice can be employed and these are reviewed in Chapter 9. Practice, however, is not sufficient for skill acquisition, since trainees also need to receive **feedback** on the efficacy of their responses to enable them to monitor and fine-tune their performance. A range of feedback methods and procedures are therefore detailed in Chapter 10.

In Chapter 1 various general approaches to training in interpersonal communication were outlined. In particular, such approaches can be divided into those which emphasize either 'thinking', 'doing' or 'feeling'. CST combines elements of all three. The skill analysis step is broadly concerned with the cognitive component of skill learning, the skill discrimination and skill practice steps involve both observing and carrying out skilled performance, while at the feedback stage discussion encompasses the affective experiences of those involved in practicals.

The third stage of CST is evaluation. The instructor may wish to evaluate the outcome of training for a number of reasons. As part of student assessment, decisions may be arrived at as to competency to progress in the course, or ultimately to practise. Here, two types of procedure can be considered. Firstly, trainees can be assessed by direct, observational methods, perhaps dealing with patients in either real or simulated practice situations. Secondly, indirect methods can be implemented such as the use of questionnaires, written tests, essays or analyses of simulated consultations. The advantages and disadvantages of such options are discussed in Chapter 11.

Evaluation exercises are sometimes conducted with the intention of reaching decisions not about those who have undergone training but about the programme itself. The overall quality of instruction can be assessed or the contribution of particular elements subjected to a more analytical scrutiny. Such feedback may take the form of formal or informal comments from trainees either immediately following CST or after a period of fieldwork at which juncture judgements about the relevance of the CST programme may more easily be made – especially in courses for pre-service trainees. Feedback can also be gauged from observation of trainees during interactions with patients, either by college tutors or fieldwork supervisors. By obtaining feedback from various sources, refinements to the CST programme are possible in order to strengthen its potential.

Identifying communication skills

7

7.1 INTRODUCTION

The first phase of the CST process has to do with preparatory matters. This chapter addresses a key aspect of such preparation, i.e. identifying the most appropriate skill content to meet the needs of the particular group involved in training. Other wider issues of programme planning and design which must also be resolved as part of preparation will be taken up in Chapter 12.

The quality of practitioner–patient communication is fundamental to effective health care and the level of communicative ability of the practitioner can either help or hinder it. But what constitutes successful interpersonal communication? What distinguishes good performance from poor performance? How can skilled performance be recognized and analysed so that training programmes can be instituted to develop interpersonal competence? What are the elements of the interpersonal process which, when integrated, form a co-ordinated whole and result in the goals of each party being achieved? What are the interpersonal skills required by health-care personnel? What are the main skill deficits within different professional groups? Are there specific situations that require special skills?

This chapter is devoted to considering some of these issues and in particular to describing ways in which trainers can begin to identify key communication skills within their own professional domain and, as a result, design and implement appropriate training. The approach used will essentially be practical, thereby encouraging readers to reflect on, observe and undertake more extensive investigation of their own practice fields in order to establish a valid and clear picture of effective professional communication.

7.2 ESTABLISHING NEEDS

Producing a cogent learning experience can be thought of as representing a sequence of distinct stages. While there are variants on the basic theme, according to Cork (1987) most programme planning begins with what students need to learn. From this the aims and objectives of training are derived. Agreement on these matters enables the content and process of instruction to be selected. Relevant learning experiences are then contemplated and finally methods of evaluation are affirmed.

It is, however, important to point out that embedded in the above process are in fact two cycles, the training cycle and the learning cycle. The training cycle takes as its starting point needs identification and then rotates through the phases of planning, implementation and evaluation. The learning cycle moves from concrete experience to reflecting upon the experience and from that drawing conclusions which can subsequently be applied and tested in new situations. The following definition of training by Buckley and Caple (1990) links the two together: 'a planned and systematic effort to modify or develop knowledge/skill/attitude through learning experience to achieve effective performance in an activity or range of activities' (p. 13).

Three aspects of the definition are worth emphasizing: firstly, the systematic character of the process, which provides a counter to the all too frequently *ad hoc* nature of training; secondly, the provision of learning experiences implies variety and exposure to real or simulated situations; thirdly, the most valued outcome is effective performance, the emphasis being on the practical, real-time benefits for the consumer.

Clearly, the quest to identify the communicative content of training must begin with the recognition of a need for change. Present levels of knowledge may be regarded as inadequate, existing abilities deficient or current skills outmoded and incapable of meeting the demands now being placed upon the practitioner, or anticipated in the future. This is strongly endorsed by Ross, Bower and Sibbald (1994) in their analysis of the workload and training needs of practice nurses. Similarly, in a questionnaire survey of the communication skills training required at the continuing education level, Lubbers and Roy (1990) report that nurses want ongoing training in the following areas, ranked in order: listening, relationship building, instructing, motivating, exchanging routine information and giving feedback.

It is the realization of such states of affairs that produces the impetus for, and gives direction to, change through instruction. But the concept of 'need', even from a curriculum design perspective, is by no means simple and unproblematic. On the contrary, it has produced considerable debate among educationalists. This has partly stemmed from imprecision in common usage, which neglects subtle semantic distinctions between it and similar concepts such as 'wants' and 'interests' (Jarvis, 1983).

'Need', in terms of learning may be thought of as a deficiency that can be remedied by the help of some educational process. Often the recognition of this deficit emerges from practitioners themselves because they feel themselves to be poorly equipped to adequately provide the levels of care called for. This could be due to skills, which have atrophied through lack of use, now being required, or the introduction of innovative techniques and therapeutic procedures necessitating new practices. Alternatively, the practitioner's role may have changed, again making the acquisition of novel skills necessary.

If, however, total reliance was placed upon needs felt and expressed by learners as the sole criterion for instituting educational interventions, many who could benefit from such provision would be denied it. Some practitioners can be completely oblivious to their shortcomings. Learning needs are frequently defined by others including, for instance, administrators, professional bodies, educationalists and senior staff. Indeed, Armstrong (1982) has drawn attention to the fact that they are often 'imposed' from above in this way by postulating an ideological dimension. Nevertheless, and regardless of how they are arrived at, learning needs must be accounted for in the aims and objectives of the training intervention.

Against this background it is wise to 'stand back' and try to obtain a more objective view of any particular situation. The following questions are useful in an attempt to gain a broad view of existing needs or potential needs facing any health-care professional group.

- What have been the findings of national reviews (e.g. the Audit Commission)?
- What are the emerging trends in practice?
- What do the findings of current research programmes suggest?
- What is Government policy for the service?
- What does the legislation require?
- What new technologies are impacting on the service?
- What do consumer reports indicate?
- What are the deficiencies or gaps in the service? – gaps in What? Who? How? When? Where? Which? and Why?

A further characteristic of 'needs' is that ultimately they reflect the uniqueness of the individual. It is highly unlikely that the requirements of any two learners will coincide entirely. The instructional implications are obvious. In this regard, Ellis and Whittington (1981) distinguished between clinical and curriculum approaches to skill identification and training. The former enables a tailor-made skills sequence to be derived from a focused assessment of the areas of strength and weakness of the individual trainee. 'In contrast, [the curriculum approach] produces an off-the-peg predetermined list thought appropriate for an entire group of trainees' (Ellis and Whittington, 1981, p.49). The rationale here is, presumably, that if a general deficit has been identified amongst a particular professional group, and this subgroup belongs to that profession, then this subgroup is likely to share the deficiency and could consequently benefit from appropriate training.

CST programmes for health-care personnel are typically based on the curriculum approach although within the training process there is sufficient flexibility to cater, to some extent, for individual idiosyncrasies. It is therefore unusual for an individual assessment of each prospective trainee to be conducted, for entry into the programme to be determined on this basis, or for training to operate on a one-to-one basis. Rather CST is typically undertaken by a cohort of students in the same way as all other elements that are likely to constitute their course of study.

7.3 FORMULATING AIMS AND OBJECTIVES

Establishing learning needs is a prerequisite for deciding upon the broad aims and objectives of training. This in turn facilitates the subsequent task of arriving at the most appropriate skills to form the substantive content of the programme.

Aims are general statements of intention and purpose characteristically expressed in abstract terms (Jarvis and Gibson, 1985). With regard to CST, they should relate to the defining features of communication competence presented in Chapter 1 (e.g. to promote relevant knowledge of, for instance, self, others, situations and/or interactive processes and techniques; to increase the ability to put such knowledge to use, and ultimately to improve communicative performance).

Objectives are more refined operational statements of the manner in which the preordained aims will be met. Their importance for training activities cannot be over-emphasized. They guide the learning, act as a means of structuring the event which is to be organized but also, and more importantly, provide the basis for evaluating the success of an event. They do this simply by linking the training to the prior needs analysis, ensuring appropriate selection of content and methodology. At the same time they provide participants with accessible targets and encourage motivation. In this regard they are better written as learner-oriented statements, as opposed to teaching-oriented statements. Thus, learning objectives can be seen as expressions of what a participant will know, understand or be able to do as a result of attending a course or event.

Focused more clearly, objectives seek to specify the performance that trainees must emulate in order to demonstrate that mastery has been obtained and the need met. Performance objectives consist of:

- the behaviour to be displayed, (e.g. trainees will be able to **demonstrate**. . .);
- the content of the task, i.e. the subject or object to which the behaviour refers (e.g. inhaler technique).

Furthermore, objectives fall into three main categories:

- those that depend upon assimilating new knowledge;
- those that embrace new behaviour;
- those that may note an attitudinal/affective change.

Taking each of these in turn and linking them to a hypothetical course on 'Communication Skills', we could say that:

- **knowledge objectives** are those based upon the participant's understanding, recalling or embracing new information or being able to problem solve on the basis of newly acquired information (e.g. 'By the end of this course participants will be able to list all the elements that make up a simple model of interpersonal communication');

- **behavioural objectives** are based upon the capacity of the participants to do something they could not do before (e.g. 'By the end of this course participants will be able to demonstrate the skill of active listening in a simulated patient consultation');
- **attitudinal/affective objectives** suggest ways in which a participant will change in disposition towards an important aspect of the course (e.g. 'By the end of this course participants will value the importance of interpersonal skills to competent practice').

Related to a specific aspect of communication, Smith (1986) set out a list of competencies which the effective listener should be capable of demonstrating. From these a set of learning objectives relevant to the skill of listening, and at this level of specificity, can be deduced (Table 7.1).

Table 7.1 Specific objectives of training in listening (Source: based on Smith, 1986)

At the end of the training programme, the group should be able to:

- Attend with an open mind
- Recognize main ideas
- Perceive the speaker's purpose and organization of ideas and information
- Recall basic ideas and details accurately
- Discriminate between statements of fact and statements of opinion
- Distinguish between emotional and logical arguments
- Detect bias and prejudice
- Recognize the speaker's attitude
- Synthesize and evaluate by drawing logical inferences and conclusions
- Recognize discrepancies between the speaker's verbal and non-verbal messages
- Employ active listening techniques appropriately.

Such precision may be impossible however, under circumstances where it is by no means certain, at the onset, how best to achieve general objectives. In some specialized interactive contexts, for instance, little may be known initially as to how appropriate communication is effected at the practitioner–patient interface. Greater precision may have to await the identification of the skills content of training (Miles, 1987). It is to this that we now turn.

7.4 TOWARDS IDENTIFYING COMMUNICATION SKILLS

Clearly any attempt at determining social adequacy must be firmly grounded in the conceptual analysis of skilled communication outlined in Chapter 1 and extended in Chapter 3. A number of features were illuminated that have special significance for the task of identifying skills and which, therefore, merit further consideration at this juncture.

7.4.1 Content and consequences

Content refers to those observable aspects of behaviour which are believed to contribute to effective communication. They may be verbal or non-verbal but it is a somewhat arbitrary decision whether they are significant components of skilled performance. Thus, on its own, the content approach to analysing performance is limited. The consequences approach, in contrast, stresses the reactions to the behaviour by others. Here the emphasis is on eliciting positive reinforcement such that behaviour that produces such reactions is considered socially skilled. However, this perspective on its own is also inadequate in that a nurse taking a principled, but unpopular, stand on a moral issue in contrast to peers would be considered to be socially unskilled when in fact that would not necessarily be the case. It is therefore important to take both content and consequences into account in defining skill. As Arkowitz (1981) pointed out, 'at a clinical level it is important to assess both what people do and the reactions which their behaviour elicits from others' (p. 300).

This particular issue is well illustrated by reference to the work of Schneider and Tucker (1992). These workers attempted to develop an instrument to relate personal communication and patient satisfaction. In its final form it comprised a series of statements under four identified communication headings: relationship maintenance, professional competence, waiting time and social etiquette. Examination of individual statements not only indicated large differences in the interpersonal aspects of the communication and indeed the skills components, but the emphasis on consequences. This is highlighted in the following four statements taken respectively from each of the above categories.

- 'I feel better when doctors explain medical terminology.'
- 'I like doctors who are organized and familiar with my case.'
- 'I get irritated if I have to wait a long time to see the doctor.'
- 'It is important for doctors to dress professionally.'

Street (1992) has further argued for the use of coding and analytical schemes that examine responsiveness and adaptation in the course of a consultation. What he proposed is the use of indices of 'dyadic exchange' which can be created by computing some features of the patient's behaviour relative to that of the practitioner, or identifying co-existent behaviours (i.e. types of patient responses that tend to co-occur with certain practitioner behaviours).

7.4.2 Single and sequenced behaviour

Discussion of the components of social situations prompts the question: in the analysis of social performance, should actions be assessed in terms of frequency of single elements of behaviour or as coordinated behavioural sequences? Similarly, how appropriate was the action within the actual context of the interaction? Measurement of the frequency of specific actions may lead to a misleading appreciation of a social encounter. Using a simple frequency criterion, an individual may be considered socially skilled because of the ability to initiate a large number of questions in rapid succession, yet the flow and expression of the questions within the context of the interaction may have produced a feeling of interrogation in the other person.

Arkowitz (1981) also pointed out that in measuring social skill, frequency counts of behaviour imply that it is better to have more of a 'good' behaviour (e.g. eye contact) and less of a 'bad' behaviour (e.g. speech disfluency). Yet an individual in any encounter who stared continually but spoke fluently may be considered less skilful than another person who gave less eye contact and an average amount of speech disruption. Thus, in identifying skilled behaviour there may well be a balance to be struck in assessing particular aspects of performance in that there may be optimal levels of certain behaviours in particular situations which simple analysis of frequency counts does not take into consideration.

Consideration of frequency counts of behaviour raises the issue of time. If time were not a constraint, how different, if at all, would be both practitioner and patient behaviours? Thus any analysis of skill must take account of the factors that impose constraints, or indeed particular freedoms on the consultation. Equally, what skills must be used to make the most effective use of the time available? Even so, patient satisfaction levels may still be disappointing, despite the efficiency of a consultation, because patients want more time with their doctors (Buetow, 1995).

With regard to the sequencing of behaviour it will be recalled that Argyle, Furnham and Graham (1981) suggested that social encounters usually follow a five-episode behavioural sequence structure:

1. Greeting
2. Establishing the relationship and clarifying goals
3. The task
4. Re-establishing the relationship
5. Parting.

In their analysis of 2500 doctor–patient consultations, Byrne and Long (1976) presented a six-episode behavioural sequence to characterize the consultation as follows:

1. Relating to the patient
2. Discussing the reason for the patient's attendance
3. Conducting a verbal or physical examination or both
4. Considering the patient's condition
5. Detailing treatment or further investigation
6. Terminating.

Such a sequence may not, of course, always follow all of these steps in a fixed or set order. For example, the reason for the patient's attendance at surgery may be a follow-up to a previous visit such that part of the consultation is implicitly known by both parties. However, the classification of behaviours into a progressive sequence is not only important but instructive in demonstrating how effective social interactions can be viewed as a series of appropriate, integrated and co-ordinated verbal and non-verbal actions, intelligently carried out, with the purpose of achieving particular goals.

7.4.3 Skills and situations

In any analysis of social skills it is important to consider the social context in which behaviour occurs, as outlined in Chapter 3. That social situations exist as regular events in society is due to the fact that they allow common needs to be met. The rules, roles, repertoire of elements and other features of situations are functional in this sense. For example Argyle, Furnham and Graham (1981) suggested that the repertoire of elements in social situations is composed of four main units: verbal categories, verbal contents, non-verbal communication and bodily actions. Thus questioning as a behaviour would be considered as a verbal category or as a content free utterance whereas the question 'How has this medicine been affecting you?' could be described in content terms.

Viewed from the patient's perspective, Beisecker (1990), for example, has summarized the range of situational factors important to patient assertive behaviour during the medical consultation (Table 7.2).

Table 7.2 Important situational factors affecting patient assertive behaviour during the medical consultation (Source: after Beisecker, 1990)

- Types of illness
- Reason for visit
- Home versus office visit
- Length of interaction
- Presence of a companion
- First versus repeat visit
- Physical
- Particular doctor
- Doctor behaviour

She also argued that the research evidence into the sociodemographic factors that affect patient power in the medical encounter suggests that high-status patients (i.e. those with high income, greater education and gender, and cultural congruence with their physicians) tend to ask more questions and receive a greater amount of information from doctors. However, Beisecker and Beisecker (1990) have indicated that patient assertive communication and information-seeking behaviour was better explained by situational than by sociodemographic factors, patient attitudes or the effects of different doctors. The most important explanatory variables were diagnosis, reason for visit, presence of a companion, first versus repeat visit and the length of the interaction.

Thus the characterization of the components of situations is an important aspect of the identification of social skill in the health-care context. Moreover, it means that generalizations will tend to be avoided, recognizing that individuals may be skilled in some situations but not in others. Consequently, communication skill trainers must be specific in their diagnosis of skill deficit, allied to the specification of which skill in which situation is most in need of training (Furnham, 1983b).

7.4.4 Skills and strategies

Reference has been made in Chapter 1 to the defining features of communication skill. However, it is important to point out that published research into skill identification adopts what may be termed both macro- and micro-descriptors of communication behaviour.

In a recent review of interpersonal communication between nurses and patients, Garvin and Kennedy (1990) grouped communication behaviour under four main headings: empathy, self-disclosure, support and confirmation, with, particularly for the latter two, several subskills being delineated. This means that the levels at which skill is categorized are very variable. As pointed out in the preceding section, in any analysis of social interaction it is important to think in terms of skills and strategies, the latter describing the integrated organization or categorization of specific, more discrete skill elements.

7.4.5 Overt and covert behaviours

In the examination of communication skill the focus of attention has tended to be on behaviours that are openly displayed. If the exclusive emphasis is placed on behavioural output, however, there may be a consequent neglect of the perceptual and cognitive processes involved. As described in the model of communication (Chapter 3) our cognitions and perceptions of social situations are crucially important, since behaviour is influenced by our knowledge of social norms, knowledge and understanding of response cues, attention within any interaction and ability to process information, and predict and evaluate the consequences of particular types of behaviour.

Against this background it is therefore possible to classify unskilled behaviour as due to a genuine behavioural deficit, misperception, perceptual bias or a lack of knowledge of the situation. Indeed, someone who cannot 'read' a situation accurately will not be able to perform skilfully regardless of their behavioural repertoire. Thus, in analysing practitioner–patient interactions, it may well be valuable to try to identify why particular behaviours occur in order to ascertain the specific cognitive or perceptual processes which mediate them. Equally it may be important to examine with trainees particular mental frameworks that are likely to produce inappropriate behaviours (Exercise 7.2). As Kagan, Evans and Kay (1986) stated: 'It is important for us to bear in mind some of the sources of bias in person perception, and what our own tendencies to be consistent and/or to generalize are, if we are to begin to be able to make realistic observations, assessments and appraisals of our own interpersonal behaviour' (p. 81).

Exercise 7.1 Person perception

Instructions

Show a picture of an individual to a group of trainees. Then ask the following questions and compare the responses.

How would you describe the person in terms of age, personality, occupation, marital status, interests, beliefs, values and attitudes?

On what basis did you make these judgements?

For discussion

- Did the conclusions reached concur? Why/why not?
- How does this exercise translate to the practice situation?
- Is it possible to identify any mental frameworks we have adopted?
- What actions do we need to take in order to achieve accurate and objective social perception?

7.4.6 Personal characteristics

Personal factors have a bearing on skilled performance, as pointed out in Chapter 3. For example, the strategies that extroverts may use successfully in interpersonal interactions may not be effective for the introvert and *vice versa*. With respect to gender, recent work in the medical domain (Meeuwesen, Schaap and van der Staak, 1991) has indicated the different ways male and female patients elaborate their complaints, and the more imposing and presumptuous stance of male GPs as distinct from the more attentive and non-directive approach of their female colleagues. Female patients ask more questions than men and female patients appear to receive more positive communication than men (Roter, Lipkin and Korsgaard, 1991). These factors have implications for CST. Indeed, Hargie and Morrow (1989) have indicated that the personality differences exhibited by practitioners will need to be taken into account when designing programmes of CST.

7.4.7 Validity and generalizability

Included here are a number of other factors impinging on the analysis of social skill. Firstly, there is the rigour–relevance argument concerned with what are the best ways in which to study the subject. Gelso and Fassinger (1990) succinctly summarized the issue: 'The rigor–relevance continuum is reflected in an emphasis on experimental control and manipulation of independent variables, allowing for strong causal inferences with internal validity placed at a premium. The relevance side of the continuum, however, emphasizes clinical realism and research that is readily generalizable, with external validity placed at a premium' (p. 372).

Secondly, and linked to the whole aspect of generalizability, is the nature of samples and the sampling process. Obviously, atypical subjects are likely to produce atypical findings and conclusions. Similarly, because empirical research in this field is invasive, it is possible that those practitioners willing to be involved may be a self-selecting group (Hargie, Morrow and Woodman, 1993). Added to this is the validity of the small sample sizes that tend to be reported in skill identification studies.

A third related factor is concerned with the extent to which control groups are used in any experimental design of analysis of skill performance. This, of course, would only be necessary where some 'treatment' element had been instituted (e.g. training), and its effects measured. However, the constitution of control groups is extremely difficult and raises ethical problems in terms of, for example, allocation of patients to 'trained' or 'untrained' personnel.

A fourth factor is that of multiple measures. Like a cut diamond, which exhibits diverse hues and colours depending upon the angle from which it is viewed, so any analysis of the interpersonal process will produce different conclusions depending upon the manner in which it is examined. Some of these differences, as has already been stated, are due to the standpoint of the individual analyst(s) involved. However, the differences can also be attributed to the analysis measures that are employed. While it is possible to accurately identify the level of a drug in the body, through a proven analytical technique, the complexity of human behaviour defies any such simple measurement. Multiple measures are, therefore, required to get nearer the 'truth' and, by extension, to allow greater confidence to be ascribed to the results by virtue of a more composite and internally consistent picture. Thus, it is not surprising to find that increasingly a wide range of variables is being used to chart and measure the communication process (Roter and Hall, 1989; Street, 1992).

7.5 APPROACHES TO SOCIAL SKILL IDENTIFICATION

Over the last 15 years there has been a more concentrated focus within the health professions on the communicative ability of practitioners. This has prompted a closer examination of what actually happens at the practitioner–patient interface not only the clinical elements of the interaction but also the communication behaviour of all those involved. The one is concerned with communication as a product while the other emphasizes the process elements of interpersonal interaction. In essence, the approaches to social skill identification fall into two main sections – the trainer identifies the skills either by reflection or by observation. However, Ellis and Whittington (1981) have proposed three styles of approach, the empirical, the analytical and the intuitive.

7.5.1 The empirical approach

This can be thought of as the traditional scientific method, in that skill identification involves systematic observation, recording, categorization and analysis of interpersonal interactions. It may also involve experimentation to determine the relative importance of skill components and, after training, measurement of outcomes. Obviously, one of the difficulties within such an approach is the establishment of a framework wherein objective analysis can be carried out. Indeed, as has been previously iterated, our perceptions of social interaction are coloured, at least in part, by our cognitive framework, such that in reality empirical analysis is more likely to be carried out within traditionally accepted skill categories that have been determined by reflection rather than observation! Thus, as Ellis and Whittington (1981) pointed out 'the pure application of the empirical paradigm has been tempered not only by pragmatism but by the logical necessity for pre-empirical analysis and theorizing' (p. 29).

7.5.2 The analytical approach

This can be described as the theoretical approach to social skill identification. In essence it demands no observation or measurement but is the result of deductive processes based on the objectives of interpersonal communication. Thus, it may be considered that effective patient communication in the nursing context is to promote trust and confidence, and encourage patients to fully disclose their needs and problems. From this, rational discourse may produce a number of skill concepts (e.g. questioning, listening, empathy), which would be important elements to address within a skills training programme. Although this method is not considered ideal for social skill identification, often the lack of empirical evidence has prompted its use.

Fletcher and Freeling (1988) suggested that the skills likely to help in conducting effective and efficient patient consultations fall into four broad groups:

- creating an atmosphere conducive to effective communication;
- encouraging the patient to volunteer information;
- conducting the interview systematically;
- identifying the patient's goals in making the consultation.

These, however, may be better described as the broad purposes of the consultation, within which 10 interviewing behaviours have been discriminated to form the focus for teaching and evaluation (Kendrick and Freeling, 1993).

These include asking open-ended questions, explaining purposes, asking closed questions, noting non-verbal cues, defining meanings, appearing to listen, clarifying inconsistencies, interrupting (inoffensively), insisting on precision, and making notes while still maintaining attention.

7.5.3 The intuitive approach

This is very much the experiential approach (i.e. 'I've been in the situation and I found. . .'). It is therefore reflective in style and to some extent inductive, in that, as experiences are collated, possibly shared and discussed, it is possible to build up a picture of what are generic key skills and also what situations demand special skills. Moreover, the results of the intuitive approach are often confirmed by empirical analysis. In the skill identification process there is therefore justification in using each of these methods depending on the facilities, time and personnel available. Indeed it is possible to produce useful lists of skills without necessarily undertaking empirical observation and analysis.

This is perhaps well illustrated with reference to the dental profession. Relatively little has been done by way of communication skill training for dentists, particularly in the UK, but some attempts have been made to identify the needs of dentists in this respect. The process of skill identification has been largely based on analytical and intuitive paradigms. Furnham (1983a) suggested that there are two different types of patient, who have quite different attitudes to, and expectations of, their dentist and who by inference require different approaches in respect of interpersonal consultations. On the one hand there is the 'preventive' patient, who is normally of high socioeconomic status, is knowledgeable about dental health matters, has confidence in the dentist and is looking for professional dental skills and accompanying social skills. On the other hand there is the 'restorative' patient. These patients are usually of low socioeconomic status, poorly informed and motivated about dental health and have negative attitudes to the dentist. During the consultation they seek primarily friendliness, reassurance and sympathy rather than professional dental skills.

Jackson and Katz (1983) presented a list of skills that need to be taught to and mastered by dental students prior to qualification. These fall into four main categories:

- giving patient attention;
- accepting and not judging the patient;
- reducing patient anxiety;
- presenting patient information.

The authors suggested a number of behavioural patterns that need to be adopted to achieve the above objectives. For example, reduction of anxiety may be effected by giving patients a source of control (i.e. hand raising, keeping the patient updated in what he/she will experience in the course of the treatment, talking at an even, relaxed pace and moving slowly and deliberately, keeping hands in sight).

7.6 METHODOLOGIES FOR COMMUNICATION SKILL IDENTIFICATION

Arising out of the three paradigms discussed above are the more specific investigative methodologies which can be employed to identify skills. These are outlined below, together with a description of specific research initiatives that have been conducted within several health professional groups.

7.6.1 Task analysis

This is essentially a competence-based observational strategy designed to identify what the practitioner does. It involves a researcher literally following the practitioner around for a period of time and carefully noting what is being done. It therefore provides a detailed description of what actually constitutes, for example, nursing, medical or pharmaceutical practice. Obviously it would normally go beyond the interpersonal dimensions of practice but could be geared more specifically to the whole gamut of communicative behaviour. While this appears an attractive approach it suffers from the major disadvantage that it refers only to functional tasks and not to the level of skill with which people perform them. Thus task analysis items might specify 'interviews patients' 'advises on medicine administration' yet there is no indication of what is involved in these tasks or indeed what is required to perform these activities effectively. As Dunn and Hamilton (1984) state: 'it tells what is done but gives no indication of how it is done' (p. 138). Another disadvantage of this method is that it is likely to produce a long list of activities without any indication of their relative importance within the practice domain. On its own, therefore, its value in communication skills determination is rather limited.

7.6.2 The Delphi technique

This technique uses a panel of experts or 'wise men' and is a useful and successful method of obtaining answers to questions which are issues of uncertainty, particularly professional behaviour/competence. It is regarded as a systematic procedure aimed at arriving at a reasoned consensus. A review of the technique, together with some of its modified versions in nursing is offered by McKenna (1994). The Delphi technique involves the following main elements.

Selection of experts

It is essential to attempt to bring together a panel of individuals who are most likely to have the relevant knowledge and experience concerning the objectives to be met. It should be recognized, however, that as far as social skill identification in a particular profession is concerned there may be no 'experts' in that field simply because the knowledge and experience of reputable individuals may be, and in many cases is, rooted in the cognitive and technical skills inherent in the profession and not in its social skills. Rapport (1983) has discussed the choice of experts and concluded that it is 'usually made on the basis of what may vaguely be called their reputations' (p. 164).

Formulation of competencies

Having selected a group of experts it is necessary to ask them firstly to define or formulate the general areas of knowledge, skills and attitudes necessary for effective interpersonal communication in the professional setting, and secondly, to identify the specific competencies within this area. This is carried out individually and anonymously by postal survey of the panel members and therefore eliminates committee activity. It also avoids the psychological influences of face-to-face debate.

Compilation of expert opinions

From the data generated by the group of experts the researcher is responsible for collating the information into a single composite document. All the information included in the returned lists should be included even if only one expert has entered a particular competency. Where specific competencies have not received unanimous support they should be marked with an asterisk.

Revision of opinions

Here the competencies compiled should be sent to all the experts with instructions to refer only to those asterisked and state briefly why in their opinion each of these competencies should be included or excluded in the final list. In addition, any new estimates of competency should be stated. Again the revised responses of the panel would be returned in confidence to the researcher for compilation. This process of listing, distributing, replying and collating competencies should be repeated until a consensus is reached and a final list of competencies is drawn up, based upon the additions and deletions.

Evaluation of competencies

The final list of competencies should be returned to the experts and each of them individually should be asked to score on a five-point scale how important each one is within the practice situation. The ratings should then be analysed, and the results obtained should indicate the principal competencies that a practitioner should possess in order to practise effectively. From this basis training strategies can be formulated to produce the competencies delineated.

These are the main elements of the Delphi technique, which is characterized by its anonymity, independent participation with controlled feedback and statistically grouped response. For further information on this technique the reader is referred to the work of Linstone and Turoff (1975) and McKenna (1994).

Duffield (1993) reported the use of this technique to identify the competencies required by first-line nurse managers. What is interesting about this work was that two panels of experts were used and the results were compared. Out of 168 competencies identified and evaluated by both panels a 93% consensus was achieved between the two in either retaining or omitting individual elements. Interpersonal competencies identified within the final list included both communicative strategies and skills.

7.6.3 Critical incident survey

This technique is a more sophisticated method of collating behavioural data about the ingredients of skilled performance in the actual practice context. Here practitioners are asked to reflect on incidents in which they have been personally involved or which they have observed, which constituted good or poor performance. Focusing upon specific incidents facilitates recall and enables respondents to identify and clarify behaviours and attach meanings or interpretations to these behaviours. Exercise 7.2 is a suggested schema for recording details of such incidents.

Exercise 7.2 Identification of critical incidents in practice

Instructions

Each practitioner should think of an incident or incidents in practice where poor/good interpersonal communication was apparent. The incident should be described below. The following questions serve to aid a full description of the event.

- Where did the event take place?
- Who were the individuals involved?
- What features of the individuals involved were important in the interaction (e.g. deafness, emotionally upset, etc.)?
- What actually occurred in the interaction?
- What was the outcome?
- Why was the interaction considered to be effective/ineffective?
- Finally, consider the implications of this incident for interpersonal communication performance.

Table 7.3 illustrates a critical incident described by a pharmacist during a CST course.

Table 7.3 A critical incident report

Pharmacist	A lady came into my pharmacy and complained that she had received the wrong tablets. As she was obviously quite concerned and upset I brought her into my dispensary to deal with the matter. In fact she hadn't received the wrong tablets but had, in accordance with her GP's prescription, been dispensed a generic form of her medicine, which was coloured differently from the proprietary brand she normally received. I explained to her that although the tablets were coloured differently they still contained the same drug. However, she did not understand this. At the same time a local council worker was removing some empty cartons from my pharmacy and overheard the conversation. He politely interrupted and spoke to my patient: 'Mrs, if you go down the street to Coulter's garage you'll see five new Ford Escorts in the showroom. They are different colours but they are still Escorts. Your tablets are just the same.' My patient understood the analogy perfectly and left the pharmacy satisfied that she had received the correct medication. I thought 'Why couldn't I have used an illustration like that?'

It should be remembered that such a technique is not designed to identify incompetent practitioners. Rather, the emphasis is on the incident as opposed to the individual. As the number of incidents reported increases it is possible to perform some content analysis on them in order to cluster the information and thus predict essential areas of competence.

A recent study in nursing employed a variation of this technique to chart consumer views of a Macmillan nurse's work as provided by 20 respondents (eight patients, five carers, five district nurses and two GPs) coming in contact with this specialist professional (Cox, Bergen and Norman, 1993). Using a structured interview approach, these individuals were asked to reflect on their encounters with the nurse, with particular emphasis on positive and negative experiences. The most positive and frequently quoted aspects of the nurse's role included:

- specialist knowledge in the area of terminal cancer care;
- provision of psychological and emotional support for patients and carers;
- liaison skills;
- having time to talk and listen to patients.

Any negative comments related primarily to structural issues rather than process elements of the service. This technique was also employed by Wetchler and Vaughan (1991) to bring to light the interpersonal skills of primary family therapy supervisors during supervisory incidents with trainees. Skills involved in providing adequate direction emerged as being of particular significance.

One specific example of the critical incident technique that has value in skill identification or training need determination is those situations where litigation is involved. Hirsh (1986a, b), using exemplar malpractice suits, examined the professional duty of health-care providers, particularly doctors and nurses, to gather information from and about the patient, appropriately examine the patient and communicate with the patient and other professional colleagues. He pointed out that 'the failure to recognize the importance of information, the failure to elicit it, the failure to communicate it either verbally or by documentation, and the failure to respond appropriately all fall below acceptable standards of care' (Hirsh, 1986a, p. 460).

Condon (1992) focused upon a number of psychological factors, based on case experience, which may cause patients to embark upon legal proceedings. He suggested that the most frequent form of psychological mismanagement is the failure to share information openly with the patient and also to provide explanations that are perceived by the patient as adequate. Even 'reassurance or sympathy if offered in the absence of adequate explanation, can have a patronizing quality and engender considerable anger, the expression of which may take the form of a formal complaint or legal action as a means of retaliation' (p. 769).

Within an 'expert systems' approach subjects are required to formulate and identify component elements of the field of inquiry under analysis (Caves, 1988). This, as the name suggests, relies on the contributions of experts, usually practitioners, as distinct from clients, and involves both empirical and intuitive paradigms. Thus, the expert system is characterized by its emphasis on knowledge governed by facts and rules, facts being 'declarative statements that give specific knowledge about a specific case of class', while 'rules give knowledge on how to reason in a domain' (Caves, 1988, p. 210). It could be argued that it is a specialized form of critical incident survey, in that it is anchored in specific experiences or incidents in practice.

Within the pharmaceutical discipline, Morrow and Hargie (1987a; 1992) have used such an approach to identify key aspects of interpersonal communication in pharmacy practice. The former study was undertaken: firstly, to generate from pharmacists a comprehensive itemization of the interpersonal difficulties in the practice situation; secondly, to discriminate and conceptualize these difficulties into discrete categories; and thirdly, to investigate from the pharmacists' perspective the nature of the central interpersonal problems that they encountered.

From the data collected it was possible to undertake a qualitative analysis of pharmacist–patient interactions. A total of 25 different types of 'problem' patient who present communication difficulties for the pharmacist was reported. These included drug addicts, confused patients, handicapped people and illiterate individuals, among others. A closer examination of patient problems revealed that embarrassing, emotional/psychological and handicap situations together with terminal illness and financial problems appear to offer substantial challenges to the pharmacist in terms of satisfactory communication.

A content analysis of the actual communication difficulties suggested that these fell within four broad but overlapping categories:

- non-verbal communication difficulties (e.g. interpreting non-verbal behaviour, establishing and maintaining eye contact, using sign language);

- difficulties in gathering and giving factual information (e.g. questioning, explaining, listening, providing reassurance);
- evaluative difficulties (e.g. recognition of patients' needs, assessment of patient understanding);
- miscellaneous difficulties including ethical conflicts, diplomacy, alleviating embarrassment and imparting confidence.

Finally, several other factors that influence pharmacist interactions were identified, including 23 features of the pharmacist (e.g. age, gender, integrity, friendliness, accessibility), 11 features of the practice environment (e.g. decor, layout, privacy, lighting) and seven miscellaneous factors (e.g. time availability, lack of training in interpersonal communication, the prescription form).

Thus this investigation represented a first step in beginning to identify and analyse what actually happens at the pharmacist–patient interface, allied to the highlighting of generic skills relevant to the pharmacy context (i.e. questioning, explaining), and also of the individual situations where special skills are required for a successful outcome. Exercise 7.3 is an adaptation of the self-reported methodology used by these workers.

Exercise 7.3 Identification of factors influencing practitioner–patient interactions

Instructions

The trainer should prepare worksheets based on each of the three headings below. Each worksheet should be divided into two columns, one to chart the types of difficulty encountered and the other to list the actual communication problems that these difficulties pose. Each practitioner should complete an individual inventory and the pooled responses can then be collated, analysed and subjected to further peer review if required.

Types of 'problem' patient

Column 1: Identify as many types of 'problem' patients as you can, e.g. the aggressive patient.
Column 2: Identify the central communication difficulties that these people present, e.g. difficulty in reasoning with patient.

Types of patients' difficult problem

Column 1: Identify as many types as you can and give two or three examples to illustrate types, e.g. embarrassing problems: impotence, stammering, psoriasis.

Column 2: Identify the central communication difficulties that these problems present, e.g. establishing a common language of understanding.

Miscellaneous factors

Column 1: Identify as many factors as you can relating to the nature of the practitioner, e.g. personality, attitude.

Identify any factors other than the above which may influence practitioner communication, e.g. environment.

Column 2: Show how the factors identified opposite can influence the communication process, e.g. the shy practitioner finds difficulty in interacting with clients, or privacy may allow a patient to express his/her problem more freely.

In their second study (Morrow and Hargie, 1992), pharmacists were asked to itemize all those situations in practice where they thought counselling was indicated, and then identify the most common difficulties that these situations presented. They were asked to ensure that what they listed represented discrete aspects of their counselling experience. The individual responses were then collated to produce a total series of elements as expressed by the pharmacists themselves. This produced two inventories, one comprising 46 situations and the other, 45 difficulties. Each participant was then asked to evaluate the lists and individually rank in order of importance the 15 most important counselling situations and the 15 most common counselling difficulties. In this way subsequent training was able to be tailored to the actual practice situation.

The main disadvantage of the expert systems approach is that the analysis of the data into distinct clusters tends to be somewhat subjective. However, this can be overcome by submitting the analysis to a group of practitioners to test its appropriateness as a behavioural model of the work situation.

7.6.4 Behavioural event interview

The behavioural event interview is an adaptation of the critical incident survey. In this approach practitioners in a given health profession are identified as being 'good' practitioners as judged by their peers. They are then interviewed in depth and asked to describe in detail some of the most critical interpersonal situations they have faced in practice. The interview should cover questions such as: 'What led up to the event?' 'Who were the individuals involved?' 'What was the purpose of the interaction?' 'What actions did you/the patient take?' 'What motivated your actions?' 'What were the outcomes for the parties involved?' 'How satisfied were the individuals concerned with the consultation?' Here the interest is focused on the goals of the individuals, the practitioner's perception of the event and the people involved, their thoughts, feelings and actions and the overall outcome, including any follow-up or future associated contact.

Following the interviews the practitioner should be asked to itemize the most important interpersonal skills required of a competent person engaged in that profession. One of the benefits of this approach is that it tends to highlight a wide variety of important and relevant situations, which can be used for practical learning in the training situation by way of simulation exercises or case studies.

The second step involves repeating this exercise with a similar number of practitioners who are regarded as average performers. The final step involves an analytical treatment of the material generated through the behavioural event interviews in order to distinguish those competencies that are present or absent in the interview records of good, as opposed to average, practitioners. Because of the complexity of the task, skilled analysts are needed. However, the results can produce a detailed mapping of interpersonal communication in the professional setting, thereby describing the competencies that predict performance.

7.6.5 Constitutive ethnography

This method, broadly defined, uses an empirical paradigm to identify and analyse the actual processes involved in interpersonal communication. It involves capturing a range of consultative events on video. Through subsequent rigorous analysis and description by the participants themselves, salient patterns and regularities in interactional behaviour are revealed. In this way, tacit knowledge is illuminated which professionals possess but which they may not be able to articulate. It is therefore possible to identify, for example, sequences in behaviour such as (1) asking a question, (2) clarifying the question if the response is inadequate, (3) prompting, (4) probing for further information, etc. It is also possible to begin to identify useful strategies for patient consultations which make the interaction more effective and more satisfying for the participants. Moreover, the importance of the non-verbal elements of behaviour can be determined and specific cues which moderate, control and facilitate interactions can be elicited, thereby giving direction to the elements of skilled performance which need to be developed or trained. Overall, then, the ethnographic technique, in relation to CST, is directed to analysing and identifying aspects of interpersonal behaviour which occur in social interactions in order to chart those skills and strategies that go to producing skilled performance.

Saunders and Caves (1986) used some of the characteristics of the constitutive ethnographic approach to chart the communication processes within the speech therapy discipline. Here speech therapists were videotaped during actual patient consultations, with the recorded sequences subsequently subjected to peer analysis.

The analysis yielded a detailed category system of behaviours exemplified by speech therapists during consultations together with the number of instances when these behaviours occurred. The categories delineated were presented either in terms of the function of the behaviour or as a more fine-grained analysis of the types of behaviour subsumed under a global category. (Table 7.4)

Table 7.4 Examples of categories of behaviour in speech-therapist–patient interactions

Global category	*Subcategory*	
Use of eye contact/ facial expression	To regulate the flow of interaction To maintain and demonstrate interest Modelling appropriate eye contact to monitor the patient's speech Maintaining eye contact to avoid underlining the patient's disability	Functional
Counselling – where patient shows stress or frustration	Methods of stress alleviation	Functional
	Pause in therapy task Humorous or light comment Instruction to relax Alerting to possible difficulties Explanation of reasons for difficulty	Methodological

Furthermore, the analysis revealed, firstly, the importance of using skills appropriate to the particular context of interaction. This was particularly true in the use of the generic skill of questioning in the process of encouraging patients to self-monitor their own speech patterns. Here the importance of asking specific kinds of open questions was highlighted allied to the actual timing of the questions. Secondly, the investigation indicated how one professional group can use a skill in a highly differentiated way. Speech therapists used some 15 different types of cue in order to encourage patient participation in the therapy, as well as using cueing techniques frequently during sessions. Similarly, positive reinforcement techniques were used widely to provide support, give praise and otherwise encourage patients during the treatment programme.

Using the constitutive ethnography approach to skill identification, Hargie, Morrow and Woodman (1993) videotaped 350 real pharmacist–patient consultations in 15 community pharmacies. Aimed at identifying the core skills inherent in effective interactions, these recordings were subjected to a detailed peer review procedure. As a result a comprehensive inventory of 45 key behaviours, categorized into 11 main skill areas, was produced. The range of skills and subskills charted in this research is of particular importance since it is the first comprehensive, empirically validated list of communication competencies in the pharmacy setting. The study revealed a number of notable features.

Firstly, the integrative nature of interpersonal performance was underscored by the fact that, in a number of instances, the same behaviour was categorized under more than one skill area. Secondly, some behaviours were described in communication process terms (e.g. reinforcing, politeness, use of humour) while others were classified by virtue of their verbal content (e.g. questions on symptoms, previous action taken, other medication used). Thus a distinction between the 'construction' of communication and its 'content' was made. Interestingly, some categories were subdivided predominantly into one or other of these two dimensions. For example, questioning was viewed as a content-based skill, whereas explaining was much more a construction-based skill.

Thirdly, it would appear that pharmacists regard the relationship element of practice as particularly powerful, such that many strategies are required to initiate, maintain and enhance relationships. This was evidenced by the fact that building rapport had by far the largest number of behavioural subcategories. There is little doubt that community pharmacy is somewhat unusual in that it operates as a helping profession within the realities of business practice. Thus there are two motivations for maintaining patient rapport: the demonstration of a caring practitioner, and the creation and preservation of patient loyalty to achieve business success.

Fourthly, as the frequency of positive skill use increased so did ratings of communication effectiveness. Equally, an extended skill usage operated in consultations where the dispensing of a prescription was not involved. Indeed the skill of suggesting/advising was evident only in these consultations. This is worthy of note, since this is a dimension of communication which has not received any real attention in the health communication literature and may indeed be a particular feature of community pharmacy practice.

Fifthly, based on a frequency of use pattern, building rapport, explaining and questioning emerged as the core skills adjudged to be central to pharmacy practice.

Finally, an extension of this research involved a microanalysis of the questions used in the consultations of five of the participating pharmacists (Morrow *et al.*, 1993), as discussed in Chapter 4. On the basis of the results these workers conclude that 'the training of pharmacists not only needs to address the content issues of questioning, including both factual and feeling aspects, but also the process dimensions, that is the construction, sequence and flow of questions' (p. 94).

Procedures used by Saunders and Caves (1986) with speech therapists and Hargie, Morrow and Woodman (1993) with community pharmacists have also enabled Adams *et al.* (1994) to illuminate the verbal and non-verbal features of skilled communication used by physiotherapists with different patient groups. Thornquist (1992) also provided a snapshot view of communication in physiotherapy practice. Based on the analysis of two videotaped consultations and post-consultation interviews with the therapists involved, this author has demonstrated the impact of the reference points or professional constructs adopted by individual practitioners. With one physiotherapist the focus was on the patient's physical health and functional ability of the body, where the patient was largely treated as the object of the therapist's attention. In the other a holistic approach to the patient's health was adopted, with the therapist encouraging patient co-operation and involvement in his/her care management.

While the ethnographic technique in its purist form demands the video recording of interactions, variations of the methodology have been used. Primarily, these employ audio recording of events, simply because it is easier and less invasive. However, it must be remembered that substantially the non-verbal elements of behaviour are lost.

The disadvantages of the constitutive ethnographic method are predictable. Firstly, there are the logistical problems of being able to videotape actual practitioner–patient consultations. Secondly, there are major ethical issues to be faced when 'invading' what are normally very private interactions. These will be discussed later. Thirdly, there is the lack of adequate safeguards against the investigator's subjective biases determining the aspects of interaction highlighted. Fourthly, there is the difficulty in obtaining consensus from peer review and analysis of the data. Fifthly, the problem of selecting individuals capable of interpersonal analysis of practice situations may be considerable, and finally, the objectivity of analysis may be impaired because of the psychological influences existing in group debate and discussion. While these factors constitute risk to the whole skill identification phase, Saunders and Caves (1986) have argued that 'this risk may be worth taking as long as subsequent attention is given to the reliability and validity of the interaction sequences which emerge' (p. 32).

7.6.6 Communication audit

In the previous edition of this book the emphasis on skill identification was substantially placed on experts evaluating observed or recorded practitioner performance and theorizing about performance, or practitioners reflecting on personal or others' performance. Less attention was directed to consumer expectations or experience of health-care professionals in terms of the style, content or duration of communication as an alternative way of eliciting skills or their lack. Similarly, little attention was paid to what might be called the wider structural elements of communication.

However, the last 6 years have witnessed an important development concerned with the issue of quality as applied to health services. Not only does this focus upon the structure, process and outcomes of what a practitioner does, but what a client (patient) expects from that practitioner. Such a movement has been particularly strong in the UK, where the Government's published Patient's Charter (Department of Health, 1992b) highlighted the health-care provisions to which members of the public are entitled. The Audit Commission (1993) has followed this up in order to evaluate the whole gamut of communication practice in the National Health Service.

Hargie, Morrow and Woodman (1992) have argued that 'because communication and client satisfaction must form important elements of any quality assurance programme, more needs to be done to determine what the actual standards of practice should be, as distinct from the activities to be engaged in, or indeed, how practice should move to meet the desired standards' (p. 688). This introduces the concept of audit, the idea of looking at what you do, learning from it and making changes. Investigation of the communicative aspects of practice has borrowed from the audit approach to produce 'a comprehensive and thorough study of communication philosophy, concepts, structure, flow and practice' (Emmanuel, 1985, pp. 2–3).

The best known audit system is that developed by Goldhaber and Rogers (1979) for the International Communication Association. This system permits the researcher to:

- describe individual, group and organizational patterns of actual communication behaviours;
- determine the amount of information underload or overload associated with the major topics, sources and channels of communication;
- evaluate the quality of information communicated from and/or to these sources and the quality of information relationships;
- identify the operational communication networks and determine potential bottlenecks and gatekeepers of information;
- identify categories of recurring positive and negative communication episodes;
- identify how and in what ways communication processes and procedures can be improved.

Communication audits have proved to be extremely beneficial in two main ways. Firstly, they offer the opportunity to comprehensively chart the actual patterns of communication that occur in any particular context. Secondly, they allow all those participating to express their views concerning how these could best be improved (Downs, 1988). It is therefore a method of gaining information in order to solve communication problems and create efficient and effective ways of communicating. Obviously the approach to gathering information can be multifaceted. For example, questionnaires can be administered to all participants asking them to evaluate current communication practices and to identify areas of strength and weakness, and suggest opportunities for improvement, as well as indicating any barriers or inhibitors to enhancement. Similar information can, of course, be obtained from interviews with participants. Other methods for collecting information include actual observation, recording and analysis of interpersonal encounters, use of *agents provocateurs*, diary analysis to ascertain with whom individuals have interacted and how often over a given period of time, and self-recording of interactions by participants on paper following each interactive episode.

Reports of communication audits often concern communication within an organization, concerned to improve the quality of working relationships by evaluating the health or otherwise of the organization's internal communication systems (Hargie and Tourish, 1993; Tourish and Hargie, 1993). Bland and Jackson (1990) suggested that this form of audit tells organizations:

- who you **should** communicate with;

- who you **actually do** communicate with;
- what you **should** be communicating;
- how you **should** communicate with them;
- how you **actually do** communicate with them (p. 142).

At the more personal level and within the health domain, Hargie, Morrow and Woodman (1992) have carried out a questionnaire-based audit of community pharmacy services as perceived and experienced by members of the public. This audit identified a range of issues reflected in the attitudes of the public, namely, patronage, privacy, time access, pharmacist image, caring approach and the tension between the health and business dimensions of community pharmacy practice.

In a more fine-grained analysis of the data, Morrow, Hargie and Woodman (1993) showed that in relation to the advice-giving role of the community pharmacist, a number of important changes needed to be made in order to satisfy consumer expectations. These concerned the provision of unsolicited advice, prescription-related explanations, checking for patient understanding and the adequacy of demonstrations.

7.6.7 Other approaches

The methodologies described above use both qualitative and quantitative assessments of communication behaviour allied to the health-care context. Obviously, adaptations of these general themes can be employed in order to identify communication skills. For example, in a study of the closing phase of the medical consultation, White, Levinson and Roter (1994) analysed the audiotapes of 88 consultations using a modified version of the Roter Interactional Analysis System. These workers found that patients introduced new problems in this closing segment in 21% of cases. These were associated with lower levels of exchange of information, fewer assertive statements by physicians and higher patient affect scores. Those closures which were more prolonged correlated with doctors asking open-ended questions, laughing, demonstrating responsiveness to patients, offering self-disclosures and engaging in psychosocial discussion with patients. The authors indicate ways in which communication could be improved during closure to decrease the number of new problems being raised (e.g. orienting patients to the interview, assessing patient beliefs, checking understanding, addressing emotional and psychosocial issues early in the consultation).

Similarly, in an investigation of doctor–patient communication, Meeuwesen, Schaap and van der Staak (1991) attempted to answer three main research questions:

- What are the communicational characteristics of patient and physician in the various phases of the medical interview?

- Does the type of complaint (somatic or psychosocial) influence the communicational pattern of the medical interview?
- Does the gender of the patient and physician influence the communicational pattern of the medical interview.

These workers audiotaped and transcribed 85 medical interviews and subjected them to the Verbal Response Mode (VRM) coding system. This system focuses upon the intent or relational aspect that an utterance has on communication as distinct from its verbal content, and consists of eight mutually exclusive and exhaustive categories: acknowledgement, edification, question, disclosure, reflection, confirmation, interpretation and advisement.

What these workers found was that there was a clear asymmetrical relation between physician and patient, evidenced, for example, in the relative number of utterances by each during the history-taking, examination and concluding segments of the interview. Secondly, interviews with psychosocial patients took more time than those of somatic patients, and psychosocial patients tended to try to exert more control in the interviews. Thirdly, women patients presented their complaints differently from men. Finally, and most strikingly, there were differences between male and female GPs allied to their style of consultation and the time spent on each consultation.

Ridderikhoff (1993) used video recorded interactions between doctors and patients to examine the nature and quantity of information exchange within the consultation. This study involved the use of simulated patients to present consistently to the different physicians participating in the research. What the investigation uncovered was that doctors under time constraints look for broad diagnostic pictures and are relatively ineffective in eliciting specific data. Thus the ability to interview effectively, in terms of the gathering of adequate and accurate information without missing key leads or cues, is crucially important.

In another investigation, audio recordings were made of over 700 pharmacist–patient interactions in community pharmacies in the London area. It was found that the average duration of consultations was 2.5 minutes (Smith, 1992a). However, in a subset of these consultations dealing specifically with coughs, the contact time fell to 1.6 minutes, with pharmacists asking a mean number of 3 questions and giving an average of 4.4 items of information or advice per consultation (Smith, 1992b).

Against this background it would be possible to draw from wider research in interpersonal communication by listing a number of communicative strategies. These could then be submitted to professional review in order to determine which strategies work most successfully in given practitioner–patient situations. An alternative technique is the 'What would you do next?' approach. Here practitioners are presented with part of a written dialogue of a patient interaction, or shown a portion of a video sequence of a patient consultation, and asked how they would proceed with the interview, or alternatively how they would have conducted it from the outset. Exercise 7.4 is an example of this approach. From the responses it should be possible to chart an effective, situationally appropriate communication strategy, which could be used as a basis for communication skills training.

Exercise 7.4 What would you do next?

Instructions

The following is the initial part of a conversation between a nurse and a patient. The patient had originally been admitted to hospital for investigation following the discovery of a lump on her breast. It was found to be malignant and a mastectomy has been performed. Follow-up chemotherapy has also been instituted. Based on this, trainees should be challenged to identify ways in which the overall interaction should be handled and the skills required to do so.

Nurse: Hello, Mrs X. How are you feeling today?
Patient: Not too good.
Nurse: Sister said you were feeling sick.
Patient: Oh, it's not the sickness. I wish that was all – (bursts into tears). What am I going to do? I never thought it would ever come to this. . . .

7.7 ETHICAL AND CLINICAL CONSIDERATIONS OF INVESTIGATIVE METHODOLOGIES

Obviously in carrying out some of the above techniques there are a number of practical considerations to be taken into account. These include, for example, technological factors concerning the choice and actual use of audio and video recordings (Chapter 12) and also the time, personnel and financial commitment that may be required to undertake a major empirical research initiative. More important, perhaps, are the ethical and clinical issues that confront the investigator using audiovisual methodologies to examine the dimensions of interpersonal communication at the practitioner–patient interface. It is therefore essential that the researcher be aware of these elements in order to afford 'protection' to all parties involved.

Any form of recording that makes the consultation between a patient and practitioner a matter of permanent/semi-permanent and possibly public record, raises fundamental ethical questions. Moreover, any access to this relationship through the use of recordings for teaching or analysis purposes endangers its integrity. Thus, firstly, do these methods, while providing potentially rich resources of material for research and instruction, violate privacy and confidentiality? Secondly, while 'informed consent' is a process whereby patients accept a certain level of risk, do they fully understand the implications of this commitment? Thirdly, does the act of recording a consultation affect the nature, content and outcome of the interaction itself? This has two dimensions, the first relating to the behaviour of the practitioner and indeed the patient within the context of the consultation; the second to the possible 'clinical' ramifications of the use of these techniques in relation to patient health/illness behaviour following the consultation.

Obviously, videotaping is a more comprehensive form of recording than audio recording, and therefore by its very nature more revealing, such that ethical guidelines developed for this form of recording will undoubtedly cover the audio situation. Block, Schaffner and Coulehan (1985) suggested that the fundamental ethical principles underpinning a practical approach to videotaping patients are those of autonomy, non-maleficence, beneficence and justice. Autonomy is concerned with respect for persons and recognizes the self-governing nature of the individual. Non-maleficence is a principle which serves to protect the individual and literally means 'do no harm'. Beneficence refers to a duty to confer benefits or further the wellbeing of others as well as helping them advance their important and legitimate interests. Finally, justice is concerned with affording others their 'rights or dues'. Thus any derived ethical principles, rules, guidelines, policies and practices should seek to reflect these underlying values.

The whole area of privacy and confidentiality is substantially governed by the principle of autonomy, where the individual has the right to control personal information to the extent of who knows it. Thus patients may share intimate information with their doctor, pharmacist, health visitor, etc., but would not want that information to go any further. However, patients may also authorize information given in a consultation setting to be used for research and educational purposes. This becomes informed consent and the practitioner must ensure that in giving such consent the patient is truly autonomous. It is therefore important that patients are fully aware of what they are consenting to. For example, videotapes used purely for analysis in research are much more easily controlled in terms of who will view them, etc., whereas the consequences of using them for educational purposes are much more open and unpredictable, and indeed potentially harmful if individuals are recognized. Patients have therefore a right to know and be made aware of these situations.

Against this background it is crucial to ensure the voluntary and informed consent of the patient and prevent unauthorized access to the tapes and the information they contain. Within the patient care setting it is possible for patients to feel coerced into participating in such activities, and therefore, it is important to create a situation where the patient is free to say 'No'. Patients should not be allowed to feel under obligation to any of their health-care practitioners to do them a 'favour' by participating in any research or teaching project. Indeed, Martin and Martin (1984) reported that patients were less likely to refuse video recording of their consultation if they were asked by the doctor for their verbal permission on entering the consulting room than if they were asked to sign a consent form prior to the interaction. Patients were also more willing to express their reservations about video recording if asked to fill in a questionnaire at home rather than immediately at the surgery. Furthermore these workers found that even 11% of those who consented to recording later admitted that they actually disapproved of the technique.

Consequently it may be better if voluntary informed consent is obtained by someone other than the practitioner. As far as informed consent is concerned the patient needs to know exactly what is being recorded and to what use it will be put. This extends to knowing who will see the tape– other health workers, students, the public – and what the risks are of being recognized. Finally, tapes should be stored securely and access to them should be limited to those legitimately authorized to use them.

Following on from this, practical guidelines need to be formulated which can serve to establish a code of practice for the making and showing of practitioner–patient recordings. In addition a consent form will be required whereby all participants must give written consent to the use of the recording(s) in which they took part. Dowrick (1991) has outlined the primary items that should be included in such a consent form:

- Communication of the general purpose of the project;
- Statement of specific purpose concerning the participant;
- Clear indication if the purpose is research;
- Statement of the steps that will be taken to protect confidentiality;
- Rights of the subject to withdraw at any time, for any reason and without jeopardy;
- Description of how and when the tapes will be disposed of after they have served the stated purpose.

One further associated feature of the ethical issues surrounding video or audio recordings is the effect that they have on the actual consultation itself. Pringle, Robins and Brown (1984), in a comparison of video recording alone, as opposed to a general practitioner trainer sitting in on a GP trainee consultation, showed that video recorded consultations more closely related to the 'normal' situation than did the two-doctor consultation, when stress levels of patients were measured. They also reported that patients who refused consent to be filmed were more highly stressed than those who agreed. Similarly, Martin and Martin (1984) reported that patients with anxiety, depression or problems relating to the breasts or reproductive tract were more likely to withhold consent.

Herzmark (1985), in a study of 295 videoed doctor–patient interviews compared to a control group of 185 patient interviews which were not filmed, concluded that the actual videoing process did not appear to affect the consultation to any great extent from the patient's point of view. However, he reported, in some instances, lower rapport ratings between doctor and patient and also recognized the potential doctor anxieties of being seen to be 'doing the right thing'. The level of refusal to be recorded by patients was also reported, 10% in one practice and 2% in the other, one of the implications being that if large numbers of patients decline to be recorded in any investigation the resulting sample will be less representative of the population and thus the credibility of the results will be undermined. Furthermore, Servant and Matheson (1986) demonstrated that if the coercive elements of obtaining consent are reduced then the consent rates are substantially decreased, thus reinforcing the ethical dilemmas of this sort of investigation, confounding the representativeness of the study sample and strongly pointing in the direction that patients do mind being videotaped.

Although this section has concentrated on the ethical and clinical issues surrounding the consultation from the patient's perspective, it is interesting to note that a recent study 'offers no evidence that awareness of video recording has an effect on objective measures of doctors' consultation behaviour' (Pringle and Stewart-Evans, 1990, p. 457). Indeed, these workers claim that it provides support for the use of video as a tool in teaching and research.

7.8 FURTHER CONSIDERATIONS

The results of research into skill identification within the health professions raise a number of issues. Firstly, are the findings from the samples reported typical, in general, of practitioners within individual professional domains? It might be argued that research that used an exclusive empirical paradigm is more likely to reflect the true situation. Yet only by resubmitting the data to further independent professional review and testing its reliability with new samples of patient–practitioner consultation data can the accuracy and precision of skill identification be guaranteed. Meta-analysis of reported studies is increasingly being used to give 'power' to individual findings by offering collective, statistical analysis.

Secondly, the skills identified for effective performance often have been those primarily generated by professionals themselves and therefore represent only one view of the situation. This raises the question as to who is best positioned to analyse communication behaviour and how valid are the judgements made. Thus, communication behaviours may be assessed differently, depending on the analyst. Bensing (1991), however, has shown that it is possible to correlate quality of communication assessments made by general practitioners with satisfaction levels recorded by patients, although the correlations were relatively weak. Street (1992), in an analysis of paediatrician consultations, produced data on differing levels of correlation between behavioural measures of physician performance and measures of patients' perceptions. For example, doctors' use of patient-centred statements was predictive of the perceptions parents had of the interpersonal sensitivity and partnership-building behaviours displayed by physicians, but the amount of information doctors provided to parents was not related to their judgements of doctors' informativeness. For this reason Street (1992), argued persuasively for the 'use of measures generated from both observers **and** participants' (p. 986).

It may be expected, therefore, that patient perspectives will unveil more about practitioners' interpersonal communication than would be revealed by more traditional analysis methods. Bensing (1991) goes on to assert that:

> the quality ratings are a reflection of common conceptions and norms of practice among physicians, and thus build a good case for the (face) validity of the communication skills under study, particularly 'affective behaviour' and 'patient-centred behaviour. As a result, this study provides us with indications as to what types of behaviour are useful for training purposes in medical and postgraduate education.
>
> *Bensing, 1991, p. 1307*

Thirdly, there must be the recognition that the training needs of one professional group may be markedly different from another, such that training initiatives need to be custom developed to retain face validity with practitioners as well as optimizing the potential for patient gains during consultations.

7.9 OVERVIEW

This chapter has sought to explore the area of skill identification within the health professions. The content of training must reflect the aims and objectives of the programme, which, in turn, emerge from the established needs of trainees. Attention was drawn to the nature of interpersonal skill and the various factors which influence identification procedures. Three major paradigms were described, together with specific methodologies that can be used in skill identification studies, and consideration was given to the ethical and clinical ramifications of such investigations. The practical applications of these techniques were illustrated from within the health disciplines, together with a brief outline of the findings of this research. Finally, the implications of these results were presented, particularly in relation to the reliability and validity of the data. Once skills have been identified training proper can begin. The following three chapters are devoted to the training phase of CST.

The sensitization phase of training

8

8.1 INTRODUCTION

Following preparation, training considerations constitute the second stage of the CST process. Here attention is devoted to the provision of a sequence of learning experiences designed to promote the acquisition of those skills identified using the techniques detailed in the preceding chapter. In keeping with the reductionist principles underlying CST, the complexities of interpersonal encounters are reduced by breaking the overall communicative performance down into a number of constituent skill elements. From a training point of view, students are typically introduced to these individual skills in a structured, systematic and progressive fashion until gradually, at the end of the programme, the repertoire of skills established can be synthesized or integrated into a complete and effective reconstitution of the targeted interaction.

The initial step in this training procedure is termed 'sensitization' and is the focus of this chapter. At a broad level the process is intended to sensitize trainees to the characteristics and rationale of the instructional nature of the particular CST programme which they will follow. More specifically, by means of skill analysis and discrimination techniques, including modelling, an understanding of the central features, functional properties and theoretical bases of each of the skills is created. Furthermore, the sensitization process aims to promote trainees' ability to successfully operationalize this knowledge in interpersonal performance.

8.2 PRELIMINARY CONSIDERATIONS

Before embarking on a training programme it is important for trainers not only to think of the detail of **what** they should cover in any course but also **how** particular issues will be addressed. Two pertinent, but seemingly dichotomous questions, need to be asked. 'What has been demonstrated to be the nature of skilled performance extending beyond a specific professional group?' and 'How can training be made uniquely relevant to the training group?' The first question concerns the issue of learning from others and preventing 'reinvention of the wheel'. The second is concerned to ensure that training fits the context in which it is to be applied.

Several practical approaches have been used to inform course content but also to guide the way a particular course is delivered (Morrow and Hargie, 1995; Hargie and Morrow, 1995). In addition to the direct observation methods discussed in the previous chapter, these include:

- a literature search to identify tactics, skills and strategies employed during particular types of interpersonal encounters (e.g. negotiating situations);
- video analysis (where available) of sequences of practitioner–patient encounters to note effective and ineffective displays of communicative performance allied to the programme of training to be instituted;
- direct pre-course consultation with trainees to identify situations where particular skills are required and the problems associated with those encounters;
- experiences of comparative training where it exists.

8.3 COMPONENTS OF SENSITIZATION

Essentially, sensitization is the instructive phase of the CST paradigm, prior to practice, where trainees are provided with information that allows them to develop concepts of effective behaviour and set performance standards. Instruction therefore involves, firstly, the transmission of substantive information or salient features about social behaviours (e.g. the labelling or description of behaviour) and, secondly, the identification of performance goals or standards as a means of inducing or guiding trainees' subsequent performance.

Sensitization comprises two main components: sensitization of the trainees to the actual programme of CST itself, and sensitization to the specific skill components that form the substance of training. This latter dimension of the process can be further characterized in terms of skill analysis and skill discrimination. In addition, skill discrimination represents the behaviour-modelling component of sensitization, of which descriptive and demonstrative models are the instructive agents. For some courses, however, a third component can be introduced, that of sensitization of trainees to their current level of skill, thereby providing a personal baseline from which to work and assess progress (Figure. 8.1). Each of these aspects will be discussed.

Figure 8.1 also indicates the various processes through which sensitization is effected. These processes incorporate both pedagogical and andragogical models of education. In the former it is the teacher who takes primary responsibility for delivering the tuition, with the learner being the passive recipient of instruction. This is sometimes referred to as the 'jug and mug' approach. The andragogical model, on the other hand, 'treats the learning–teaching transaction as the mutual responsibility of learners and teacher. In fact the teacher's role is redefined as that of a procedural technician, resource person, coinquirer; more a catalyst than an instructor, more a guide than a wizard' (Knowles, 1980, p. 48).

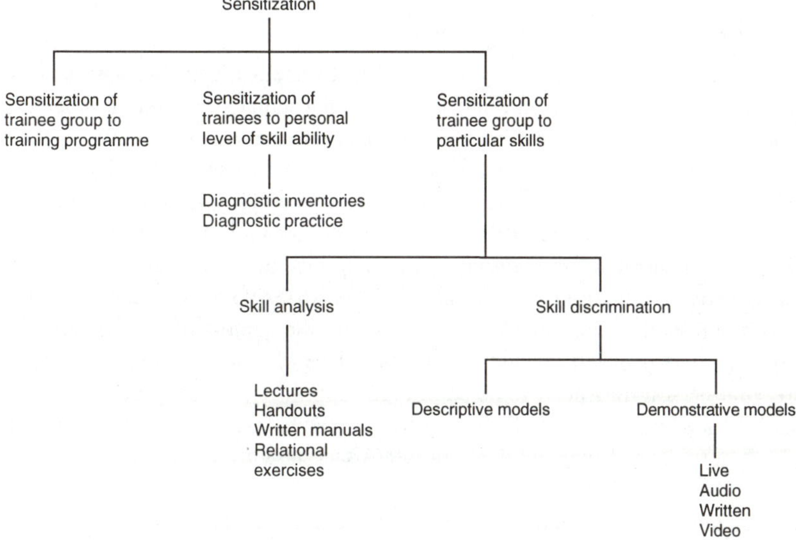

Figure 8.1 Components of the sensitization process.

8.3.1 Sensitization to the training programme

At this stage trainees are alerted to the actual methodology of the training process in which they are about to participate including the theoretical antecedents that underpin the training techniques and strategies employed. Aims and objectives of training need to be established and agreed in order to provide trainees with a clear view of what they should achieve, and also to provide personal assessment markers during the CST course. Central to this aspect of sensitization is the fact that trainees need to be made aware that a participatory learning approach will be a key feature of the overall programme. Thus efforts should be made to encourage trainees to contribute to the process through, for example, group discussion, requesting and asking and providing homework assignments.

In addition, practical exercises that sensitize trainees to various dimensions of the communication process, within the context of health care, can be used to initially produce non-threatening participation. For example, exercises that explore the various dimensions of health and their implications for interpersonal communication can be used in this regard (Chapter 2). Another aspect of this phase is, for example, the use of video to film and then replay some group discussions, in order to allow trainees to assimilate how they look and sound on film prior to role-play with CCTV. The use of video for such purposes is discussed further in Chapter 9.

8.3.2 Sensitization to current skill level

At the outset of a course it may be possible to use a diagnostic approach to allow participants to gauge baseline ability in a particular skill area, or indeed to provide the trainer with some background data on each trainee relative to their perceived level of skill. For example, written test measures that include an established and validated inventory of items can be employed to permit trainees to compare their skill status with existing test norms and with a peer group.

While the majority of trainees enjoy the challenge of such inventories and are keen to know the outcome, care must be taken to explain the meaning of the results and how they are to be interpreted within the context of practice and the training course itself. If an individual should receive a particularly negative score, that person may need some additional support or encouragement, or have concerns or anxieties to be allayed by the trainer before training can proceed. Thus trainers need to have worked out in advance how they are going to handle such situations should they arise.

As an alternative, a diagnostic practice method can be used for the same purpose. Morrow and Hargie (1995), in a course on presentation skills, commenced training by giving participants a set topic on an everyday issue and asking them to give a 2 minute talk following 5 minutes of preparation. Each person was videotaped and the presentation was replayed and analysed to identify the pre-course strengths and weaknesses of individual performance. This also permitted participants to become familiar with the idea of seeing and hearing themselves on video and gave them insights into their ability to give an 'impromptu' presentation. Furthermore, it demonstrated the inherent difficulties of such performances and acted as an advance organizer for further practical exercises that featured in the course. Again, it must be stressed that in using the latter approach care must be exercised to ensure that feedback is supportive and not destructive.

8.3.3 Skill analysis

At this stage of sensitization the skill is described to trainees in verbal form, involving the use of live or recorded lectures, handouts and background reading. Here the purpose is to provide the trainee with some theoretical understanding of the skill, outline its functions in designated contexts, present relevant research findings, and analyse the behavioural components (e.g. the skill of non-verbal communication would include the behavioural components of positive facial expressions, touch, etc.). It should again be emphasized that this material needs to be presented within the framework of contemporary professional practice.

Lectures

Despite the fact that CST is often regarded as a 'high-tech' mode of instruction, being commonly associated with the use of CCTV and video recording facilities, the basic mechanism of skill analysis is undoubtedly the traditional lecture or lecturette. Although frequently maligned, Bligh (1971) concluded from available empirical evidence that this time-honoured teaching method was as effective as any other, with the possible exception of programmed learning, in the transmission of information. Several variants have been proposed by Jarvis and Gibson (1985) as appropriate for teaching health professionals. The extremely teacher-centred nature of the 'straight lecture' may reduce its appeal for more mature groups of practising professionals. The 'lecture-discussion' tends to be a more attractive option. This may involve creating discussion groups to consider pre-selected questions arising from the preceding address. However, 'if the trainer's presentation is too expository there will be little learner participation' (Law, 1991, p. 336). Alternatively more informal 'buzz' groups may be set up at different junctures in the course of the lecture to give trainees an opportunity to share their experiences, compare their understanding or air their opinions on some issue central to a targeted skill. Different audio-visual aids, including 'trigger' audio or videotapes, are a useful catalyst in promoting discussion among students and are used extensively as part of the sensitization procedure in CST.

Handouts and other readings

Often, because of time constraints placed on CST, it may be necessary to provide trainees with preparative reading prior to attending the course. Even if this is done it is necessary to review the material at the outset of training to consolidate its understanding. In addition it is helpful to prepare a checklist of the main features of the handout as an *aide memoire* and also as a reference guide for subsequent analysis of exemplars and role-play situations. Care is also required in producing reading material in that psychological and sociological terms need to be adequately defined, especially for those trainees who have not had any previous background in the social or behavioural sciences. Further, it is important to introduce students gradually to what for many will be a new area of training, otherwise they may feel overwhelmed by an unfamiliar topic.

Relational exercises

Relational exercises may be regarded as participatory activities that sensitize trainees to the actual components and use of skills without any recourse to professional knowledge or interactions. Essentially, they may be described as games, puzzles, brain teasers, skill tests or creative exercises, which, by their intrinsic nature, vividly portray elements of the communication process. They are not designed for skill practice but rather to create awareness of the actual components of an individual skill. In this respect they are relational, since the trainer can use these generic exercises to draw parallels with the actual practice situation. Thus, for example, in Exercise 4.2 the trainer can clearly illustrate the problems of listening within the context of an experiential, non-professional situation. The value of this approach is fourfold. Firstly, it is highly motivating for trainees in that they are keen to be seen to be successful in what appear to be quite straightforward exercises. Secondly, because the exercises do not directly draw on or test professional knowledge they are non-threatening and trainees can involve themselves fully in the experience. Thirdly, they are a potent method of ensuring that trainees actually remember core elements of the topic under discussion. Finally, this form of experiential learning allows trainees to pinpoint its relationship to their own professional practice, by drawing links between simulated and real interpersonal communication. Simulation exercises are considered more fully in Chapter 9.

8.3.4 Skill discrimination

This involves providing trainees with practical examples of the skill in action, thereby enabling them to critically analyse its behavioural components, evaluate its effectiveness and be prepared, in a particular practice context, to operationalize that information. This can either involve 'live' modelling, where the lecturer enacts the skill in class, or, more usually, videotaped models of the skill being used. Alternatively, audiotaped models could be used or written transcripts of patient–practitioner dialogues could be introduced to exemplify each skill. Such models form the focus for group discussions during this phase and their use will be described in greater detail later in this chapter. That the acquisition of social behaviour is facilitated by imitating or modelling the behaviour of others has been well established. However, there is considerable work involved in preparing suitable exemplar models for a CST programme, the practicalities of which will be discussed in a subsequent section of the chapter.

8.3.5 Modelling

Modelling may be defined as the process whereby an individual (the model) serves to illustrate behaviour that can be initiated or adapted by another individual (the observer). Essentially, it serves three basic purposes. Firstly, it stimulates the learning of new skills or behaviours and secondly, it encourages the strengthening or weakening of previously learned behaviour through disinhibition or inhibition of performance. Thus, at one level, it is creative in that it exposes the learner to a range of skills not previously known or practised. At another level it is actually therapeutic or developmental in that 'good' behaviour can be enhanced or refined while negative behaviours can be attenuated. A third purpose is that of response facilitation. The effect of this latter objective 'is to increase behaviours that the observer has already learned and for which there are no existing constraints or inhibitions. The effect of the model is simply to provide an information cue that triggers similar behaviour on the part of the observer' (Perry and Furukawa, 1986, pp. 69–70).

Modelling theory and practice is based on the principle that people are influenced by observing the behaviour of others. Thus in viewing others, learning or reading about them, we gain information about their behaviour, which may mean that our own behaviour is modified as a result. Baum and Gray (1992), in an experimental study of the effectiveness of various methods in acquiring basic listening skills, showed that the contribution of an 'expert' appears most influential in skill gain terms. In their investigation, 48 female college students were divided into four equal but randomly assigned study groups. Following a recorded pretest with a model client and subsequent evaluation, all students were given handouts on listening skills and each group was subjected to one of four videotapes:

- an experienced therapist giving a didactic explanation of the use of the skills, with examples of therapist–client interactions (expert lecture group);
- an experienced therapist talking with a client, demonstrating the target skills during the consultation (expert model group);
- a novice interviewer talking with a client and including both appropriate and inappropriate communication behaviours (novice model group);
- the videotape of her own pretest (own model group).

Following their exposure to teaching, each student was given a post-test similar to the pretest but with a different client. Again both student reaction to the interview and the interview itself were formally evaluated. Statistical analysis of the results showed that all the training approaches used resulted in a significant increase in the use of facilitative responses, but the group observing the expert model improved more than any of the other groups. These workers strongly advocate the use of such models in the training of practitioners.

Bandura (1977) has suggested that modelling requires an individual to attend to the behaviour of another, to remember what has been observed, to have the capacity to imitate that behaviour and to be motivated to subsequently enact it. Thus, attention, retention, reproduction and motivation represent four crucial stages in the modelling process, and ways of maximizing each must be considered by the trainer.

Attention

Although attention alone does not guarantee that new behaviours will result, it is a necessary condition for modelling to occur. The characteristics of the observer and the setting influence receptivity to the modelled behaviours. Thus, the observer needs to be aware and comprehending of the modelled performance in an environment conducive to such activity. Dowrick and Jesdale (1991) pointed out that 'observation requires capable and alert faculties, and the development of abilities to learn from modelling opportunities. . . . An optimal level of arousal, as in most learning settings, is to be stimulated moderately above rest, with minimal distractions, and supportive company' (p. 66).

In order to focus attention it is important that the observer is not swamped with learning points, but that those which are made are clear and vivid. It is also important to note that the availability of models who exhibit a certain type of behaviour will influence what is learned. Thus, in a one-to-one training situation, trainees will tend to imitate the behaviours of senior colleagues, on the basis that there are no other models available. This, of course, may pose difficulties, in that there will be a limited repertoire of behaviours from which to learn, and what will work for one individual may not necessarily work for another because of differences in personality, style, attitudes, etc. As a result, in any training programme a range of models displaying competent behaviours should be depicted, thus enhancing the likelihood of the trainee identifying with at least one of them. It is imperative, though, that multiple models are broadly consistent.

The functional value of any behaviour as observed by a trainee will also affect attention. The outcomes of interactions are important in that behaviours which, for example, gain patient confidence, produce new clinical information or enhance therapy are more likely to be attended to and remembered. Linked to this is the idea that if behaviour is rewarded or praised it will be observed more closely. In addition, research evidence suggests that the attractiveness of the model to the observer affects attentiveness. Models are more effective when they are similar to the observer in terms of gender, age, class, culture, knowledge and experience (Hargie and Saunders, 1983). Identification with the model is therefore important, and it is for this reason that students are more likely to identify with newly qualified practitioners than with more mature ones. At the same time there is evidence to suggest that higher-status models may produce greater modelling efficacy (McCullagh, 1986). The reasons may be due to their ability to mediate attention and retention, provided they do not detract from the replicability of demonstrated performance (Dowrick and Jesdale, 1991).

Retention

As well as attending to displayed behaviours, trainees must remember them if they are to be reproduced. Bandura (1977) posited that retention processes contribute to the learning of modelled responses and their accurate reproduction. Essentially the retention process involves the representation and cognitive organization of behaviours (i.e. they are represented in the memory in either an imaginal or verbal form). With skill elements that are primarily non-verbal, the former system is likely to be particularly important. In addition, this process also includes observers visualizing or imagining themselves performing the behaviours that were previously seen performed by another individual. This is termed covert rehearsal (Goldstein and Sorcher, 1974). Overall, then, the moves in any sequence of behaviour are labelled and catalogued, providing a cognitive base from which performance can ensue. It is therefore important to involve trainees in analysis of modelled behaviour in order to develop more comprehensive frameworks from which interpersonal communication can be understood and self-performance modified to ensure more effective outcomes.

It should, however, be remembered that trainees come to the modelling process with already established views on interpersonal communication, such that there may be a refusal to accept any alternative other than the cognitive framework from which they already work. This may mean that the retention process is hampered. For example, a doctor may refuse to accept that interviewing patients across a surgery desk is in fact 'distancing' them, justifying it on the grounds that there have never been any problems with doing it that way, or that it allows greater control over consultations.

Reproduction

The reproductive stage of modelling concerns the capacity to perform the behaviours which have been observed. It therefore involves converting symbolic representations into appropriate action. Behavioural enactment can be viewed as comprising three separate but associated phases: (1) cognitive organization of responses, (2) their actual initiation and (3) their monitoring and refinement on the basis of informative feedback. Thus an individual moves from mental organization and rehearsal of behaviour through to critical appraisal of action whereby flaws in behaviour can be identified, excluded or modified to improve the overall performance. External reinforcement may also be provided for positive behaviours.

At this point it is important to emphasize three points. Firstly, observational learning does not mean that observers can carry out any given behaviour perfectly first time, or that they necessarily become replicas of the model. A combination of practice coupled with feedback may be necessary before performance is perfected, and indeed each person brings something of him or herself to each behaviour, such that it is subtly different from the actual model. Secondly, the amount of observational learning exhibited behaviourally partly depends on the availability of component skills. This means that if deficits exist in the basic skills required for complex performances these must first be developed by modelling and practice before moving to more complex routines (Baldwin and Baldwin, 1981). One implication for CST might be that basic skills (e.g. questioning) need to be mastered before introducing trainees to higher-order strategies such as counselling. Thirdly, reproduction will only occur where the observer or trainee is sufficiently motivated to imitate the modelled behaviour.

Motivation

The motivational process is important to the concept of modelling. Individuals are more likely to adopt modelled behaviour if results are valued rather than if they are accompanied by unrewarding or punishing effects. Thus greater modelling will tend to occur, for example, where the model controls rewards or resources desired by the trainee (i.e. is of higher recognized status, is better paid, has more power, etc.). However, Bandura (1977) suggested that imitative learning can occur without reinforcement, in that people may observe, code and retain patterns of behaviour that can be reproduced at a later time even when not rewarded. Such behaviour is unlikely to emerge, though, unless there is sufficient incentive. While reinforcement is not a prerequisite for learning to take place it can have a facilitating effect at each of the stages of the modelling process. Anticipation of reinforcement can influence what is observed and behaviours that have been seen to have positive consequences will be more likely to receive increased attention. The prospect of reinforcement can also promote retention by inducing the observer to implement effective symbolic procedures and engage in rehearsal. In designing models it is therefore important to incorporate motivational features in order to enhance and facilitate learning.

From the trainer's perspective it is important to guide and support the trainee through each of these stages of the modelling process, in order to maximize the potential for acquiring effective repertoires of behaviour in given situations. Failure of an observer to match the behaviour of a model may result from:

- not observing the relevant behaviour displayed;
- inadequately coding modelled events for memory representation;
- failing to retain what was learned;
- physical inability to perform;
- experiencing insufficient incentives.

8.3.6 Types of model

As has been indicated (Figure 8.1), models have been characterized as either descriptive or demonstrative. Ellis and Whittington (1981) have differentiated between the two, suggesting that while the latter present, by means of videotape, audiotape or in written form, the original verbal and non-verbal behaviour, descriptive models operate at a more abstract level by presenting an account of that behaviour. As such, descriptive models are one step removed from the communicative performance they represent.

Descriptive models

Descriptive models, as the name implies, are written or verbal analyses of communication behaviour. They describe or label the behaviours both in terms of what they are and their effects and outcomes in any interaction. Thus, for example, statements that reflect back to a patient in alternative language what he/she has previously said may be labelled as reflective listening, but also could be described in terms of demonstrating interest, concern or understanding, and also facilitating additional patient expression. To some extent, therefore, descriptive models are both evaluative and interpretative in their presentation, and by their very nature seek to enhance the trainee's awareness and understanding of communication behaviour in various situations. At the same time, evaluative and interpretative statements of behaviour on their own may be inadequate to produce imitative behaviour. The ability to reproduce particular behaviours depends fundamentally on knowing what those behaviours actually are. Thus, descriptive models should ideally be used alongside examples of performance, thereby providing both account and analysis.

Descriptive models may be provided orally during lectures and also by means of written handouts, either as prior reading material or as summaries of the lecture input. An elaboration of the handout approach is the production of self-instructional packages whereby trainees undertake independent, self-paced learning in communication skills. Such written material can be accompanied by model videotaped sequences, thus incorporating demonstrations from the practice situation in a recorded form. Chandler (1989) described the use of an instructional videotape to teach medication interview techniques with older people, incorporating labelled behaviour and triggered discussion and supported by a written manual.

Demonstration models

As indicated in Figure. 8.1 there are two main types of demonstration model: live models and recorded models. In both cases, the actual behaviour to be acquired is presented. For the purposes of discussion a third subsection has been incorporated, that of interactive video. In practical terms this approach bridges both model approaches and is an increasingly used medium in the training field.

Live models

In this situation the trainer, a trainee or a third party enacts the behaviour to be modelled in front of the class. In the health-care context this is likely to be a portrayal of a practitioner–patient consultation designed to sensitize trainees to the behaviour of the professional and the outcomes of such behaviour. It also facilitates an understanding of patient behaviour in such situations. Live models offer flexibility in the sensitization phase and are usually inexpensive to produce. They do not, however, offer the same degree of control as can be obtained with a recorded scenario, where the action can literally be stopped and discussion can ensue before proceeding with the remainder of the interaction. However, standardized patients, trained to present a simulated clinical situation for teaching or testing purposes, can provide extremely valuable insights to the understanding of consultation behaviours. Swanson and Stillman (1990) have reviewed the use of standardized patients, noting their particular value in teaching medical interviewing.

In addition, live modelling may be less controlled, in that responses are totally reactive to a situation, while recorded models do offer the opportunity to script the action in order to more specifically programme learning. Another factor here is the lack of exact reproduction of live role-play. A further consideration is the environment in which the modelling takes place, since a classroom setting does not necessarily mimic the actual practice situation and to that extent may not create face validity with trainees, who may be well aware of, for example, various forms of distraction occurring in the workplace.

Recorded models

Recorded models come in three forms, written transcripts, audio recordings and video recordings. It is, however, now more common to have video recordings of modelling behaviour than audio recordings. Moreover, in a review of research into clinical interviewing, Carroll and Monroe (1980) reported that standardized presentations of illustrative patient interviews are more effective as teaching aids than live, spontaneous demonstrations of patient consultations. As Morrow (1986) pointed out, 'the use of videotaped exemplars is likely to be more consistent and efficient than live unrehearsed interactions designed to illustrate certain skills or concepts' (p. 343). The potential uses of video exemplars for modelling may be summarized as follows:

- presenting information for observational learning to trainees;
- highlighting models of positive and negative interpersonal skill use;
- stimulating group discussion;
- giving trainees a common learning experience;
- illustrating self-instructional modules/units/packages;
- stimulating trainee self-awareness;
- stimulating trainee awareness of patients' goals and feelings;
- providing insights into the real-world environment.

Written dialogues of either real or fictional practitioner–patient consultations can also be provided for trainees, thereby allowing skill discrimination to be effected. Here it must be remembered that the non-verbal aspects of communication are substantially excluded, so that learning will be more limited than if a video recording had been used. Written materials are obviously cheaper to prepare than video recorded models, as well as providing a more permanent record for the trainee to return to for subsequent revision, clarification and consolidation of learning. Exercise 8.1 is an example of how a demonstrative model in the form of a transcript may be used to critically analyse and evaluate the effectiveness of particular practitioner behaviour in a health-care setting.

Exercise 8.1 Skill discrimination using a written demonstration model

Instructions

The trainer should provide trainees with a written dialogue of an actual practitioner–patient interaction chosen for its portrayal of particular behaviours (e.g. interviewing technique). The following questions, aimed at examining questioning behaviour, can be used to guide discussion of the key elements of the interaction.

1. Count the number of questions asked by both the patient and practitioner.
2. Identify and categorize each of the practitioner's questions as being either closed, open, leading or multiple. Then judge whether the question is also a probe and identify the type of probe.
3. Describe the implications of the various types of question and evaluate their influence upon the consultation.
4. Determine to what extent the consultation focused upon physical or psychosocial issues.
5. Identify how and in what ways the questioning approach of the practitioner could have been modified to improve the consultation.

This approach can be expanded to analyse other forms of behaviour within the same interaction (e.g. listening, self-disclosure, reinforcement, etc). The technique can equally well be applied to the analysis of audio- and video-recorded models.

As has been indicated, recorded models offer more control to the trainer in conducting trainees through the different learning elements. Indeed because of the editing opportunities that video presents it is possible to use visual cueing techniques to label individual behaviours on the TV screen throughout a given scenario for the benefit of trainees. Furthermore, it is possible to use such cues on screen to alert trainees to particular elements in the action. The greater control that video models give also permits trainers the facility to 'freeze' the action to draw attention to some feature of non-verbal communication, to discuss what has gone before or challenge trainees to consider how best the professional should respond. Video exemplars allow the trainer to feature a wider range of models than would be easily possible through live modelling. They also guarantee reproduction of behaviour, which is not always possible with live demonstrations. Indeed, we now live in a 'television age' and people do learn readily from TV.

There are also certain disadvantages of recorded models, some of which have been identified by Eisler and Frederiksen (1980). As previously indicated, videos can be costly to produce both in financial terms and also in respect of the time commitment required. However, it should be remembered that in recording either real or simulated practitioner–patient interactions it is possible to largely accept the behaviour enacted. This is on the basis that what is being sought is not 'the perfect performance' but rather a performance that will stimulate constructive and instructive discussion. This reduces the time-commitment that may be required to produce and film 'perfect' consultations and, as will be discussed later, enhances the face-validity and impact of the whole presentation.

A second disadvantage is that in having exemplar material available there may be a tendency for the trainer to rely too heavily on this mode of learning to the extent that trainees become overloaded with taped material and fewer learning points are remembered. Finally, the production and use of audio or video recording demands that consent is obtained from those involved. The ethical issues surrounding recorded material are fully discussed in Chapter 7.

Interactive video

Interactive video (IV) is a relatively recent addition to the technology of interpersonal skills training. While its contribution to the training process is potentially broader, it is at the sensitization stage that it is presently held to be most useful (Schroeder *et al.*, 1986). As such, it holds out much promise as an efficient method of assisting participants in the task of skill discrimination. Interactive video is the product of the coming together of two powerful technologies, represented by the computer and video. The video medium contributes the realism and impact of the moving image, coupled with accompanying sound. The computer offers not only text and graphics but flexible control of the accessing of material, making meaningful interaction with it possible. Take the simple example of students learning to discriminate between open and closed questions using IV. They watch a segment of an interview between a nurse and a patient. At a certain point they are prompted to identify the type of question just used by the nurse. Having made their selection, and depending upon their accuracy, the programme may take them on through the interview or branch into a remedial sequence, which, let's say, provides further information on open and closed questions, together with opportunities to identify more obvious examples of both types, before rejoining the nurse–patient dialogue. Examples of programmes of this type have been described for improving the interviewing skills of student educational psychologists (Cummings, Hansen and Sillings, 1990) and systems analysts (Alexander, Whittingham and Peppard, 1993). *The Suicidal Adolescent* is a further example, described by Cavalier (1991), designed to help medical students interview troubled adolescents.

The original IV set-up comprised a videotape recorder, monitor and small computer, the latter being used to regulate the viewing sequence. Later developments have exploited the advantages of the videodisc over the earlier tape format, permitting the storage of substantial information in a visual database, which can be quickly, easily and flexibly accessed. The advent of CD-ROM (compact disc read only memory) opens up a whole new horizon of exciting multimedia possibilities, combining huge quantities of text, video, graphics, voice, etc. on a single disc. The complexity and ease of access of branches through the programme is also greatly enhanced.

Several detailed reviews of the outcomes of IV-based instruction have been conducted, including meta-analytic studies by Fletcher (1990) and McNeil and Nelson (1991). The results suggest that it is both an efficient and effective technique, although it seems that programme-controlled versions are more successful than those that are learner-controlled. A number of investigations have explicitly focused upon the application of IV to the acquisition of interpersonal skills. One of the most recent is that by Martin, Jones and Hearn (1994), who tested its effects in comparison to a variety of more traditional instructional techniques typically employed as part of skill sensitization. Subjects were university undergraduates improving their negotiating skills. While students who made use of IV found it an attractive way to learn, and responded positively to it, no marked superiority in actual conceptual learning was evident over students who had a more usual sensitization experience with videos and an instructor. Martin, Jones and Hearn (1994) suggested that it may be in cost-effectiveness terms that the advantages of IV come to the fore, especially in teaching simple concepts to do with basic skills.

Summary

Overall, then, demonstrative models have a crucial part to play in modelling behaviour. As pointed out in Chapter 5 one picture may be worth 1000 words but a demonstration is worth 1000 pictures. Thus demonstrative models may have greater potential to help long-term retention than descriptive models. They also foster attention and are motivating for trainees. These three factors of retention, attention and motivation contribute, as will be recalled, to the reproduction of desired behaviour in trainees.

Homework

One further way of consolidating the sensitization phase is the assignment-type approach, whereby the trainee is given homework to complete prior to the next training session. Here trainees are encouraged to continue the process of skill discrimination through written problems or observational learning. The exercises given to trainees may be structured in such a way as to cause them to think critically of the interactions to be conducted. Observation of actual practitioner–patient interactions may be used to focus attention on specific behaviours of communication and their impact on the consultation. Alternatively, written dialogues of interactions may be presented to trainees for analysis and report back at the next session (Exercise 8.1). Homework may also involve trainees writing a short essay on the use of a particular skill in their professional situation (e.g. explaining skills in patient education). A further example of a homework type assignment is given in Exercise 8.2.

Exercise 8.2 Questioning technique

Instructions

Each trainee should be asked to identify the type of leading question given below and suggest an alternative wording of the question to eliminate the 'lead'.

- 'I take it you've found the speech therapy sessions helpful, Mrs Hamilton?'
- 'You're not having any pain are you, Mr Sloan?'
- 'You would, I think, want to give your children fluoride drops to strengthen their teeth, wouldn't you?'
- 'Do you get these headaches frequently?'
- 'After your operation for varicose veins, did you take regular walks?'

For discussion

Trainees should be asked to submit their reworded questions to the trainee group for review and analysis. Trainees should seek to identify the problems and implications of the above questions and to what extent the alternative questions overcame these difficulties. The limitations of the suggested alternatives should also be identified.

Falloon *et al.* (1977) demonstrated the effectiveness of homework as a form of learning in a study of social skill training of outpatient groups. Those who were given structured homework assignments did better on nearly all of the outcome measures taken.

8.4 USES OF INSTRUCTIONAL TAPES

There are several ways in which recorded exemplars can he used during CST. It is important for trainers to consider using such material as creatively as possible, since to merely show a series of videotaped scenarios may in itself become repetitive and demotivating for trainees, especially if there is little stimulus variation to the presentation. Instructional tapes can be employed in four main ways.

8.4.1 Self-instructional packages

In this instance trainees are provided with self-contained recorded material, which can be replayed in their own time, accompanied by written explanatory literature. While this approach may be favoured, particularly in situations where the curriculum is already crowded, it does in fact suffer from serious deficiencies. In the first place, for such an approach to work successfully, sufficient playback facilities are needed. Secondly, in what is a very practical area of training the self-instructional method is primarily directed at the cognitive level at the possible expense of performative learning. Thirdly, to attempt to develop interpersonal skills in isolation appears to be a peculiar approach to this area of professional competence, in that skills can best be refined and improved through structured feedback in the interpersonal dimensions of practice (Hargie and Morrow, 1986a).

8.4.2 Brief vignettes during lectures

Here a brief episode of recorded material is shown, the object being to illustrate a point rather than to explain. Each vignette needs to be closely linked to the elements of the lecture and is specifically chosen to emphasize a particular point or issue or to provoke discussion from trainees. When used in this way it encourages participation by trainees, thereby fostering a wider exploration of the subject under discussion. Thus exemplar material can be used to stimulate and motivate participants to involve themselves fully in the training programme, while at the same time creating a valuable learning experience.

8.4.3 Opening/closing lectures

As well as interspersing taped material throughout a presentation, exemplars of this type can be used with good effect at the beginning or end of a lecture. For example, showing a tape at the start of a lecture will stimulate attention and provide a focus for the session. Similarly at the end of a lecture it can be used to recap and reinforce the points already presented, and to send the trainees away with the topic fresh in their minds. As has already been stated, it is important not to overload trainees with taped material such that a number of important points are forgotten simply because of the volume of material presented.

8.4.4 Role-play stimuli

Role-play as a popular method of skill practice will be discussed in detail in the following chapter. It is relevant to mention here, however, that an effective technique of introducing a particular role-play scenario and stimulating participation in it is through the presentation of appropriate videotaped material to the group.

8.4.5 Model tapes

These are positive instances of practice shown with the intention of illustrating for trainees what to do and to what standards. As mentioned earlier, there is seldom a requirement for exact replication of such performance. Alternatively, negative models can also be provided to help trainees discriminate effective practice. Baldwin (1992) reported that trainees exposed only to positive models performed significantly better in terms of their ability to reproduce the modelled behaviour than did a similar group of trainees who viewed both positive and negative exemplars. However, the latter group were significantly better in the transfer or generalization of their learning to contexts outside the learning environment. On the basis that generalization from specific to widely varied situations is a desirable outcome of skills training, the use of positive and negative models would seem the most appropriate.

8.4.6 Trigger tapes

While model tapes can be used in the ways described above, it is important to distinguish them from what are known as trigger videos. These are shorter video recordings, often only a few seconds long, designed particularly to stimulate discussion on particular behaviours or to initiate the 'What would you do next?' challenge. As such, in themselves they do not usually provide models of performance. Indeed Biggs (1991) draws the distinction between modelling material, which shows instances of appropriate behaviour, and triggers, which often portray difficult situations involving the use of inappropriate behaviour. He goes on to point out that the use of triggers 'should promote recognition of the problem but not subsequently encourage participants to copy or to act out the scene' (p. 207).

8.5 SOURCES OF INSTRUCTIONAL TAPES

Model tapes are available from a number of sources. In the first instance a wide range of commercial tapes are available to trainers on topics such as interviewing, handling bereavement, dealing with aggression, counselling and negotiating, among others. Some of these are generic in nature in that they do not focus specifically on any professional group (e.g. Hargie and Bamford, 1993). Others are produced to directly address the needs of a particular profession (e.g. Morrow and Hargie, 1988a).

Commercial tapes may not always be appropriate for the trainee group in that there may be differences in culture between the people and situations depicted on the recording and the trainees. For example, material produced in the USA may not mirror a European situation, and indeed within countries there may be wide regional variation such that it will be important to present model videos with which trainees can easily identify.

Consequently, we would recommend that trainees give consideration to producing their own tapes, since regional variations in culture, dialect or practice can be depicted, thus enhancing the face validity of the recordings. While it does require a certain level of expertise and time commitment to produce one's own tapes, the results are usually well worth the effort.

A third source of practice-related video recordings is role-plays that have been video recorded during training. However, before using such material it is imperative that the trainer obtain written permission from those involved in the role-plays before showing them to another audience. Even if permission is given, the trainer, in using these tapes, should always alert other trainees that the performance of the individual recorded was in the context of a training situation, and that it does not necessarily mirror real practice. This is especially true if the exemplar shown depicts poor communication performance.

8.5.1 Self-produced instructional tapes

Mention has already been made of the value of the trainer producing model tapes specifically designed to meet the requirements of a particular trainee group. It is possible to produce these exemplars using a minimum of equipment and it certainly does not require the involvement of a professional production team. All that is required is a camera, a video recorder, two clip-on microphones (or one omnidirectional microphone), a spotlight (optional, depending upon the camera) and a television monitor. Of course a second camera would allow an alternative perspective of the interaction to be filmed but it also means that the material either needs to be 'mixed' as it is shot or edited at a subsequent date in the studio. The latter procedure is both expensive and time-consuming and is usually employed only if the material is subsequently to be marketed.

For those embarking on the production of model tapes, the five Cs of cinematography elaborated 30 years ago are worth noting (Mascelli, 1965). These are:

- Camera shots, the basic unit of communication;
- Continuity – the principles governing how individual shots are linked together to produce a logical flow of the story over time;
- Cutting or editing – the procedures for placing the shots in the finished tape;
- Close-ups;
- Composition – the framing of shots.

Although such exemplars can be produced with relative ease there are a number of important practical points that any trainer should carefully consider before embarking on filming. The first thing required is a detailed plan of all the interactions to be enacted. At one level it requires the trainer to have prepared 'loose' scripts of all the encounters by way of a guide to role-play participants as to how the interaction should be developed. Alternatively, what may be required is a more formal presentation of a script including detailed notes for the setting up of each individual shot, the duration of the action, props, etc. However, this would only tend to be necessary where very discrete elements of performance were being recorded, the intention being to edit these together into an overall scene.

At a second level, a timetable needs to be prepared of the order in which scenarios are to be filmed so that a rota can be worked out among the actors as to when they are required. A second factor that needs to be considered in the planning stage is that all recordings in one area should be completed before moving into another location (e.g. ward situation to office situation). A third factor to address at the planning stage is to identify what props or dress (e.g. uniforms) will be required in order to make the role-play completely authentic. Failure to do this will inevitably mean that the scenario, no matter how good it may be, will suffer from a lack of credibility and will be open to criticism by trainees.

The selection of actors is also an important factor in preparing model tapes, since the quality of the finished product is dependent upon their acting ability. It is possible to use professional actors in such circumstances but that is usually costly and there may also be difficulties in these people conveying, without considerable rehearsal, real credibility, especially in the practitioner's role, where technical language and know-how may be involved. The use of naturally good performers within the profession or individuals who have undergone CST is perhaps the ideal as far as choice of actors is concerned since these people will appreciate the nuances of the communication process and will have a ready understanding of what is required of them. Those who have undergone CST will also have already experienced role-play and to that extent will not be camera shy. They should be able to 'get into roles' quickly and adapt any written scenario to fit their own personalities and previous experience in the real practice environment. Furthermore, in contrast to professional actors, these individuals are totally convincing in their practitioner's role in that they are literally 'playing themselves'.

Scripts are, however, useful in determining the overall pattern of any interaction, and the more structured role-play approach (Hargie and Morrow, 1986a) is likely to produce the best results. Here the nature of the interaction, based on a loose script, is worked out in detail and discussed with all the actors. At the same time spontaneity is encouraged so that, as indicated, 'stiffness' in acting or the 'script-bound' phenomenon is reduced.

With regard to the technicalities of filming, little detailed knowledge is required to produce tapes of reasonable quality. Obviously, it is important to ensure satisfactory sound levels, which can often pose most difficulties, and also that the camera operator focuses upon the relevant behaviours of those taking part. Spotlights are also useful, but with a light-sensitive camera this may not actually be necessary. Finally, the environment in which the recordings are made is quite crucial in order to provide face validity for trainees. Although it is often possible to simulate a real environment it usually is extremely costly to do so effectively. Thus, it is usually necessary to film interactions in the real practice context (i.e. the ward, the home, the pharmacy, the consulting room, etc.). This means that filming on location will demand careful attention to detail at the preparation stage, even down to the degree of cabling that will be required for the equipment. For further information on the production of video exemplar tapes, the reader is referred to O'Dell, 1991.

8.6 MODELLING CONSIDERATIONS

In using various forms of model tape, trainers should give consideration to a number of factors. Firstly, mention has been already made of the importance of using models with which trainees can closely identify in terms of gender, class, knowledge and experience. Secondly, it is important that models should be seen to cope successfully in the practice situation. Moreover, they should be seen to improve with time rather than being perfect at the outset. The advantage of this approach is that trainees are given realistic behavioural targets to meet, with their own performance progressively improving along with the models. Thirdly, skilled behaviour should be seen to be rewarded in that trainees are more likely to imitate the behaviour of successful people.

Fourthly, while a positive approach in modelling is important it can be useful for trainees to view scenarios of 'how not to do it' (i.e. negative exemplars). The use of negative exemplars is cautioned in that one danger of using this type of model is that the trainee can actually copy negative behaviour. As Hargie and Morrow (1986b) point out, 'this danger is particularly prevalent where the negative model is not grossly incompetent and the trainee, who is also inexperienced, actually identifies with the weak model. Where negative models are to be employed, therefore, they should be markedly incompetent' (p. 66).

Fifthly, negative models should never be shown without being counterbalanced by positive models. Indeed, positive models should be longer and be shown more often than negative exemplars. Here the object is to highlight and reinforce positive behaviour while illustrating the consequences of inappropriate interpersonal communication. This is best achieved by demonstrating positive and negative approaches to the same situation, thereby visually illustrating some of the strategies that can be used to ensure more successful and satisfactory outcomes. Consequently positive models will be most successful if they:

- depict a variety of models;
- are vividly presented and not 'hidden' within a range of other behaviours;
- are shown frequently, particularly where complex behaviour is involved;
- are explained by 'cueing' techniques which draw attention to the features of behaviour to be modelled;
- end with a restatement of the essential learning points.

8.7 OVERVIEW

Sensitization is the initial stage of the training sequence. Its functions are to provide trainees with a broad introduction to CST and the aims, objectives and content of the particular programme that they will follow. More specifically, it is intended to provide them with a theoretical appreciation and sound working knowledge of each of the skills focused upon. This is achieved through the processes of skill analysis and discrimination. Modelling is a central facet of the latter. It has been defined as the process whereby one person learns behaviour patterns through observing them being performed by another person. The process of modelling has been shown to be a critical feature of social learning. This chapter has sought to explore the dimensions of the sensitization phase, with particular emphasis on the conceptual and practical aspects of the modelling process. Moreover, guidelines have been presented for trainers relating to the preparation and use of descriptive and demonstrative models in CST, with a special focus on the production and application of recorded videotaped models.

The practice phase of training

9

9.1 INTRODUCTION

According to Johnson (1990, p. 21), 'To learn an interpersonal skill you must first see the need for the interpersonal skill, then understand what the skill and its component parts are, and finally practise, practise, practise until the skill. . . does not require conscious thought'. Sensitization can, therefore, be thought of as a necessary but not sufficient condition for the promotion of skilled behaviour. By their very nature, skills must be worked at in a practical way if performance is to improve. It is therefore to training issues surrounding skill practice that this chapter is devoted.

Following sensitization, participants should have essentially a broad understanding of the CST procedure, a realization of the structure and content of the particular programme that they will follow and an awareness of its relevance in equipping them to meet the demands on their communicative competence that they will experience, or perhaps already have experienced, in their chosen profession. More particularly, they should have a knowledge of the specific skill being concentrated upon at that point in training, its characteristics, components and functions in various relevant interpersonal contexts, together with an awareness of the principles that govern its use. These are typically derived from the theoretical underpinning of the skill. Some appreciation of the appropriateness of different behaviours in particular situations and standards of performance that pertain will also take place during sensitization. As a result, and in relation to outcome, it would be perfectly reasonable to expect students to be able to talk knowledgeably about the skill, to write an essay on it, to make judgements on the effectiveness of its use by another, indeed to make a good attempt at doing it. To anticipate a full-blown and highly polished performance at the first attempt, however, would normally be unrealistically ambitious except with the most basic of content.

Trainees must be given opportunities to practise if standards of behavioural proficiency are to be improved. A central premise of the deliberations of Ericsson, Krampe and Tesch-Romer (1993) on the acquisition of expert performance is that 'the level of performance an individual attains is directly related to the amount of deliberate practice. Hence, individuals seeking to maximize their performance within some time period should maximize the amount of deliberate practice they engage in during that period' (p. 370). Accordingly, Anastasi (1987, p. 748) advised, when conducting interpersonal training, that emphasis should be placed upon 'practical sessions in which the students practice the skill under the guidance of a skilled instructor'. Focusing more specifically on the development of counselling skills, Dryden and Feltham (1994) again advocated that sufficient training time be given over to practice.

The vast majority of the various training interventions that could readily be subsumed under the rubric of social or communication skills training reflect this axiom in their design. This was found to be the case by Kurtz and Marshall (1982) who undertook a survey of publications in this area over a 12-year period. A total of 141 studies was accessed in a variety of fields including medicine, social work and counselling. In a high percentage of cases skill practice played a central role in the instructional sequence. A similar survey conducted by Hargie and Morrow (1986a) in pharmacy schools in the UK and Ireland revealed consistent although less pronounced outcomes. Anderson and Sharpe (1991) reviewed 40 interventions designed to enhance practitioner–patient communication skills and reported that skill practice was the most frequently employed instructional technique. A further survey of communication skill training practices in British medical schools, by Frederikson and Bull (1992), likewise revealed that skill practice was a conspicuous part of the instruction provided, with role-play procedures receiving a special mention.

This chapter will cover some of the main functions of the practice component in CST, together with details of the various methods available, such as behaviour rehearsal, covert rehearsal, simulations, role-play and *in vivo* interaction. Advantages and disadvantages of each will be discussed and examples of exercises given that can be used with students. Practical procedures involved in the implementation of these methods will also be outlined. An important part of the chapter will be devoted to the use of observation and recording procedures, particularly video recording, and some of the steps that can be taken to maximize the potential of this stage and overcome common difficulties.

9.2 FUNCTIONS OF PRACTICE

A number of different objectives for having trainees practise skills during training has been offered. The more central of these have already been intimated but will be specified more explicitly in the following list. They include:

- **To facilitate the enactive element of skill acquisition**. By performing the various actions that go to make up the skill and experiencing the consequent kinaesthetic feedback, appropriate patterns of behaviour can be built up in keeping with underlying intentions. Care must be taken, though, to ensure that such procedures do not degenerate into the mere rote production of stereotypic behaviour to the neglect of the mechanisms which effect the selective application of appropriate skills in context.

- **To enable the outcomes of skill deployment to be experienced**. One possible reason for failing to make use of already acquired skills may be due to an inaccurate anticipation of negative consequences (e.g. the belief that listening to patients' anxieties and encouraging their ventilation will only exacerbate them).
- **To highlight incongruities between what trainees think they do and what is actually done**. Only through interacting and being made aware of their performance can discrepancies between trainees' intentions and actions be reduced.
- **To create a more realistic and personally meaningful appreciation of the circumstances surrounding skill deployment**. It is difficult to create this level of awareness through lectures or observing models – one has to experience it.
- **To effect changes in attitude**. By acting in a particular manner in accordance with a certain skill, more fundamental attitudinal adjustments may be created, which will serve to maintain that type of behaviour in future.
- **To enable the professional role for which the student is ultimately being trained to be 'tried out'**. The extent to which such opportunities are afforded will depend largely upon the type of practical experience provided.
- **To gain confidence**. Promoting feelings of self-confidence is an important but frequently overlooked aspect of CST. Bandura (1989) pointed out that failure to display appropriate levels of skill in a given situation may be due to the lack of a sense of self-efficacy, in other words, not having sufficient confidence in one's ability to put acquired skill to use.
- **To furnish broad insights into the complexities of certain social situations** and the rules and conventions that pertain.
- **To produce more lasting benefits from training**. It has been speculated that the outcomes of programmes lacking practice and feedback components may be less enduring.
- **To involve students more fully in the learning experience**. It is widely accepted that instruction is more successful under these circumstances and that students who play an active role in their learning generally find it more attractive and stimulating.

9.3 METHODS OF PRACTICE

There are a variety of techniques from which to choose when considering how best to provide an appropriate and meaningful practical experience as part of the training sequence. Among the most common are covert rehearsal, behaviour rehearsal, role-play, simulation exercises and games, and *in vivo* practice (e.g. interviews with actual patients or clients). The most basic distinction is between simulation and *in vivo* practice. Choices at this level lead to a series of subsequent decision points, as illustrated in Figure 9.1.

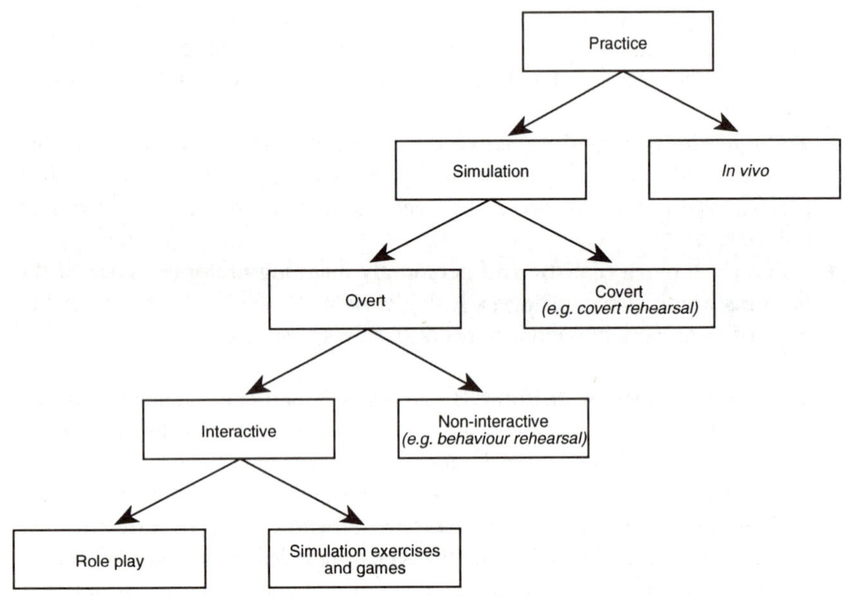

Figure 9.1 Dimensions of practice.

Simulation seeks to recreate within the classroom setting the key operational features of some actual situation from, for instance, the ward or clinic. *In vivo* practice, by contrast, makes direct use of the 'real life' encounter for purposes of instruction. It is therefore centred in the work place, perhaps with a patient, patient's relative or other health professional.

In the case of simulation, there are obvious advantages in maximizing the fidelity of the practical experience by ensuring that what takes place during it approximates to the real world equivalent in as many important respects as possible. Trainee motivation and the extent to which the effects of training carry over to the workplace increase as a result, as will be seen in Chapter 13. But this does not mean that the simulation must be **exactly** like the real event. If it did then presumably all skill practice would be best conducted on the ward, in the consulting room, the patient's home, etc. In the early stages of training, in particular, there are merits in having skill practice at one remove from the actual situation.

According to Lierman (1994) a simulation is a model of some process, event or activity. Keiser and Seeler (1987) extend this definition by pointing out that it represents a view of reality including the salient resources, restrictions and consequences of that which is simulated. Some of the associated advantages include the following.

- **Safety**. The consequences of making errors are less grave than in the real situation. Newell (1994) points to the advantages of being able to attempt skills in an environment where risk-taking is acceptable: 'Once the student nurse is involved in "practising" such skills in the ward setting, it is often too late or too threatening to experiment' (p. 3).
- **Simplicity**. The complexity of situations can be stripped away, allowing students to concentrate on those aspects that are important to immediate learning objectives.
- **Overcoming ethical problems**. These can arise when inexperienced students handle patients or clients to further their training.
- **Control**. Greater control can be exercised over what unfolds than is typically the case in the 'real world'.
- **Additional instruction**. It is much easier to provide supplementary guidance and coaching during simulation. Feedback possibilities are also enhanced, as will be illustrated in the following chapter. Newell (1994) noted that the ward environs don't provide the ideal atmosphere for quiet, insightful reflection on practice.
- **Varying the time span**. The ability to manipulate the temporal dimension of the piece of interaction can be a considerable benefit.
- **Enjoyment**. Participants can find this method of learning extremely engaging – fun with a purpose!
- **Costs**. Creating practical experience through simulation, while not without cost (Keiser and Seeler, 1987), tends to be a much less expensive option than some of the alternatives, including periods of placement in the field.

Simulation practice may be either overt or, by using mental imagery, take a covert form. Overt practice can occur within the context of an extended piece of spontaneous interaction. The use of patient simulators as a means of skill practice is a case in point. These can be: members of staff taking on the role of patient; other students; professional or amateur actors who are (usually) paid to act the part of the patient; and trained simulators who receive special instruction in how to present with certain symptoms and conditions, give a history, be examined, etc. and who, to all intents and purposes, 'become' a patient (Metcalfe, 1989).

In addition to role-play, practice through simulation may be achieved by using various exercises and games. (The use of role-play and simulation procedures in the evaluation of skill performance is considered in Chapter 11. Here they will be discussed as methods of enabling skills to be practised.)

However, non-interactive overt skill practice is another possibility, which merely requires that aspects of the targeted skill be produced separately and in isolation as part, for example, of a behaviour rehearsal exercise. It is to this sort of technique that we now turn.

9.4 COVERT REHEARSAL

To date covert rehearsal has featured more extensively in the remedial and developmental spheres of interpersonal skills training than in the specialized context of preparation for health-care delivery . However, it has been put to use, and with some success, in counsellor education (Baker, Daniels and Greeley, 1990). Simply put, this technique requires trainees to 'visualize' performing the targeted skill through mental images rather than in action. For this reason it has also been called visualized rehearsal by Nelson-Jones (1991). Trainees must imagine a specified situation and then go over 'in their mind's eye' the appropriate way to respond. Practice is therefore entirely covert, taking the form of an imagined reproduction of the skill or procedure introduced during sensitization. According to Bandura (1986) this process facilitates the temporal and spatial organization of cognitive elements into a pattern which approximates to that presented in the earlier stages of instruction, prior to behavioural enactment. Magill (1993) also speculates on effects in establishing long-term memory representations of the action together with the potential for furthering problem-solving.

Practice through covert rehearsal can be incorporated into either group or individualized training regimes and is carried out in the following stages:

1. A state of physical and mental relaxation is induced by the trainer. (Information on relaxation techniques can be found in, for example, Charlesworth and Nathan, 1984 and Morris, 1991.)
2. The scene in which the skill is to be used is depicted as graphically as possible so that it can be readily visualized by trainees.
3. Members of the class are instructed to imagine themselves responding in accordance with the targeted skill. They may be asked to respond 'internally' to a trigger statement made by a significant other in the scene.
4. They should be encouraged to picture the consequences of their covert performance so that judgements may begin to be formed as to the likely effects of really behaving in this way.
5. The scene can be gone through several times to promote the contemplation and imaginal testing out of a variety of coping strategies before attempts are made to identify the one that seems most appropriate. This stage, strongly recommended by Cartledge and Milburn (1995), is more likely to foster an understanding of effective interaction as a process demanding a flexible, decision-making approach rather than the unthinking performance of rigid, stereotypical patterns of behaviour.

6. Experiences should be discussed and general outcomes and recommendations established during debriefing.

In training groups, homework often takes the form of a continuation of covert rehearsal between sessions (Nelson-Jones, 1991).

9.4.1 Advantages of covert rehearsal

There are various advantages and disadvantages associated with this form of practice which should be appreciated by the trainer before trying it out. Among the former can be listed the following.

- The potential exists for modifying cognitions and emotions. This may well be where the real value of covert rehearsal lies. Imagery-based interventions have produced changes in, for instance, perceptual sensitivity, self-awareness, self-control and reduced levels of anxiety (Baker *et al.,* 1985; Kanfer and Gaelick-Buys, 1991).
- It may be extremely useful in cases where other types of practice would be difficult to arrange for logistical, safety or ethical reasons.
- Trainees, once familiarized, can readily use it on their own.
- Special benefits accrue in helping trainees deal with situations imbued with negative feelings such as anxiety. Given the proper expertise, there is scope for extending these exercises in accordance with systematic desensitization procedures (Morris, 1991), to help trainees deal with situations where poor performance may be due in part to feelings of unease with that type of person (e.g. homosexual AIDS patient) or situation (e.g. terminal illness).
- Some empirical evidence exists attesting to the efficacy of covert rehearsal, particularly with advanced trainees learning more complex skills (Baker *et al.,* 1985; Magill, 1993). It is an interesting speculation that, at the level of higher-order operation, competence may essentially involve the development of plans and strategies for using already acquired subskills in original ways. Such reorganization probably takes place, more importantly, at a cognitive rather than a behavioural level and, in consequence, lends itself to rehearsal which is covert in nature. Baker *et al.* (1986), reported that the combination of the two methods, overt and covert rehearsal, resulted in a form of practice which was superior to either alone in the acquisition of counselling skills. This arrangement has also been recommended by Mills and Pace (1989) who argued that, 'With complex tasks, such as communicating, mental traces must be created before meaningful motor learning can occur. Mental development appears to precede motor development' (p. 174).

9.4.2 Disadvantages of covert rehearsal

- It is a 'high-risk' option – it can flop! This technique tends to be better suited to the more mature, experienced, well-motivated and open-minded student.

- It can be viewed as silly or boring by the less imaginative.
- Some trainees find it difficult to create and sustain a conducively contemplative ambience, together with the appropriate imagery.
- The trainer has difficulty commenting on 'performance'.
- There is no guarantee that that which is imagined will be successfully enacted when it comes to actual performance.

9.5 BEHAVIOUR REHEARSAL

In the overwhelming majority of CST programmes, practice has been explicit and is often carried out within the framework of an ongoing, spontaneous interaction such as an interview, group discussion, case conference or counselling session, often in simulation. But behaviour rehearsal techniques can also be non-interactive (Nelson-Jones, 1991). Trainees may practise on their own provided that they have a concept of the targeted skill and the criteria governing acceptability of performance.

Some behaviours lend themselves more readily to non-interactive behavioural rehearsal than others. Those that do include various facets of non-verbal behaviour. In order to improve active listening and the communicative aspects of empathic understanding, for example, students may be given the task of reading a well known poem, nursery rhyme or story in such a way that different predetermined emotions are conveyed through paralanguage. Alternatively a newspaper story can be read in accordance with such underlying states as enthusiasm, boredom, sympathy, sincerity, joy and so on. If an audio recorder or camcorder is available (and most students have at least the former) these attempts can be self-recorded, played back, evaluated and, since each should not last long, repeated and improved upon as required. Exercises of this type may be extremely useful, since it has been found that one of the features that attracts patients to physicians is the latter's ability to effectively convey emotion, particularly positive emotion, in the use of voice and facial expression (Buller and Street, 1992).

9.5.1 Advantages of behaviour rehearsal

Among the recognized advantages can be listed the following.

- The focus is upon objective behaviour. Trainees must be able to translate their understanding of the skills material into practice.
- Trainees can practise on their own. It can therefore be used as homework.
- Some may feel less inhibited, during initial practice attempts, when others are not involved.
- It is easier to devote full attention to a specific aspect of behaviour unhampered by the complexities surrounding ongoing interaction.

9.5.2 Disadvantages of behaviour rehearsal

- It may be regarded as silly or childish. A thoughtful introduction can often overcome these attitudes.
- Trainees must have a firm and accurate realization of what constitutes acceptable performance.
- Opportunities for checking progress by drawing upon the views and comments of others may be lacking.
- Little appreciation can be gained of the consequences of implementing the skill during interaction.
- Emphasis is upon the production of a particular behaviour to the possible exclusion of such vitally important matters as the circumstances determining expediency of action.
- Concerns about skills training promoting artificiality and indeed disingenuousness can be heightened.

Some of these drawbacks can be overcome by including other trainees in the process. Thus in the exercise described above, the poem or passage could be read to another, or to a small group, rather than into a tape recorder. They could then have to guess the emotion 'behind the words'. An alternative along these lines, which could also be used in connection with the skill of reflection of feeling, is suggested in Exercise 9.1.

Exercise 9.1 Reflective statements

Aim

To help trainees in their use of reflective statements

Organization

Divide the group into pairs. Depending upon numbers, groups of four can be created, with members joining in pairs.

Instruction

Participants on their own or, in the case of foursomes in pairs, write out a list of about five statements that a patient might say to a nurse while being prepared for an operation. Pairs (or foursomes) then come together and take it in turns to read out their statements. Before reading a statement, they must stipulate whether it should be responded to with a paraphrase, reflection of feeling or overall reflection. The other participant/s respond accordingly. After each attempt, the accuracy of the response can be discussed.

Discussion

More general discussion can centre upon difficulties in differentiating between fact and feeling messages; appreciating which feelings were meant to be expressed; and problems in formulating accurate and appropriate responses.

Group-based methods of behaviour rehearsal, if suitably introduced, can be fully enjoyed by trainees. Group involvement means that feedback from others is available and the individual is not forced to rely solely upon his own, perhaps idiosyncratic, notions of acceptable performance. Nevertheless, while these techniques do enable closely targeted and highly concentrated practice to take place, what they can provide is necessarily limited by their inherently restricted nature.

9.6 ROLE-PLAY

The origins of role-play tend to be traced back to Moreno (1953), who introduced it as a means of improving the general social skills of a group of delinquent girls in anticipation of their release from the institutional setting in which they had been living. It has subsequently acquired a remarkably wide range of educational applications and is eminently suited to the training of professional groups (Dickson, 1995b). Role-play, for example, has been described by Parathian and Taylor (1993) as not only an effective but a natural method of learning in nurse training. Furthermore, it is one of the most common forms of simulated interactive practice in CST. Trainees role-playing take on and behave in accordance with a role not normally their own or, if their own, one that would not usually be played in that situation. The role may be that of an imaginary person or someone who actually exists and is known to them. The others taking part in the interaction may likewise be indulging in role-play and what transpires can be largely predetermined or completely improvised.

Role-play is eminently suited to CST interventions for several reasons:

- It affords the safety and control of simulation.
- The experience provided of a situation can closely replicate that of the 'real world' equivalent, as demonstrated by Maerker, Lisper and Rickberg (1990) in a research setting, and Hargie and Gallagher (1992), in counselling.
- Trainees generally find it attractive when properly introduced and organized.
-]It offers substantial opportunities for concerted feedback.
- Situations that occur infrequently in reality can be arranged as required.
- Since students are also involved as role-play partners they gain some insights into what it is like to be in the position of 'the other' in the encounter. Opportunities exist, therefore, for improving awareness and sensitivity. This

is seen as one of the advantages of having student nurses (Parathian and Taylor, 1993) and undergraduate medical students (Sanson-Fisher *et al.*, 1991) role-play patients.
- A meaningful appreciation can be gained of the complexities of the professional role. Rhys (1992) reported how a role-play exercise with student health visitors served to illuminate issues of power and control associated with the professional role.
- It engages the totality of the learner and changes can be effected not only in behaviour but in beliefs, attitudes and feelings, including those which are self-focused (Jupp and Griffiths, 1990). Based upon a meta-analysis of some 26 studies, McGregor (1993) affirmed that role-playing minority group members was an effective attitude change technique for curbing racial prejudice amongst students.

The latter point is worth elaborating upon. While the primary objective of role-play, as a means of CST practice, is to produce improvements in particular pre-established facets of performance, it can make more extensive contributions. Some of these have been mentioned by, for instance, Cooke (1987) and Shooter (1992). They include:

- affording learning opportunities for observers;
- facilitating the integration of theory and practice;
- promoting greater awareness of self and others;
- improving problem-solving abilities;
- focusing upon difficult situations and contentious issues.

9.6.1 Types of role-play

Teasing out the objectives to which role-play may be put leads naturally on to thinking about the different types of role-play available. The objectives that one has in mind will be more or less successfully met depending upon the type of role-play selected. The most common basis for distinguishing between types of role-play is that of structure. Some role-play exercises are highly circumscribed affairs while others are much less constrained.

Structured role-play

Here the goals and circumstances of the role-play are preordained. The general scenario is presented to the students at the outset and key characteristics of the roles involved, such as status, personality, knowledge, disposition, etc., are settled. The relationship which each participant shares with the others is also clarified. The lines along which the role-play will develop tend to be envisaged beforehand, together with the particular issues to be brought forth. The main purposes of the exercise typically revolve around experiencing the inbuilt tensions and influences that emerge and arriving at acceptable solutions.

This type of role-play tends to be provided by the trainer, especially in more elaborate cases requiring quite detailed information in written form. Trainees, however, may also be given the task of formulating examples perhaps based upon real situations previously encountered.

Distinct similarities exist between structured and what has been referred to by Wohlking and Gill (1980) as method-centred role-play This approach is particularly suited to skills training when the skill in question is simple and easily broken down into a series of steps, and when the social process involving the skill is quite short and largely ritualistic (e.g. admitting a patient, conducting a hearing test).

Unstructured role-play

Here what takes place is much less preformulated. While initiated with an explicit aim in mind the unfolding interaction depends largely upon the improvisation of those taking part. Although roles and a particular situation are established in advance, details of the scenario and its eventual outcome are left to be worked out by the participants as it unfolds. Students are frequently involved in devising these exercises based upon their experiences or concerns. What Wohlking and Gill (1980) call developmental role-plays are of this sort. A challenging problem, for example, may be presented and students are encouraged to formulate and test various strategies in dealing with it. A special feature of this approach is that it facilitates the exploration of feelings and motives underlying action. It can also be used successfully in the training of advanced communication skills that are part of more complex interactive processes such as counselling or negotiating.

Semi-structured role-play

The essential characteristic, as the name implies, has to do with the intermediate level of constraint imposed upon the interaction. In practice, this type of role-play is often trainer-initiated but it permits greater scope for trainee interpretation than its more structured equivalent. Consequently, it often proves more attractive to trainees.

9.6.2 Stages in role-playing

The likely success of this type of simulated interactive practice depends largely upon the trainer being aware of the various stages involved, the particular requirements of each and how they should best be handled.

Preparation

A lack of adequate preparation is probably the most frequent cause of those taking part in role-play failing to benefit from the experience. A useful starting point is in establishing the learning objectives to be accomplished. These stem from the educational needs of the group and may be quite narrowly focused (e.g. specific skill improvement, mastery of a certain technique) or more general and abstract such as effecting a tighter integration of existing knowledge. They need not be mutually exclusive, of course. While several objectives may be pursued in the course of a single role-play, being overly ambitious in this respect, can de-focus the exercise leaving students confused and uncertain.

Having identified appropriate learning objectives, thought has to be given to the type of role-play best suited to achieving them. Features of the group, including maturity, familiarity, motivation and experience, must not be overlooked since these will have an important bearing upon what is likely to work. As a crude rule-of-thumb, less structured, developmental role-plays tend to be more successful when:

- the objectives are to increase awareness, change attitudes, explore feelings or illuminate underlying issues;
- trainees are more mature and experienced;
- trainees are more familiar with and trusting of each other;
- the interactive process featured is highly complex;
- the programme is well advanced. Nelson-Jones (1991) identified a trend, over the course of training, from more to less structured role-plays.

In some instances it may be useful to increase students' awareness of the problems faced in a certain situation by having them take part in a developmental role-play based around it during sensitization. When the general purpose is to refine skills, especially those which are quite basic, then more structured variants should be contemplated.

In addition to determining the degree of structure there are a variety of other techniques which can be used and which should be considered at this stage. Among these are the following.

- **Multiple role-play**. This involves dividing the group into subgroups each of which then enacts the scenario concurrently. Everyone is involved and some members may be designated to act as observers, recording what takes place for the purposes of feedback. Multiple role-play is frequently associated with the more structured, method-centred approach.
- **Fish-bowl technique**. In this case several trainees enact the role-play in the centre of the room with the rest of the group looking on – hence the name. This is arguably the most common technique, being particularly suited to exploring the complexities of situations and gaining insights into underlying issues. As a means of skill practice, though, it is more limited.
- **Role rotation**. Here a number of trainees take it in turn to play the main role, usually the 'health professional'. Other roles may also be rotated, although not to the extent of seriously compromising the continuity of the interaction. Role rotation is one method of offering at least some skill practice to a number of trainees in a short space of time.

- **Role reversal**. The essential feature of this technique is that participants have an opportunity, at some point during the interaction, to switch roles so that, for example, 'the GP' now becomes 'the patient' and *vice versa*. This can be a very effective way of developing self-awareness, changing attitudes and encouraging empathic understanding. By having student nurses play the role of patients with various problems and handicaps, a greater appreciation of the special needs of these groups can be brought about (Parathian and Taylor, 1993).

There are two more specialized techniques for surfacing feelings and attitudes.

- **Doubling**. This derives from psychodrama and is particularly effective in focusing attention on the emotional dynamic of the chosen situation. It involves each role-player having a 'double' who acts as a mouthpiece for those inner voices that seldom get expressed during normal interaction, but are nevertheless highly influential (Duryea, 1990). The double typically speaks to the partner doubled, but just loud enough for the rest to hear as well. For example, in the context of a GP–patient role-play scenario in which the patient has been kept waiting for an excessive period before the consultation, the GP may begin:
  GP: 'Good morning Mr Green – sorry for the delay.'
  (**GP Double**: 'I'm not really sorry at all!')
  Mr Green: 'That's perfectly OK.'
  Mr Green Double: ('I'm bloody furious. Because you kept me waiting for 45 minutes, I've just missed my lift home.')
- **Sculpting**. Here participants convey their experiencing of the situation and the other role-players, together with commensurate feelings and attitudes, in non-verbal actions rather than speech. Students are encouraged, in physical positions taken up towards the others, through posture and gesture, etc., to do what seems to flow naturally from how they react to the situation. Feelings and actions then form the content of subsequent discussion. Faulkner (1993) has described the exercise being put to use with health-care workers, and the benefits which it has to offer.

Once issues of learning objectives and types of procedure have been settled, the trainer must give thought to actually providing a suitable role-play. Here there are three possibilities.

- Borrow or purchase existing material from sources such as Brandes and Philips (1978) and Burnard (1992).
- Trainees establish the role-play, with proper guidance from the trainer.
- Trainer creates the role-play.

Writing role-plays is not difficult and has the advantage of more completely meeting the requirements of the particular training programme. There are benefits, however, in adopting a systematic approach to the task, using the following guidelines.

- Identify the background situation or scenario. It should be meaningful to the group and in keeping with the established learning objectives.
- Write the scenario, establishing the location of the action together with the salient events which have led to it. This should be done simply and concisely.
- Decide upon the roles. It may be imprudent at the beginning to specify roles that depart radically from those familiar to trainees. Faulkner (1993) refers to this as the 'own skin' approach, in that trainees keep their sex, rough age, social circle, etc. She suggests that it not only reduces the chances of the procedure being seen as artificial or silly, but has the added advantage of freeing participants from the superficial features of the role to focus upon more significant aspects.
- Write role-briefs. Producing role-brief cards is a useful way to do this. These should document the relevant motives, beliefs and abilities of the player together with the major influences to which they are subjected. Again, one has to consider how much each player must know about each of the others and what information should be private.
- Decide upon a time-frame. This can vary widely depending on the purpose of the exercise, but 10–20 minutes is usually adequate for skill practice.
- Decide upon setting, props, etc. Role-play is not acting and there is seldom need for an elaborate arrangement of props. Occasionally, though, some may be invaluable. Having a large doll, for instance, is an extremely useful aid when a trainee health visitor is explaining to a 'young mother' how to bath baby!
- Have your role-play material checked. Despite careful attention to detail, it is extremely easy for vagueness and confusion to be written into the material produced. It is advisable, therefore, to have a colleague read over the scenario and role-play briefs before turning up with them to the practical. Any minor residual uncertainties can, of course, be ironed out during the briefing.

Some of these points are illustrated in the semi-structured role-play provided in Exercise 9.2.

Exercise 9.2 Semi-structured role-play for listening

Aim

- To give practice in the skill of listening.
- To create an awareness of some of the circumstances that can get in the way of effective listening.

Preparation

Make copies of role-play scenario and role-briefs.

Scenario: The Brown family comprises Mr Brown and Mrs Brown (Junior), both in their early forties; the children, Joan (8 years), Samantha (6 years) and Colin (5 years), and Mrs Brown (Senior), who is in her late seventies and moved in following the death, 4 years ago, of her sister, with whom she had been living. She has been bedridden for the past year as a result of an extensive stroke and her condition has slowly but steadily deteriorated until she now needs constant attention.

Mr Brown, a primary-school teacher, has an elder brother who lives in London but with whom he has little contact, and two younger sisters, both married, who live nearby but have little to do with their mother. Having attended to Mrs Brown's pressure sores, during a visit, the community nurse came downstairs to find the daughter-in-law in tears with her husband trying to console her. Mr Brown asks the Community Nurse if she could help to find out what is wrong and Mrs Brown (Junior) begins to explain how she is finding it all too much. . . .

Mrs Brown: Recently you have been finding it increasingly difficult to cope with looking after the house, the children, your husband and your mother-in-law. Although you have a good relationship with your husband, everything seems left to you to deal with. No one seems to recognize how much you are expected to do. While you get on well with your mother-in-law and would hate to have her feel rejected, you find that you can no longer tend her. What about her son and daughters, don't they have any responsibilities. . .?

Mr Brown: You owe your mother a lot and are very fond of her. Your father left when you were young and money was scarce, but she went without so that you would not be denied. You simply can't have her dumped in a geriatric ward or nursing home. She was always there when you needed her – you can't let her down now . . . yet there is your wife and children. At the time your aunt died, both sisters objected strongly to you taking your mother to live with you and a family quarrel ensued. Although they visited your mother in hospital, at the time of her stroke, they have not done so since she was discharged. You think that, regardless of their feelings towards you and your wife, they should come to see her. But they, like you, have a stubborn streak!

Community nurse: This has come as something of a surprise. Of course you had been alert to the possibility, but Mrs Brown (Junior) had appeared to be managing without apparent difficulty. Indeed, you had admired her resolve, fully appreciating the demands that this sort of situation can make. When your own mother fell ill you had nursed her at home until she died, giving up work in order to do so. Indeed, in many ways, Mrs Brown (Senior) reminds you of her. . .!

Organization

Divide the group into subgroups of three members each, or four to five if observers are used. Role-plays should last about 10–15 minutes and should, if possible, be video recorded. At the end, feedback should be provided within subgroups. The main points to emerge can be raised with the whole group.

Instructions

Introduce the role-play, establish appropriate climate, allocate roles and rehearse the major characteristics of the skill of listening.

Discussion

Following the enactment, discussion should involve feedback from video recordings and/or observers, and should centre upon:

- the extent to which both the husband and wife were listened to and the verbal and non-verbal bases of those judgements;
- characteristics of the situation that made listening difficult;
- factors which, in general, detract from accurate listening and how these can be overcome.

Introduction

This involves orienting trainees, both procedurally and affectively, to the technique. The latter can, on occasion, be much more difficult but unless an accommodating disposition can be created the exercise is doomed to failure from the beginning. Depending upon the group, role-play may be introduced either directly or indirectly. The former involves presenting the notion, explaining what it entails and dealing with any misgivings or resistances that may arise (e.g. belief that it requires acting ability, is too artificial to be useful, is childish). This is generally the most common approach and the one which tends to be most frequently described in the literature. With the indirect alternative, the topic of role-play is little mentioned as such. Rather the group is gradually brought to a stage where they are doing it. Rhys (1992) described how, during a workshop on communication skills with student health visitors, a discussion on asking clients questions gave way to an invitation to participants to illustrate their ideas practically.

Regardless of the strategy invoked it is imperative that a facilitative climate be created. This is typified by a freedom from anxiety, an openness to change, confidence to experiment while accepting that mistakes may happen, and the assurance that, should things go wrong, participants can bring the role-play to an end without losing face. Such a situation is more likely to be created, in the view of Knowles (1987), if the trainer espouses values of mutual respect and trust, encourages collaboration rather than competition and supportiveness rather than judgementality, and stresses the 'fun with a purpose' nature of the learning exercise.

The procedural aspect of the introductory stage has several facets.

- **Providing a rationale**. For motivational reasons, participants should understand why they are role-playing. When the role-play is designed to facilitate skill practice, recapping on the major features of the targeted skill is also sensible. This need not take long and indeed may be omitted when the practical follows on directly from the sensitization phase.
- **Allocating roles to trainees**. This can be done by asking for volunteers although there may be merit in having particular members play certain roles. Doing so on a counter-to-type basis can be a valuable way of changing attitudes and promoting interpersonal sensitivity (e.g. having a rather assertive member play the relatively powerless role of patient).
- **Establishing and briefing observers**. This is especially important if the interaction is not being video or audio recorded. Observers should be in no doubt as to what exactly it is that they are required to focus upon. Various types of recording schedule, some of which will be reviewed in the next chapter and in Chapter 11, can help in this respect and make the procedure more thorough and systematic.
- **Warming up**. As pointed out by Nelson-Jones (1991), some recommend brief warm-up exercises designed to get the group doing things rather than merely sitting talking, in preparation for the enactment. Whether or not they are thought necessary, though, is a matter for the trainer and the type of group.

Videotaped material can also be used as a means of effectively introducing trainees to role-play. Several strategies may be adopted. A short segment of an interaction can be played and trainees can then be asked to demonstrate how they think the interaction should proceed. This can be a particularly successful way of 'triggering' a piece of developmental role-play. Alternatively, a quite short but complete practitioner–patient interaction may be presented where the interpersonal performance of the practitioner is rather poor. Trainees can then be asked to role-play the same scenario, demonstrating improved performance on the part of the health professional. Exemplars should be carefully chosen to reflect the training needs of the group and to present situations which they will find challenging. The resulting role-plays are, of course, much more structured in this case. Students tend to find this approach highly motivating. Moreover, trainers can have a positive model of the same situation prepared in advance, thereby allowing the group the opportunity to compare their efforts against alternative strategies during feedback.

Interaction

Participants should now be ready to commence. Once the role-play gets under way the instructor's job (assuming no direct role-playing involvement) is largely one of monitoring. The temptation to constantly intervene to ensure that things happen exactly as was intended should be curbed. It spoils the coherence of the enactment, makes it difficult for roles to be played convincingly and is generally demotivating. A number of occasions when intervention is warranted, however, have been identified (van Ments, 1983; Faulkner, 1993; Dickson, 1995b). They cover the following.

- **One or more player persistently dropping out of role**. This may be due to poor preparation and not getting adequately into role, or reflect feelings of vulnerability.
- **'Hamming' roles**. This can stem from inexperience, overexuberance or, more insidiously, may be a deliberate attempt at sabotage! Negativism can suggest flawed preparation and/or inadequate introduction.
- **Stultified performance**. A common cause is anxiety or insufficient time to get into role.
- **Over-involvement of players**. This is the opposite of the previous difficulty, with role-players investing too much of themselves in their roles and becoming over-emotionally involved. The trainer should be on hand to defuse the situation.
- **The breakdown**. Here a tactful rescue is called for. The trainer should always be mindful of the potential embarrassment which can result from a player 'getting stuck' or 'drying up' and try to minimize it.
- **Off target**. If it appears unlikely that any useful learning points will accrue from its continuation the enactment should be abandoned.
- **Utilizing the 'teachable moment'**. The trainer may feel justified in occasionally interrupting to draw attention to some important event which, if let pass, would be lost.

The trainer also acts as a director during the enactment, ensuring that a time schedule is adhered to and that things happen more or less when they should.

Feedback and discussion

In many respects this is the most valuable stage of the role-play process and typically requires from two to three times as long to complete as the interaction itself. During it, the events of the interaction are analysed and clarified, underlying causes of what happened are identified and general principles governing interpersonal communication are arrived at. Since these issues more properly fall within the ambit of the following chapter, which deals with the feedback phase of training, they will not be further elaborated upon at this point.

One further function of this final part of the role-play exercise has to do with 'de-roling' or easing participants out of the roles played. Its salience increases in relation to the depth of immersion achieved – especially in roles demanding a strong emotional involvement. Cooke (1987) described several techniques that can be used to help participants 'finish unfinished business'. This can be done by facilitating the ventilation of residual feelings and progressively relating to these individuals more obviously as students rather than the characters of the roles. If need be, participants may be asked to repeat their names, proper roles, true circumstances, etc. It is not always necessary to go to these lengths though, and indeed, some find this quite superfluous. Faulkner (1993) simply recommends being alert to signs of lack of disengagement and taking this up privately with the individual/s concerned.

Role-play is probably the most common method of practice in CST. Through it a reasonable facsimile of the sort of situation within which the trainee will have to operate can be created in the safety of the classroom. It does have limitations, nevertheless, as pointed out by Cooke (1987).

- Some trainees find it difficult to accept, regarding it as artificial or merely play-acting.
- Some trainees, while acknowledging its value as a learning technique, experience difficulty in taking on and sustaining a role.
- On the other hand, some participants can become over-involved emotionally. Shooter (1992) describes dropping a particular scenario from a workshop for carers dealing with the dying and bereaved upon learning that one of the group was actually living through a similar experience.
- Role-play can pose a threat to certain students, who may prefer the anonymity of a less personally involving form of learning.
- It may reinforce stereotypes and degenerate into the caricaturing of individuals and categories.
- Outcomes may not carry over from the training environment to the real world. This important topic will be returned to in Chapter 13.

9.7 SIMULATION EXERCISES AND GAMES

The relationship between role-play and simulation exercises and games is complex and the dividing line between them tenuous. For a start, all of the practice methods already covered in this chapter rely upon simulation to some extent. In this broad sense, 'simulation is a technique which enables adult learners to obtain skills, competencies, knowledge, or behaviours by becoming involved in situations that are similar to those in real life' (Gilley, 1990, p. 272). It provides a rubric that subsumes a variety of techniques, each with features which enable loose distinctions to be made. Some of these take the form of games and exercises.

Simulation exercises are structured affairs, which depict the salient parameters and vectors of some real or hypothetical event and require the student to operate in accordance with them in reaching a decision or completing a task. Although they may involve an element of role-play they tend to be distinguished from it on a number of counts. These have been neatly encapsulated by Jones (1985, p. 5): 'Although simulations have roles, they do not have play, but are concerned with a job and a function, not a new personality.'

Simulation exercises are often group-based. They are incorporated into training to create an awareness of, for instance, role relationships and conflicts, the various constraints and influences that can impinge upon different positions within a social structure, and to provide the individual with an experience of how an organization or system works. It is possible on the other hand for these exercises to be carried out in dyads (Exercise 9.3). A central objective in this case is to provide a skill practice opportunity within a context that can frequently be remarkably similar to 'the real thing'.

Exercise 9.3 Interviewing

Aim

To offer practice in conducting a medical history-type interview.

Preparation

- A content sheet. This should outline the various areas of content to be covered during the interview. A copy should be provided for each student.
- A process sheet. Here the different skills and processes of the interview which are being practised should be included.

Organization

Divide the group into dyads or, if it is necessary to use observers, triads.

Instructions

Identify interviewers, interviewees and observers. While interviewers and observers are being briefed, interviewees can have a coffee-break. Distribute content and process sheets and familiarize interviewers with them. Interviewers should be given some time to plan and prepare, realizing that a complete history, which will probably necessitate note-taking, is required. Observers should be clear what they are to look for and how it is to be recorded.

While interviewers and observers are getting ready, interviewees can be briefed. This should be minimal. All they need to know is that they will be required to give their medical history to date. If there are facets of it that they would rather not disclose, these can be withheld, but they should try to make it as genuine as possible. Interviews should last about 15 minutes. Given time, each student can have the opportunity to interview.

Discussion

Discussion can focus upon the following issues:
- How effectively were the pre-established skills and procedures implemented?
- How complete was the history? Were there areas that were ignored?
- Were some areas easier to explore than others?
- What did it feel like to be interviewed in this way?

Keiser and Seeler (1987) chart the origins of gaming as an educational and training technique, and comment on its current popularity in a variety of areas including business and management schools. A game can be thought of as a 'structured activity in which two or more participants compete within constraints of rules to achieve an objective' (p. 460). The distinguishing feature of games, therefore, is the element of competition, which is inbuilt. Here participants have goals that they strive to achieve. There is frequently the possibility of some being able to facilitate or thwart others in their quest. In any case it is important that, at the end, there is a winner, clearly identified through pre-established criteria.

The trainer should approach simulation exercises and games with the same four stages in mind as those that typify role-play.

- **Preparation**. Here aims and objectives are often quite broad, such as illuminating a concept, or providing initial experience of a novel situation or insights into how some complex system operates. But they can also be quite specific and personally oriented (e.g. increasing awareness of personal involvement in a given situation or improving levels of skill in it). When it comes to getting hold of games and exercises of this type, the two main alternatives are either to use ones already developed or design your own. Those intending to pursue the former option may find worthwhile sources in Horn and Cleaves (1980) and Johnson (1990), amongst others. Trainers who prefer to construct their own will find useful advice in, for instance, Jones (1985), Thatcher (1990) and Lierman (1994).

- **Introduction**
- **Interaction**
- **Feedback and discussion**.

Much of what was discussed under these points in relation to role-play is of relevance here and will not be repeated.

9.7.1 Advantages and disadvantages of simulation exercises and games

Again many of the advantages and disadvantages of this method of practice have already been mentioned, particularly in relation to the comments made about simulation in general as an approach to practice.

Advantages include the following.

- Little of consequence hangs upon mistakes being made. Gilley (1990) commented on the vulnerability of the adult learner and pointed to simulation as an approach which is practical and realistic, yet with little threat to the self-esteem of the participant.
- What takes place can be largely predetermined and is capable of being closely controlled by the trainer.
- The intention in using simulation exercises and games, is frequently to reduce the complexity of the actual situation by extracting only the salient features or influences from it.
- The possibility of ethical concerns being raised as a result of having trainees practise in the real situation are eliminated.
- Additional instruction during the interaction is easier to give although the trainer must recognize the dangers of violating the integrity of the simulation in so doing.
- There are extensive opportunities for providing detailed information on what took place during the interaction.
- Simulation exercises, and particularly games, if properly prepared, carefully chosen and adequately introduced, can prove extremely popular with trainees, who often find them less threatening than role-plays. This is particularly the case with exercises which have, as the major focus, the operation of systems rather than the performance of a particular individual.
- Use of evolving technology. Keiser and Seeler (1987) have mentioned the enormous contribution which computer technology has made to the popularity of simulation and games. With the advent of virtual-reality technology, a whole new and exciting vista of possibilities opens up. While still in its infancy, one could imagine the student on a CST course of the future practising their influencing skills with, let's say, an alcoholic patient, in virtual reality!

Nevertheless, drawbacks also exist.

- Some trainees, failing to appreciate the benefits to be derived from this technique, may see it as grown-ups 'playing games' and therefore regard it as ridiculously childish.
- In order for it to succeed, considerable thought and careful planning must go into the design of the simulation. Even so it is often impossible to anticipate all weaknesses at this stage. These often surface for the first time during the enactment and can spoil it.
- These techniques, especially when group-based, can take up considerable time. They can be completed in several hours or go on for literally days!

Time can create practical problems of two sorts. Firstly, a disproportionate amount of the total time given over to this part of the course may be used up. Secondly, it may be logistically difficult to find a suitably large slot on the typical student's timetable to accommodate this type of input. It is often necessary, therefore, to spread the exercise over several sessions, although the enactment should usually be completed in a single one.

- Compared with role-play, simulation exercises and games tend not to be used as much for in-depth analysis of particular relationships; the illumination of the intrapersonal factors, including feelings and attitudes, which subtend social behaviour; or the promotion of profound levels of self-awareness.
- As with role-play, there is always the possibility that learning which takes place in the simulated environment will fail to be applied in the situation for which trainees are being prepared.

9.8 *IN VIVO* PRACTICE

It will be recalled from Fig. 9.1 that simulation and *in vivo* practice are the two basic alternatives when it comes to devising some sort of practical exercise that will permit trainees to attempt to put their knowledge of the targeted skill into operation. The majority of practice techniques available in CST, including those already discussed, rely upon simulation in some form. On the other hand, there are exceptions, which are not premised upon the essential 'as if' requirement of this approach, where 'make believe' is not a condition and where uncontrived interaction is engaged in. It is to these *in vivo* methods that we now turn.

This procedure necessitates, firstly, participants acting in accordance with the roles that they would typically play in those situations in which they are located – in other words 'being themselves'; secondly, what transpires between them being natural rather than contrived; and, thirdly, this interaction being grounded in an appropriate situational context. *In vivo* practice is overt rather than covert, with the skill being implemented during the course of an ongoing interpersonal encounter. Thus the student operates in the normal work setting, whether that be a ward, pharmacy, health clinic or client's home, with an actual patient, client, relative or health practitioner, about some genuine concern in order to meet a real need or achieve a proper goal. The much greater demands placed upon trainees as a result will be readily appreciated. Not only do they have to perform the skill or procedure focused upon but there is often a more general, but very real, expectation that they 'be a member' of the profession to which they aspire. Great care must, therefore, be taken to ensure that the individual is adequately prepared for what, potentially, can be a tremendously beneficial learning experience.

Some considerations surrounding the use of *in vivo* practice have been outlined by Metcalfe (1989) and Faulkner (1993) and should be taken into account by the trainer before using this approach. In the training procedure detailed by Maguire (1984b) for instructing medical students in interviewing procedures, *in vivo* practice was given. Apart from the fact that patients were, to some extent, hand-picked on the basis of their willingness to cooperate and the likelihood that they would not prove too difficult to deal with, this exercise was, to all intents and purposes, what these students would be required to carry out as part of their routine duties if, once qualified, they chose to work on that ward.

In vivo practice also featured in the programme designed by Schofield and Arntson (1989) for preparing general practitioners. Likewise the workshops described by Faulkner (1993) on communication and counselling in cancer and palliative care had participants interview patients on audiotape for later feedback and discussion.

9.8.1 Advantages and disadvantages of *in vivo* practice

Some of the strengths and weaknesses of this method have already been attended to in other contexts. Due to the nature of their relationship, the disadvantages of simulation techniques often coincide with the advantages of *in vivo* procedures and *vice versa.*

Advantages can include the following.

- Greater realism. There can be no motivational difficulties due to charges that the exercise is false or artificial, if trainees are adequately prepared to undertake it and are made aware of what they are trying to accomplish.
- Problems of transfer of training, associated with simulation practice, are removed.
- More general experience of the work environment is gained, in addition to practising aspects of communication.
- Trainee self-confidence can be promoted through the successful accomplishment of an exercise of this sort.
- It affords a strong locus of integration for the many elements that comprise the health professional's training course.

Disadvantages which should be recognized are as follows.

- Reduced control over what takes place. It is always difficult to anticipate and legislate for the many problems, even crises, which can occur in the real situation.
- Students who perform badly due either to lack of preparation, or perhaps a rather difficult patient, can find the experience quite traumatic and confidence can suffer as a result.
- Ethical considerations. Patients may have their confidence in the level of care that they are receiving shaken following an unsatisfactory encounter with a weak trainee.
- The exercise may become defocused. There is a greater possibility that, in the added complexity of the real situation, where predicting what may take place is much more hazardous, trainees may lose sight of the specific objectives of the exercise.

- Difficulties in providing detailed levels of feedback may occur.
- Organizing *in vivo* practical experience may be much more difficult than any of the alternative forms of practice already outlined and may incur greater financial cost.

9.9 SUMMARY OF METHODS OF PRACTICE

By this stage, two points should be obvious about choosing methods of practice to include in training. The first is that there is no 'best' one in any absolute sense of the word. All have strengths and weaknesses which must be appreciated and taken into account. Given such factors as the level of ability, competence, experience and confidence of the group, the facet of the communication process under consideration, and the specific learning objectives, some of these characteristics will weigh more heavily than others in reaching a decision.

The second point is that any choice made should not be arrived at on an 'either–or' basis. It is seldom a case of selecting one to the exclusion of the rest. Rather, different combinations and sequences of exercises can be put into effect, some serving as preparation for others. *In vivo* practice is often used at the culmination of a programme whereas behaviour rehearsal exercises are incorporated in the earlier stages. Taking a more cross-sectional perspective, some methods may build upon others. With a difficult skill to master, covert rehearsal may precede role-play, for instance, during the practice phase and indeed this arrangement has been recommended by Mills and Pace (1989).

9.10 OBSERVATION AND RECORDING OF PRACTICE

Options for observing and recording the skill practice exercise become relevant when thoughts turn to the subsequent stage of feedback and analysis. There are several techniques that can be exploited when obtaining a permanent record of what transpired during the practical. These make use of observers, together with audio or video recordings. The discussion of these options in the present section will be restricted to the recording implications which they pose for the practical session *per se*. Other aspects will be raised in the following chapter and in Chapter 12.

9.10.1 Observers

The possibility of involving one or more of the group as observers of the interaction has already been mooted. With multiple role-play methods requiring trainees to work in triads, a 'round robin' procedure can be followed in which each takes it in turn to act as an observer for the other two. It may be advisable to have a plurality of observers involved when the exercise is more extensive in numbers of participants, duration and learning points. Regardless of the particular method of practice, before commencing, observers should be thoroughly briefed about what to attend to and how to record it. They may be physically present while observing, although watching from behind a one-way screen or over a CCTV link is less intrusive.

9.10.2 Audio recording

It is now common practice to replace the observer with an audio recorder or video recorder. An audio recording of an interaction can represent an invaluable permanent record of interaction upon which to base later analysis and discussion. Indeed it seems to be the option favoured by Ann Faulkner and her co-workers when running communication training programmes in palliative care (Faulkner, 1992). It is especially valuable when the focus is upon the verbal domain of communication with a skill which is essentially verbal in nature, such as questioning or reflecting, being practised. Its big disadvantage, of course, is that all non-vocal aspects of non-verbal communication are lost. Further strengths and weaknesses, together with guidelines for making the most of audio recording, are offered by Bell (1991). These include ways of maximizing the quality of the sound reproduction, an achievement that is not always insubstantial!

9.10.3 Video recording

Without doubt this has become the most popular method of providing a permanent record of the practice stage of training, providing as it does the 'actual data' of interactive sessions (Feltham and Dryden, 1994). But while it has the potential to be of tremendous benefit in this regard it can also have a detrimental influence in the hands of an insensitive, over-zealous trainer. Considerations which should be acknowledged can be grouped under two headings; firstly, those that precede recording proper and have to do with introducing trainees to it, and secondly, recording procedures themselves.

Introducing video

The trainer must contemplate how best to expose trainees to being video recorded. Trainees react to the prospect differently. Some positively relish the opportunity. These tend, in general, to be young, attractive, confident extroverts with high levels of self-esteem. At the other extreme distress may be engendered among a small minority who are typically older (late middle-age), female, less attractive, introverted, anxious and with poor self-concepts. The majority frequently experience various levels of apprehension at the thought of having their practice attempts observed and recorded in this way. For example, in a lecturing improvement staff development programme which involved the videotaping of lectures, as many as 75% of the small sample of lecturers included expressed apprehension at the prospect (Cryer, 1988). Trainers should be aware of this concern and take steps to deal with it so that the training process is not impaired.

Advice offered, including that by Cryer (1988) for making videoing less daunting, covers:

- explaining to participants why they are being videoed and the importance of the feedback information which it provides for overall learning – in essence, video simply affords an extremely informative feedback channel on practice;
- showing students how to use the equipment and encouraging them to take responsibility for this aspect of the practical session;
- assuring students that they will not be recorded without their knowledge and permission; this is a ground rule which should be established at the outset with the group (ethical issues of this type have already been raised in Chapter 7);
- acknowledging feelings of apprehension and being prepared to talk them through with the group;
- recording participants initially in a group setting rather than individually or in dyads; this can be while carrying out an introductory exercise or perhaps just discussing some agreed topic;
- being friendly and trustworthy;
- encouraging mutual support within the group;
- familiarizing students with role-play and simulation beforehand, if these are to feature in the interactions to be video recorded;
- letting members see recordings of others doing what they are about to attempt, perhaps through use of model tapes.

Using video

Making the video recording is invariably governed by the necessity to achieve a balance between two frequently conflicting requirements. One is to produce as accurate a representation of as much of what took place during the encounter as can be achieved. The other to distort that encounter as little as possible in the process. The former can be best carried out in a studio which lends itself to multicamera arrangements and where levels of light and sound can be carefully controlled in order to optimize technical quality. Unfortunately, this environment tends to be maximally reactive. Trainees typically complain that it makes them feel nervous and that practice seems artificial and unnatural. What takes place during interaction is distorted as a result and is regarded by those taking part, rightly or wrongly, as being entirely unrepresentative of how they would normally behave in a more familiar setting.

When such recordings are being made for feedback purposes only, rather than for demonstration, it is best to resolve this dilemma in favour of making the recording process as unintrusive as possible. Most of the pertinent detail can usually be obtained from productions that fall far short of the high levels of technical excellence required when, for example, broadcasting. Such a reduction in quality is, therefore, an acceptable price to pay if it means that participants can, during the subsequent stage of the training procedure, readily identify with and 'own' their performances. A corollary is that video equipment can be effectively employed in CST even though the trainer may not have access to the rather specialized facilities of a recording studio.

When a recording is being made, the trainer must be alert to any possible signs of distress by the participants being taped. Sometimes an interactor will 'dry up'. If it isn't possible to prompt and if it seems unlikely that they will readily resume, the recording should be brought to a premature end rather than subject the individual concerned to further stress or embarrassment. While remaining sensitive to the need of someone to whom this has happened to talk about the experience, such incidents should be largely played down. Time permitting, the opportunity to carry on and finish should be given once a more composed state has been regained.

Recording procedures and the range of skills and artistic techniques that go to make for quality video production are a further matter. While much can be gained from a basic static, single camera arrangement, more elaborate recording effects can add a further dimension to the instructional use of this medium. They tend to be more important, however, when it comes to the making of high quality model tapes and will not be gone into here. Further information can be found in Wetzel, Radtke and Stern (1994), for example.

9.11 OVERVIEW

The opportunity for trainees to put the material covered in the preceding phase of sensitization into practice is seen as a central feature of CST. Why practice should be thought to be of such importance can be attributed to a plurality of sources. When considered in combination with complementary techniques which typically go to make up a CST package, the practice component has generally been found to make a positive contribution to training outcomes (Baker, Daniels and Greeley, 1990).

Survey data has certainly demonstrated the ubiquity of the practical element in programmes implemented to improve levels of communication within the health professions. Some of the objectives which trainers have had in mind when requiring trainees to practise have been quite narrow and specific, others much broader. Perhaps the most common has had to do with furthering the behavioural reproduction aspects of skill performance. Others include:

- enabling consequences of performance to be experienced;
- highlighting discrepancies between what is thought to be done and what actually is done by students;

- providing practical knowledge of the interpersonal complexities of situations and the operation of different social structures;
- facilitating the restructuring of beliefs and attitudes;
- creating a greater awareness of self and others;
- permitting new roles to be tested.

These can be accomplished by means of one or more of a range of options, some of which make use of simulation. They include covert rehearsal, behaviour rehearsal, role-play and simulation exercises and games. Using patient simulators is one variant that has become particularly popular, especially in the training of medical students. Alternatively, *in vivo* practice can be provided. The choice will largely depend upon a complex of considerations, the most important of which have to do with the learning objectives specified, characteristics of the group and the particular point that the programme has reached. These aspects will be further considered in Chapter 12.

Although observing and recording performance during practice can be potentially disruptive, and steps must be taken to minimize this possibility, it is typically carried out in order to facilitate subsequent feedback and discussion. This can be done by members of the group who have been designated to act as observers and briefed accordingly. More frequently audio or video recordings of the interaction are made, the latter being the most popular. The instructor must always be mindful that videotaping can cause some trainees varying degrees of unease, especially in the early stages and should be used with sensitivity.

The feedback phase of training

10

10.1 INTRODUCTION

We have seen that sensitization is necessary for effective skill acquisition to take place but is not sufficient on its own. Practice opportunities are necessary. Likewise, while practice is necessary, it in turn is not sufficient to bring about improvements in performance. It is practice coupled with feedback that works. Ericsson, Krampe and Tesch-Romer, (1993) believe that, 'In the absence of adequate feedback, efficient learning is impossible and improvement only minimal even for highly motivated subjects. Hence mere repetition of an activity will not automatically lead to improvement' (p. 367). For progress to take place there must be an awareness on the part of the performer of the characteristics and consequences of action enabling judgements on appropriateness to be reached and adaptations to be effected as required. In other words, as intimated in the preceding chapter, practice must be accompanied by resulting feedback to enable increased levels of skill to be attained. This phase is, therefore, crucial to the success of the whole training sequence and it is to it that we turn our attention in this chapter.

It has been pointed out by French (1994) that feedback is a concept borrowed from information theory. It refers to a process whereby a system undergoing change has information available to it on the nature and extent of that change so that the change process can be regulated. In a situation where learning is taking place leading to improvements in performance, the centrality of feedback has long been recognized. Bartlett (1948, p. 86) declared that 'the common belief that "practice makes perfect" is not true. It is practice the results of which are known that makes perfect.' Little has happened in the intervening years to confound this dictum and the belief that feedback is conducive to heightened achievement is now regarded as essentially axiomatic. Indeed many theorists regard it as 'the single most important variable controlling the acquisition and performance of motor skills' (Kamal and Blais, 1992, p. 203).

As a component of the CST procedure, the role of feedback is also stressed (Rosenfarb, Hayes and Linehan, 1989). Reviews of training practices in this facet of health-care delivery, some of which were referred to in the previous chapter (e.g. Anderson and Sharpe, 1991), have specified feedback as featuring prominently in many of the interventions included. Indeed, Kurtz and Marshall (1982) found it to be the most commonly used training technique. Of the 27 UK university medical schools surveyed by Frederikson and Bull (1992), all but six made use of video feedback for this part of the course. Similarly, Carroll and Monroe (1979), when deriving instructional principles based upon the results of their earlier survey of CST in US medical schools, stipulated that 'a crucial variable is the provision for direct observation and feedback on students' interviewing behaviour. The feedback principle is so fundamental to the design of instruction that it may often be regarded as merely an educational platitude' (p. 498).

But popularity does not necessarily equate with efficacy. The effects of this component have also been the subject of empirical investigation. While a comprehensive review of the work that has been carried out will not be attempted, the general finding to emerge is largely confirmative. For instance, as part of the microtraining package, feedback was found to have made a highly significant contribution to skills acquisition, based upon the meta-analysis of some 23 studies undertaken by Baker, Daniels and Greeley, (1990). Although Mills and Pace (1989) found video feedback on its own to be an effective medium for improving listening behaviour, it seemed that long-term benefits were more likely when it was combined with practice.

The bulk of this chapter will outline the major functions served by this phase of the training regime, together with a range of possible modalities and sources that can be exploited to provide performance-related detail for trainees. This will include discussions of the features and use of audio, video, written and oral feedback provided by trainers, trainees or indeed those who have partnered trainees during the practice interaction. Consideration must also be given to organizing and conducting the feedback tutorial, including practical advice on how to avoid some of the problems and pitfalls that can confound this stage of the training procedure. We will continue, though, by considering alternative conceptualizations of feedback and the differing forms it can take.

10.2 THE OPERATION OF FEEDBACK

In the CST literature it is common to find terms such as 'reinforcement' or 'knowledge of results' used instead of 'feedback'. Although these, for the most part, are used interchangeably, they do have slightly different connotations, which are reflections of contrasting views of the *modus operandi* of this aspect of instruction. The fact that feedback has the potential to facilitate learning and improve performance is commonly accepted – how it functions to effect these outcomes is open to several interpretations.

There are broadly three theoretical interpretations of feedback (Fitts and Posner, 1973). These have been discussed by, among others, Adams (1987) and Magill (1993) in terms of motivation, reinforcement or information. Those who regard feedback as a means of influencing the level of motivation of the recipient point to the fact that individuals are typically more interested in the task which they are doing, are prepared to invest greater effort in it and may feel more confident in their ability to succeed when it leads to a recognized and accepted positive outcome. Such feedback has energizing properties, serving as an incentive to strive even more determinedly. Conversely, lethargy and low morale leading to reduced effort and poor-quality output frequently result from insufficient incentive. Viewed in this way, feedback produces direct changes in performance rather than in learning and consequently its impact tends to be comparatively transient. This is not to deny, however, that it can indirectly promote learning by increasing the amount of practice that the trainee is prepared to undergo.

Alternatively, feedback can be looked upon as a means of reinforcement, acting to increase the frequency of occurrence of that behaviour which produced it and perhaps even doing so in a completely reflexive manner. Cairns (1986), argued that 'the feedback concept described in most communication theory is equivalent to the reinforcement concept of operant conditioning' (p. 129). Here strong parallels are drawn between systematically modifying some targeted behaviour of an animal in a laboratory experiment by providing food or some other reward each time it appears, and praising the trainee for displaying high levels of a particular skill during a practical. Presumably those who talk of providing reinforcement rather than feedback as part of CST have, at least implicitly, a model of this sort in mind.

Contrasting with the previous two positions is the notion of feedback as information, operating very much at a cognitive rather than an affective level. By making learners more aware of the extent to which their actions approximate some recognized standard, information that can be assimilated and acted upon is made available. If this information about the response and its outcome is accurately interpreted and implemented a new response can be generated on the next occasion that is more appropriate than the previous attempt. Here skill acquisition is very much thought of in terms of effective information processing. When 'knowledge of results' is the chosen term, feedback is often assumed to function in this fashion.

While it is relatively easy to theoretically distinguish between these three operations of the process, the practical problems of doing so will be appreciated. Any specific instance of feedback could serve to motivate, inform and reinforce at one and the same time. Most CST trainers would probably accept this eclecticism. While much of what takes place during this stage is concerned with making additional information available to the performer, the commonly held view that feedback should be essentially positive rather than negative has more to do, it would seem, with motivating and reinforcing.

10.3 TYPES OF FEEDBACK

Taking a more analytical approach to the concept, there are a number of distinctions that can be drawn when thinking of feedback, each with significance for CST. These include intrinsic *versus* extrinsic feedback, knowledge of results *versus* knowledge of performance, concurrent *versus* terminal feedback, immediate *versus* delayed feedback, positive *versus* negative feedback, descriptive *versus* prescriptive feedback and solicited *versus* unsolicited feedback (Kamal and Blais, 1992; Fedor, Rensvold and Adams, 1992; Magill, 1994).

10.3.1 Intrinsic *versus* extrinsic feedback

This is one of the most fundamental discriminations that can be made. Intrinsic feedback is available as a natural consequence of performing a task. It was this type that was mentioned in Chapter 3 as a component of the interpersonal skills model. The notion will be recalled of behaviour being responded to by the other involved in the encounter, thus providing feedback intrinsic to the task which can be acted upon in order to achieve the specified goal.

It is, however, largely with extrinsic feedback, sometimes called augmented feedback, that the present chapter is concerned. Extrinsic feedback refers to supplementary information which, while not forming an integral part of the task, enables decisions to be reached about its accomplishment. It can be supplied by observers in the form of verbal comments or by a variety of mechanical devices such as buzzers, lights or other visual displays, together with audio and video recordings. Most commonly in CST it has taken the form of trainer and peer comments together with videotaped replays of practice.

A general finding would seem to be that in many situations extrinsic feedback is an effective means of facilitating skill acquisition. It is commonly used in this context and with both anecdotal and empirical support (Magill, 1994). However, Magill also makes the point that, under certain circumstances, augmented feedback can be counterproductive and actually hinder learning. This can occur when learners become dependent on these extrinsic sources of information to the neglect of intrinsic cues available in the performance. Towards the end of training a frequent recommendation is that feedback that is extrinsic be gradually removed as levels of performance improve.

10.3.2 Knowledge of results *versus* knowledge of performance

Strictly speaking, knowledge of results conveys information on the extent to which the outcome of action matches some standard or achieves a desired goal. The trainee will have been made aware of that standard during the sensitization phase by, for example, viewing a model tape depicting the communicative element under focus. Indeed it has been speculated that the most important role of the trainer in the feedback tutorial may be to facilitate comparison by students between their own attempts and the performance of the model (Ellis and Whittington, 1981). The goal striven for may have been suggested to the student prior to practice in the context of, for instance, a structured role-play. With less structured forms of practice greater opportunities exist for students to formulate their own goals for the interaction. Either way, the trainer who helps the student appreciate the extent to which such goals were actualized makes knowledge of results available.

Where the trainee has little recollection of action or does not know how to best modify it to approximate the standard or goal more fully, knowledge of results may be of little advantage. What is required is knowledge of performance, or kinematic feedback, which deals with the sequence of action producing the particular outcome, rather than with the outcome itself. Videotape replays of what took place are one method of furnishing this type of information, which can be potentially extremely effective.

During CST, making both knowledge of results and knowledge of performance available is, of course, important.

10.3.3 Concurrent *versus* terminal feedback

Concurrent feedback is provided during the enactment, while terminal feedback is only made available upon its completion. In the vast majority of CST programmes it is the latter type of extrinsic feedback that is employed. (Intrinsic feedback is, of course, available concurrently.) Although it may be felt necessary, especially in the absence of systematic recording, to intervene during skill practice and attempt to make use of the 'teachable moment' by drawing attention to some highly pertinent happening, for the most part analysis and discussion of performance takes place after the enactment has come to an end.

Nevertheless, some training programmes have built in concurrent feedback provision. One technique made use of is called 'the-bug-in-the-ear' or BITE. This consists of an earpiece worn by the trainee, which the trainer, watching the performance from behind a one-way mirror or over a CCTV link, can use to relay messages about how the situation is being handled as it unfolds. Gallant, Thyer and Bailey (1991) reported positive results when the technique was used to promote selective therapist skills during marriage and family therapy training. Having reviewed its application in a number of contexts, including teacher and therapist training, Adamek (1994) concluded that BITE was an essentially effective method of promoting professional skills and one that was reacted to favourably, on the whole, by trainees.

An interesting extension of BITE, described by Quigley and Nyquist (1992) and called 'video coaching', takes the procedure a step further by videotaping the enactment, thus providing a record of the trainee's performance, the actual feedback given by the trainer, and the ongoing effects of the trainee's acting on that feedback. Being able to witness the beneficial consequences of adjusting performance in accordance with this concurrent information, has been described as a powerful training device.

10.3.4 Immediate *versus* delayed feedback

The length of time between the termination of practice and the provision of terminal feedback is the key factor in this case. The general consensus of opinion is to reduce the period of delay to a minimum (Hargie and McCartan, 1986; Brinko, 1993), although Pope (1986) suggested that, in the absence of any significant intervening event, feedback could be delayed for up to 24 hours and still be effective. Using video replays helps in this regard. One of the proposed advantages of this facility is that it serves to reinstate what happened during practice, including not only behaviour but also thoughts and feelings experienced at particular points in the interaction.

10.3.5 Positive *versus* negative feedback

Take the example of a student explaining to a patient how to use an inhaler. Aware of having covering all of the essential points at an appropriate pace and in a comprehensible fashion, coupled with the fact that the patient was able to effectively self-administer the medication using the piece of apparatus, constitutes objective feedback which, in this case, is wholly positive. A video or audio replay of the consultation would also afford a relatively objective source of feedback. A trainer may also be available to pass comment on what took place. If so this additional perspective represents, by way of contrast, subjective or interpersonal evaluative feedback (Jussim, Coleman and Nasau, 1989). It is characteristically the latter to which trainers implicitly refer when they extol the virtues of positive over negative feedback. As such the habit of constant fault-finding and associated criticism during analysis and discussion of skill practice should be resisted. Rather, the weight of comment should be placed upon positive rather than negative features. This is reflected in one of the recommendations offered by Brinko (1993, p. 583), that 'feedback is more effective when it contains a moderate amount of positive feedback with a selected and limited amount of negative feedback'.

Brinko (1993) offers further useful advice on how to deliver negative feedback when it is felt justified to do so. It should be:

- sandwiched between positive information such that more positive comment is given before and after;
- self-referenced rather than norm-referenced, making comparisons with that trainee's past performances or levels of ability rather than with those of others in the group;
- given in the context of a first or third person statement (e.g. 'I wasn't quite sure what your goal was for the meeting,' or 'A clear goal for the meeting

wasn't evident,' rather than 'You didn't seem to know what you were trying to do in the meeting');
- factually rather than emotionally based;
- inclusive of the offer of positive alternatives;
- sensitive to the self-esteem of the student. Those low in self-esteem can be particularly attuned to any comment that hints at criticism.

However, as already stated, negative feedback should be used with extreme prudence. Curtailing it has been advocated on two grounds, one cognitive, the other affective. According to the former, it is pointed out that in telling people that they have done something wrong, they are only being told what not to do in future! Secondly, negative feedback, particularly if persistent, can have a detrimental effect on self-esteem and lead to a lowering of aspirations (Lee and Whitford, 1992). It can also become translated into beliefs that the source does not like the recipient, or indeed is lacking in competence, if rationalized in that way (Kernis and Sun, 1994).

A related differentiation is that between constructive and destructive feedback. According to Baron (1988) constructive feedback has three defining features. It is specific, considerate of the feelings and sensitivities of the recipient and avoids attributing poor performance to internal causes such as low ability. In the notion of 'corrective feedback', Nelson-Jones (1991) acknowledged that even information on performance that is essentially negative can be packaged more or less constructively. It is, of course, important that it be so done. The topic of constructive feedback will be returned to in a later section of the chapter.

10.3.6 Descriptive *versus* prescriptive feedback

In contributing descriptive feedback the trainer concentrates on a typically factual account of what took place with, perhaps, some limited evaluation. Prescriptive feedback, on the other hand, is much more evaluative in nature, with the emphasis upon getting across to trainees in quite explicit terms how they should modify their performance in future to increase effectiveness. Although there is little research evidence on which is the better approach, Christensen (1988) discovered that, in postobservation conferences with student teachers on their teaching, university supervisors, compared with a group of actual teachers, tended to spend less time telling them what to do and more on encouraging reflection on performance. No doubt there will be many occasions with a well-informed and quite experienced group when all the trainer needs to do is to draw attention to what was done or said. Members will know without being told how the situation should have been handled. This approach, under these circumstances, can be highly successful and foster a sense of self-empowerment through creating a climate of sharing ideas amongst equals. When possible, it is often the preferred option. Indeed, one of the conclusions to emerge from the review undertaken by Adamek (1994) was that feedback that required trainees to think to greater depths about the information made available was ultimately more effective. But there may be alternative conditions of poor insight, little or no practical experience, major errors, etc. when the best course of action is more prescriptive. The stage of learning is another factor not to be overlooked. As stated by Magill (1994, p. 326), 'If augmented feedback is given to beginners, prescriptive information is important to facilitate learning.'

10.3.7 Solicited *versus* unsolicited feedback

Traditionally, recipients of feedback have been cast as totally passive partners in the process. But trainees may actively seek information of a certain type and do so in certain ways with differential effects. Fedor, Rensvold and Adams, (1992) distinguished between eliciting feedback, where performance-related detail was explicitly requested by the trainee, and monitoring, which enables information to be gleaned on the basis of assumptions derived from trainer's verbal and non-verbal cues. They charted sets of personal and situational factors that predisposed to one or other strategy being adopted. It is probably wise, therefore, to take into account the advice not to impose feedback on students. Unwanted information of this sort will have much less impact and may well be rejected. But the trainer is not a passive partner either. It is important that the group appreciate the need for obtaining feedback.

Before leaving the topic, any prospective trainer should be aware of some of the recent findings suggesting that certain trainees may be inclined to seek out information of a particular type. People with a dysphoric temperament (mild, non-clinical depression) and those with negative self-perceptions, for example, have been reported to have a greater inclination to avail themselves of unfavourable feedback even though it may make them unhappy (Swann *et al.*, 1992). However, Alloy and Lipman (1992) take a slightly difference stance on the evidence, suggesting that it only supports the conclusion that such individuals prefer negative self-focused information of this type, not that they necessarily actively seek it out. Either way, this possibility should be taken into account by the trainer.

In sum, extrinsic feedback during CST is typically immediate (or relatively so), terminal and should provide knowledge of performance as well as knowledge of results. It should be mostly positive, always constructive and, where possible, descriptive and solicited.

10.4 FUNCTIONS OF THE FEEDBACK PHASE

In broad terms, and at a theoretical level, the major functions of this part of training have been outlined in Chapter 3. They are to motivate, reinforce and/or inform. Beyond that, however, a range of more fine-grained, practical functions of relevance to training have been noted by, for example, van Ments (1983) and Bradley and Phillips (1991).

- Clarify what took place during practice.
- Promote reflection upon what ensued during the interaction.
- Establish why things happened as they did.
- Re-affirm standards of performance.
- Identify ways in which improvements can be effected.
- Facilitate self-awareness. One of the central objectives of CST is to, sensitively and non-threateningly, make participants more fully aware of their needs, attitudes, feelings, beliefs, etc.; characteristic styles of interacting; how these may be construed by others; and likely outcomes that may result. The sort of skill which this book is about is predicated upon such knowledge. The feedback process offers unique opportunities for bringing about such awareness.
- Inspire confidence.
- Develop observation skills. Effective communication depends upon accurate perceptions of situations, people and events. Observation skills, like skills in general, can be sharpened (Rosenfarb, Hayes and Linehan, 1989) and techniques for doing so have been outlined (Boice, 1983; Burley-Allen, 1995).
- Draw conclusions about interpersonal behaviour and facilitate the generalization of learning.
- Locate learning outcomes in the broader ambit of training. Feedback is an occasion when the links which bind sessions together in a programme can be highlighted, although this stage should not be thought of as the only opportunity for so doing.
- Establish action consequences. This is a prospective aspect of feedback. Based upon conclusions reached following analysis and discussion, and in accordance with suggestions and advice proffered, trainees, either individually or collectively, should commit themselves to make use of their learning in some specific and explicit way.

10.5 MODALITIES OF FEEDBACK

Attention will now be turned to the various media typically utilized in CST programmes to provide information for feedback purposes. The most common are videotape, audiotape, written material and oral comments. While each can be used independently, some combination is more often the case in actual practice. Thus oral comments tend to accompany whichever of the other modalities is selected.

10.5.1 Videotape

This method of feedback is popularly associated with CST. Its widespread use has been commented upon by Frost, Benton and Dowrick (1990), while Quigley and Nyquist (1992) asserted that its characteristics and facilities make it 'especially well suited for assisting the instructor in providing feedback concerning specific communication skills' (p. 327). Its application as an instructional medium for promoting skills in medical settings is also discussed by Parrish and Babbitt (1991). A number of features of video playback can be listed that make it attractive to trainers.

- It is potentially the most comprehensive form of feedback. As expressed by Mills and Pace (1989, p. 173), 'Video provides the most specific, informative feedback possible about verbal and non-verbal behaviour.'
- It is available once skill practice is completed, thus enabling immediate feedback to be provided.
- It constitutes a permanent record of what took place, which, if necessary, can be reviewed on different occasions over a period of time. Alternatively, a recording can be compared with earlier attempts, or with more successful attempts by self or others. Slow-motion playback and 'freeze-frame' options to facilitate the in-depth analysis of elements of non-verbal behaviour are also available.
- It is a relatively objective modality. This is particularly so when compared with the unsupported impressions of an observer. Nevertheless distortions of reality can be introduced through choice of recording techniques such as camera angles, close-up shots, amount of time the camera dwells upon a particular individual, etc. Furthermore, perception of what is depicted on tape can be affected by the vagaries of individual representational processes (Frost, Benton and Dowrick, 1990).
- Perhaps the most attractive feature of video replay is that it presents feedback in pictorial form. This eliminates the difficulty and frustration of searching for the proper expressions to adequately describe, in sufficiently graphic detail, the important nuances of some non-verbal action. It is also especially accommodating of those individuals who assimilate information most conveniently in visual form.
- Video seems to have an intrinsic appeal for trainees, who, for the most part, react positively to it (Brook, 1985), although some initial apprehension at the prospect may be engendered (Cryer, 1988).

No doubt positive features such as these are responsible for many of the exaggerated claims and unrealistic expectations that initially pervaded discussions of the effectiveness of video feedback. There has been a tendency to regard this element as the *sine qua non* of successful training outcome. Reviews of the available research have arrived at a more guarded conclusion (Hung and Rosenthal 1978; Fichten and Wright, 1983; Dowrick, 1991). Indeed, Sorenson and Pickett (1986, p.13) go so far as to say that 'when videotaped feedback is used by itself,... students make no greater gains in competency than control groups'. But they were referring to the use of what Dowrick (1991) called 'unstructured' video replay. To be effective, a degree of structure must be introduced. This can be accomplished in several ways, most notably through the organization of the critique session. In order to maximize the potential of this modality, therefore, certain circumstances should prevail.

- Trainees' attention must be directed to the pertinent features of playback. It could be to this end that students prefer to have tutors present during playback sessions.
- Video feedback should be provided within the context of a structured training sequence. There is evidence attesting to the contribution that this component can make when complementing sensitization and practice procedures (Sanders, 1982; Mills and Pace, 1989).
- The extent of exposure to self-viewing would seem to be important (Hung and Rosenthal, 1978). Unless the recording lasts long enough for trainees to be exposed to sufficient instances of the targeted feature of performance, training effects may be limited. Allowances must also be made for 'the cosmetic effect', which refers to trainees' initial preoccupation with physical features of appearance rather than the subtleties of skilled communication when seeing themselves on tape for the first time.
- Trainees should be in a receptive frame of mind. Heightened states of anxiety or feelings of threat will lessen the benefits to be derived.
- With regard to content, it has been suggested that concentrating mainly upon positive rather than negative features of the recording, during replay, may be more efficacious (Hung and Rosenthal, 1978) and is the common practice (Dowrick, 1991).
- There is some limited evidence that video feedback may be more effective when carried out with small numbers, rather than in large groups of 12 or more members (Decker, 1983).

It is likely that the more of these conditions the trainer can implement the greater the benefits to be derived from this form of feedback. Nevertheless, one must always be mindful of the fact that self-viewing may be hurtful and damaging in certain cases and can be mishandled. The trainer has to be constantly alert to this possibility and always ready to quickly intervene, if need be, to prevent it happening. While many experience mild anxiety when first exposed to video, which soon dissipates, for a small minority this reaction may be more extreme, as mentioned in Chapter 9. Distress may be caused by 'self-confrontation'. This has been described by Hargie and Morrow (1986c, p. 362) as occurring 'when the ideal self-image of the individual is challenged by the public image as portrayed on the TV screen'. It is more likely to be experienced by what Fuller and Manning (1973) termed the HOUND type (i.e. homely, old, unattractive, non-verbal, dumb) rather than the YAVIS type of trainee (i.e. young, attractive, verbal, intelligent and successful). Such a disaffected student should be treated sympathetically and given support and informal 'counselling'. In the final analysis the trainee must always have the right to forgo videoing and have an alternative feedback modality substituted.

The possibility of such a student requiring professional help from a counsellor or psychotherapist should not be overlooked in some extreme cases.

10.5.2 Audiotape

Despite the fact that the whole dimension of non-vocal behaviour is neglected, many trainers make use of audio rather than video recording to create a permanent and reasonably objective record of skill practice. For instance, and as already mentioned, Ann Faulkner and her colleagues, when running communication training programmes in palliative care for health-care workers, had participants audio record interviews with patients to be brought along to the next session for playback, analysis and discussion by the rest of the group (Faulkner, 1993). An evaluation of the approach has produced some initial results, which are described as being quite promising (Faulkner, 1992). The audiotaping of counselling sessions for subsequent feedback purposes has also been strongly advocated by Feltham and Dryden (1994).

While sharing a number of the positive features of video playback already listed, audio feedback, in comparison, has several additional advantages.

- Less information is carried, thereby reducing the risks of distracting the trainee from the targeted (verbal) skill.
- Audio feedback may be less threatening for some.
- Audio cassette recorders are generally more available than their video counterparts.
- It is more convenient to make audio recordings in the field. Obtaining high-quality reproductions can, however, be difficult!

Considerations such as these spurred some researchers to determine the relative effectiveness of these two feedback modalities. Reviewing early studies into the acquisition of teaching skills, Griffiths (1974, p. 17) concluded that 'the evidence provided does show that audiotape feedback can be as effective and sometimes more effective than videotape feedback within the verbal domain'. Maguire (1986) also reported that 'feedback of performance by audiotape replay or television was worthwhile, but audiotape alone was almost as good as television at the basic level of the skills being taught' (p. 155). Again, these skills were exclusively verbal in nature. Where measures of outcome have been more wide-ranging and have included non-verbal criteria, the results of audio replay have been less impressive (Mulac, 1974). This serves to underscore the one big drawback of this type of feedback; its confinement to the verbal and paralinguistic domains of communication.

10.5.3 Written material

As an alternative to video- and audiotapes, or indeed as an adjunct, feedback can be delivered by means of written comments. (For reviews of research see

Fichten and Wright, 1983; Brook, 1985; Serna, Schumaker and Sheldon, 1992). These may be made by selected observers during the course of the interaction or based upon a recording of it. The importance of giving focused feedback has already been stressed; in like fashion the attention of observers should be channelled to the relevant features of performance. Some form of observation schedule is often provided for this purpose and to assist in the task of recording the appropriate detail. But schedules vary greatly in the extent to which they structure these activities, with some being much more analytical than others. (For a more detailed discussion of the relative merits of global/holistic and molecular/analytical approaches see Bellack and Hersen, 1988 and Wilkinson, 1995, and in relation to the coding of doctor–patient communication, Stiles and Putnam 1989.)

An example of a schedule that is quite global and can be used for giving feedback on the skill of explaining is presented in Table 10.1.

Table 10.1 Global schedule for explaining

- Coverage of topic
- Sequence of key elements
- Pace of delivery
- Clarity of presentation
- Feedback obtained

Here the observer is merely presented with several headings corresponding to the key facets of the skill under consideration. It is left entirely to the users to decide how best to express their perceptions and judgements in written form. Consequently, there may be considerable variability in, for example, the quantity, specificity and content of information included. Some may be primarily descriptive in their comments, others essentially evaluative.

An example of a more molecular schedule, again designed with the skill of explaining in mind, is presented in Table 10.2.

Students often find that these instruments furnish increased information and are more helpful than their less analytical counterparts. Serna, Schumaker and Sheldon (1992) reported that students found global scores representing competence in various aspects of performance less desirable than a more detailed alternative which included written descriptive comments. Feedback provided by analytical procedures is both systematic and structured. As can be seen from the example, the skill is represented by a larger number of more precise items and the system for recording observations, in this case a rating procedure, promotes greater consistency. Supplementary comments can also be added. This type of schedule is particularly useful because it outlines, for the benefit of the trainee receiving feedback, a profile of performance that readily highlights areas of strength and weakness. (Further information on skill assessment can be found in Chapter 11.)

Table 10.2 Analytical schedule for explaining

	Very well done	*Well done*	*Fair*	*Could be better*	*Could be much better*	*Comments*
Introduction						
Suitable vocabulary						
Vagueness avoided						
Adequate concrete examples						
Within listener's experiences						
Fluent verbal style						
Verbal emphasis						
Non-verbal emphasis						
Use of pauses						
Appropriately paced use of audiovisual aids						
Stimulating delivery						
Suitable structure						
Main ideas clarified						
Parts linked to each other						
Concise summary						
Understanding checked						
Feedback acted upon						

Benefits would also seem to accrue for the observer from using such a schedule. Thus Sorenson and Pickett (1986) reported that those who were involved in conducting ratings of the interviews of other students subsequently evinced substantial improvements in their own interviewing skill!

10.5.4 Oral comments

This is probably the most frequently employed feedback modality. It is extremely unusual, with the possible exception of individually based self-instructional packages, not to have a feedback tutorial in CST where those involved share the responsibility of commenting upon skill practice with a view to assisting in the learning process. Discussion may be based upon a recollection of the just-completed practice interaction, but more typically is grounded in the contents of video recordings, audio recordings or observation schedules. Indeed there is evidence that the potential of other modalities, such as video, is only exploited when accompanied by some level of guiding comment from an instructor, for example (Quigley and Nyquist, 1992). But, as we have seen, oral feedback can be positive and constructive or, even if well intentioned, negative and destructive. Several writers, including Pendleton *et al.* (1984), Nelson-Jones (1991) and French (1994), have suggested ways of maximizing the former. The following guidelines draw upon their recommendations.

In addition to suggestions already mentioned in relation to positive feedback, oral feedback is most effective when it:

- deals only with what the trainee is capable of changing;
- concentrates on the performance rather than the person;
- is geared to the learner's needs (Feedback should be at a level and couched in terms that the learner can readily relate to. It should also, for the most part, be restricted to those particular aspects of the communicative process under focus rather than attempt to be all-embracing. Overwhelming the trainee with detail is one of the most common abuses of feedback);
- is specific rather than general, since commenting in vague generalities does not create the detailed knowledge upon which subsequent improvement depends;
- is always constructive;
- provides positive alternatives;
- considers links with the causes and consequences of behaviour, thus highlighting intrinsic feedback within the interaction and avoiding a debilitating reliance upon extrinsic sources;
- is two-way and takes place in the context of open discussion;
- is generalizable, enabling the wider relevance of information on a specific performance to be recognized.

10.6 SOURCES OF FEEDBACK

With the written and oral variants, the distinction between modalities and sources of feedback is much clearer than with video- and audiotape. Written and oral comments on performance and outcome are given mostly by tutors, peers, and participants in the practice interaction.

10.6.1 Tutors

Students prefer to have a tutor present during the postpractice critique session and react more favourably to CST programmes when this happens. This is partly because the instructor is recognized as having a valuable knowledge-base, together with expertise in analysing interaction and drawing comparisons with accepted standards of proficiency. Indeed, some trainees have a tendency to bestow almost mystical powers of understanding and insight in this respect! This can have both advantages and disadvantages. On the positive side, it legitimizes the right of the tutor to pass comment and increases the likelihood that feedback given will be accepted and implemented. Brinko (1993) commented that feedback is more telling when the source is regarded as credible, knowledgeable and well-intentioned. The views of fellow students may not be as readily accepted, especially in the early stages of the programme. A disadvantage is that the tutor may be pressured into a more directive style than would be wished, with participants adopting a passive role.

Tutor feedback may be more influential with less experienced trainees, especially those who, following the sensitization phase, have failed to fully grasp the nuances of the communication skill under consideration and the standards of performance that pertain.

10.6.2 Peers

As already intimated, there may be an initial reluctance on the part of trainees to accept comment from a fellow student, especially if it is negatively evaluative, and indeed there may be a hesitancy on the part of some peers to offer it. On the other hand, participants can sometimes be brutally frank! But having all the members of the tutorial group sharing their observations and opinions on what took place, if properly handled, can make an invaluable contribution to this stage of training. The instructor can take steps to maximize the potential of this source by:

- clarifying with trainees, before viewing the interaction, what exactly it is that they are meant to be observing;
- reminding trainees that feedback should be based not on personal preference but on the material presented during sensitization;
- encouraging trainees to document their observations;
- reinforcing feedback that conforms to the guidelines mentioned earlier;

- serving as a model for trainees to emulate.

In the process of providing feedback, trainees must exercise their perceptual capabilities. The feedback tutorial is therefore a setting within which much worthwhile work can be done in the development of observation skills. It will be recalled from Chapter 3 that the ability to search out, identify and accurately interpret salient cues is central to effective communication. Such skills are not intuitive but can be worked at and improved. A teaching technique advocated by Hogstel (1987) makes use of videotape analysis and is remarkably similar to what takes place during the post-practice critique session.

10.6.3 Participants

Those who participated in the skill practice exercise can comment upon what transpired from the unique perspective of having been part of the interaction – others can only 'look in from the outside'. In addition to the individual practising, there may be peers, patients or others (e.g. patient simulators) providing a particular practical experience. The special insights into the dynamics of the encounter afforded by their involvement in it should not be overlooked since they make possible an additional dimension of feedback that takes account of intrapersonal considerations such as intentions, beliefs, feelings, etc.

One way of tapping this source of information in a systematic way is by using process-recording techniques. A process recording is basically a detailed written record reconstructing the interactive sequence between the professional and patient in the context of their professional relationship. It has been described by Collins and Collins (1992) as a 'valuable tool for both learner and teacher, and compiling and analysing a process recording provides an opportunity to reflect at length about the various aspects of a piece of interaction' (p. 34). Jones (1984) outlined its role in promoting the communication skills of student nurses when working with psychiatric patients.

Different formats for recording this type of analysis exist. The one presented in Table 10.3 requires both interactors to separately record their verbal and non-verbal behaviour together with that of the other, to note what meanings they attached to the other's behaviour, to state their intended consequent reaction and to make critical evaluation of what they actually did.

Although the procedure can be time-consuming and it may not be possible to analyse all of a lengthy interaction or to provide this form of feedback for each student's skill practice, it is a useful way of gaining access to some of the processes that subtend communication. The instructor, however, must be alert to the shortcomings of a reliance upon students' reports of their own work. Amongst these Feltham and Dryden (1994) list the possibility of consciously or unconsciously 'inventing' perceptions and intentions in the interests of consistency and with the benefit of hindsight, rather than basing those parts of the recording upon what actually took place. Such distortion is more likely when the work is being formally assessed.

Table 10.3 Process recording format

Other's behaviour (verbal and non-verbal)	*Interpretation of other's behaviour*	*Intended response to other*	*Own behaviour (verbal and non-verbal)*	*Critical evaluation of own behaviour*

Place:
Significant situational factors:
Goals (long-term and short-term):
Description of the other:
Preconceptions:

An alternative method of uncovering this type of detail is by means of interpersonal process recall (IPR) (Kagan, 1980; Kagan and Kagan, 1991). Here the objective is to develop specific skills and promote interpersonal awareness through facilitating the systematic recall of thoughts, feelings, intentions, etc., that occur during the course of interaction. The procedure requires interview participants to watch a video recording of their interaction and through recall to share an understanding of their moment-to-moment influence on each other. A third party, called an inquirer, serves as a catalyst in this enterprise. The technique has been used extensively in the training of a range of professional groups. Gershen (1983) discussed IPR as an approach to developing the interpersonal skills of dental students, while McQuellon (1982) reviewed its successful application in the training of various health professionals, including dentists, nurses, dietitians and pharmacists. Its impact on the performance of emergency medical service personnel has also been assessed (Kagan and Kagan, 1991).

Where the trainee has taken part in *in vivo* practice the benefits to be derived from having the patient contribute feedback have been recognized (Maguire, 1986). Some reports of this being implemented can also be located although there seems to be little by way of formal evaluation of the outcome.

10.7 ORGANIZING AND CONDUCTING THE FEEDBACK SESSION

This topic can be approached at two levels: firstly, at the broad level of the complete session, and secondly, with regard to the review of a particular skill performance within a session.

10.7.1 The feedback session

A useful way of structuring the feedback tutorial is to view it in terms of three major processes of briefing trainees and establishing a facilitative climate, reviewing performances, and drawing conclusions and establishing commitments. While these processes roughly correspond to sequential stages there may be some overlap (e.g. conclusions and commitments may take place during practice review as well as at the end of the session).

Briefing trainees and creating a facilitative climate

Trainees should be informed at the outset how the tutorial will operate, what they can expect to happen as it unfolds and what will be required of them. A more demanding task for the trainer, and one to which special attention must be paid in the very first session, is the creation of a group syntality conducive to the mutually beneficial process of giving and taking feedback. It is not an overstatement to say that the success of the entire CST programme may well depend upon how successful the instructor is in this respect. Failing to recognize this typically leads to a number of problems encountered at this juncture.

- **Defensiveness**. Overly defensive students may react to comments by, for example, denying that the featured incident took place or construing it in such a way as to make it more personally acceptable (e.g. attributing the event to the presence of the camera). (It may be recalled, from Chapter 3, that such bias is quite common in the attributional process.)
- **Hostility**. The session degenerates into a spiral of accusation and counteraccusation – attack and counterattack.
- **Reticence**. Trainees are extremely reluctant to offer comment or do so briefly and in very general terms.
- **Collusion**. An implicit norm is established that requires all feedback to be positive – regardless of accuracy. Not all positive feedback is constructive!

In a group that is relaxed and where there is acceptance, trust and genuineness so that members feel sufficiently confident and safe to set aside defensive barriers and display an openness to the views and suggestions of others, such problems are unlikely to occur. But bringing this spirit about can be difficult. While the seeds must be sown in the first session, it is something that takes time to mature as the group evolves. The instructor can do much to nurture it, however, by, for instance:

- reminding students that the programme is essentially about learning and development rather than personal evaluation and assessment;
- being open, accepting, and genuine;
- working hard to foster a positive relationship with the students;
- presenting feedback as a means rather than an end;
- being primarily positive, especially in the early stages;
- discussing and offering guidance on how best to give and receive feedback.

Reviewing performances

When this is undertaken within the small group setting, as it normally is, rather than on a one-to-one basis with a student, there are two main organizational options. One is to review each performance before the next trainee practises. This alternative tends to be followed when video or audio facilities are not available for recording. It has all the advantages of immediate over delayed feedback in these circumstances. Again, those students practising later have the benefit of being privy to the feedback offered to those at the start. Such advantage may, however, be more illusory than real, according to Brook (1985), who documented evidence suggesting that those still to practise may be adversely affected. As far as contributing feedback is concerned, these students are often more preoccupied with their own pending practice attempts than with the one currently being reviewed. The quality of the tutorial can deteriorate as a consequence.

Video recordings afford the possibility of replaying and analysing the performances of those in the group one after the other. This is probably the more commonly implemented alternative.

Drawing conclusions and establishing commitments

As already mentioned, this can take place in relation to each individual performance following the critique. An important contribution of the tutor lies in synthesizing the multisource feedback, distilling the salient themes and presenting these to the individual concerned in summary form. Some commitment to the implementation of agreed proposals should also be sought and the trainee should be encouraged to consider the wider relevance of the learning experience to the field.

At the end of the tutorial it is worthwhile for more general learning points to be reiterated and consequences for action reaffirmed. This is also an opportunity for making connections with what has been established in prior sessions together with anticipated future extensions.

10.7.2 The practice critique

Concentrating more single-mindedly upon reviewing the performances of individual students, several approaches can be identified in terms of the style of tutoring adopted. Such style is a reflection of a multiplicity of considerations, including the way in which trainers view their role in the process and the relative weighting given to its various facets.

The role of the tutor

We have already discussed the part played by the tutor as a powerful source of feedback. Providing insights into what took place during the practice interaction, in this direct fashion, is only one of a number of functions performed. The trainer plays a multiplicity of roles as reviewed by Woolfe (1992). They include:

- **facilitator** – by eliciting feedback from group members and promoting contributions;
- **chairperson** – through organizing and conducting the discussion, preventing monopoly, digression, overtalk, etc.;
- **arbiter** – by intervening in cases of irreconcilable disagreement;
- **protector** – by preventing harm from overzealous negative criticism;
- **counsellor** – by being an ever-listening ear for students and their concerns;
- **supporter** – by providing reinforcement and encouragement;
- **judge** – by making sure that everyone has an opportunity to have their say and formulating an agreed conclusion.

How the tutor goes about the task of conducting the critique will depend upon the importance attached to each of these subroles.

The style of the tutor

Extending an earlier distinction between descriptive and prescriptive feedback, one of the most fundamental features of the characteristic way in which the tutor carries out the practice review has to do with the degree of direction and prescription offered. These qualities form the basis of a difference drawn by Bailey and Butcher (1983) between the 'directive' and the 'casual–analytic' styles of supervision in CST. They also resonate with a more profound distinction, discussed by Knowles (1987), between the andragogue and the pedagogue.

The directive style is likely to be chosen by those who emphasize the tutor's contribution as an information resource. Here the tutor is seen very much as an expert who:

- describes and interprets what took place;
- identifies instances of good and bad practice;
- explains happenings;
- establishes the extent to which intended outcomes were actualized;
- stipulates changes to bring about improvements in skill performance;
- controls and dominates the tutorial, with the other members obliged to listen passively.

Although it does have some merits, this style is perhaps more frequently associated with shortcomings. McGarvey and Swallow (1986) discovered that supervisors who manifested it were reacted to less favourably by students than counterparts whose approach was more learner-centred.

With the casual–analytic style, 'the trainer explores interview events with observers and the interviewer by seeking a description of interview behaviour and interviewee reactions, eliciting suggestions for alternative behaviours and exploring the likely effectiveness of these' (Bailey and Butcher, 1983, p. 110). In this case the roles of facilitator and chairperson are much more prominent. Rather than giving information the tutor strives to create awareness and understanding by facilitating reflection on practice. This was very much the approach taken by the university supervisors with student teachers in the study by Christensen (1988) previously cited. Self-monitoring and observation skills, together with a heightened commitment to change, tend to be promoted as a result.

Being able to implement different styles based upon an awareness of circumstances and a commitment to rational decision-making would seem to be the hallmark of success (Bailey and Butcher, 1983). Accordingly, Hargie and McCartan (1986) advocated a compromise 'listen–tell' style, with the tutor changing, towards the end of the critique, to become more directive in order to raise points and present information that would not otherwise be forthcoming.

Stages in the critique

The particular style of tutoring adopted has structural implications for the critique and how it unfolds. Writers have presented different scenarios of the stages through which it develops. Most, however, would seem to acknowledge two underlying principles.

- Establish the facts before undertaking a more profound analysis.
- Discuss positive before negative features.

To these can be added a third.

- Let the performer have first say.

These precepts are influential in the identification and sequencing of the following stages of the critique, based upon the proposals of Pendleton *et al.* (1984) and Brinko (1993).

- Observe and analyse. The whole interaction may be observed before discussion commences. With longer practices, however, it is often more expedient to stop at various points for this purpose. In may even be necessary to replay sections of the recording. Faulkner (1993) feels that there is merit in inviting the participant to do the editing if this is the case.
- Clarify what took place at the factual level.
- The individual who has practised comments upon standards of performance and goals achieved, concentrating upon positive features.
- Other group members comment upon such positive features.
- The trainee who practised comments upon standards of performance and goals achieved, concentrating upon negative aspects.
- Other group members comment upon such negative features.
- Differences of opinion are reconciled and consistencies formulated.
- Reasons for what happened are discussed. Again, those who took part in the practice session have a major contribution to make here.
- Positive alternatives to improve performance are offered.
- Main conclusions are summarized and generalized, together with the establishment of action consequences.

Content of analysis

Interpersonal communication is a multifaceted and enormously complex phenomenon. Even when a limited aspect is isolated for the purposes of training, and regardless of the style of tutoring adopted, analysis and feedback can be directed at one of several levels ranging from the purely objective and readily observable surface aspects of behaviour to the underlying dynamic of personal beliefs, values and motives that lie at the heart of the individual psyche. To be useful, the feedback discussion should at least take account of the individual's subjective perceptions of events and meanings attached to them, together with the plans and strategies formulated and pursued. However, deeper analysis should only be contemplated by well-trained and experienced instructors. Here the general ambience of the feedback session and the self-exploration encouraged becomes more redolent of some of the more psychodynamically oriented approaches to therapeutic change.

10.8 OVERVIEW

There is general agreement that the learning and performance of skill is dependent upon information on attempts at practice being made available for the benefit of the learner. Feedback is consequently indispensable to the successful acquisition and refinement of communication skills. This chapter has been exclusively concerned with extrinsic or augmented feedback, which may be provided by means of videotape or audiotape replays of what took place. Additionally, written or oral comment on appropriate facets of the performance can be supplied by trainers, peers or indeed participants in the practice interaction, including, perhaps, patients.

A typical group-based feedback tutorial combines videotape or audiotape replay with written and oral comments from peers, participants and the instructor. It is important, in organizing this tutorial, that time be spent, especially at the start of the programme, creating a facilitative climate. The review can be pitched at different levels of complexity from a description of the behaviour witnessed to a more in-depth exploration of those factors identified in Chapter 3 as constituting skilled interpersonal performance. Feedback should, at least, strive to encompass the personal meanings attached to behaviour by trainees and the intentions, plans and strategies that were operationalized to effect the skilled communication under study.

Evaluation of communication skills training

11

11.1 INTRODUCTION

This chapter is devoted to the third main stage of CST – evaluation. Evaluation is an integral part of the general education system. Indeed it is difficult to conceive the system functioning effectively without applying evaluative procedures, since success in almost every phase of the education process is based upon evaluation. At the same time it should be remembered that evaluation at the continuing education level, in particular, is comparatively weak, a reason perhaps being that continuing education deals with adults whose mere presence indicates a motivation towards learning. This latter observation is important for CST programmes offered to established health professionals who have had little or no formal CST, in contrast to more recently qualified practitioners who are much more likely to have undergone such training prior to accreditation. However, at any level it is increasingly important to demonstrate the effectiveness of the programme being offered, in that, within a climate of economic accountability, further financial resources are unlikely to be committed to a training course where positive benefits cannot be established.

In a health-care environment which is becoming increasingly business orientated the return on investment related to training will come under keen scrutiny. However, as Hassett (1992) pointed out, if the training is needed to meet organizational objectives that are not directly measured by short-term profit and loss then 'a single-minded focus on the bottom line is misplaced – instead you should consider analysing non-economic results of the programme, such as improved compliance with regulations or safety procedures' (p. 55). Even with this latter approach it may be ultimately possible to attach costs to performance outcomes; for example, savings produced through medication education programmes leading to improved patient adherence to treatment regimes.

Many of the evaluative studies in the health domain are designed to 'prove' that CST works. It may be argued that the rigour of such investigations serves the academic community best. What is more realistic and acceptable within the health practice domain, however, is not proof but rather good evidence that a training course makes a difference. Such evidence is not necessarily hard to come by. Indeed, as Gordon (1991) observed, 'good evidence is to know what you're looking for before you ever conduct the training. If you do a good needs analysis up front, evaluation takes care of itself' (p. 23). Thus for the trainer considering evaluation two basic questions must be addressed – **what** should be measured and **how** should it be measured?

Evaluation of any programme of training must be carried out against the background of previously defined objectives, since it is not possible to measure the results obtained from an educational system when the objectives have not been explicitly stated. Gordon (1991) emphasized the point that 'if you can't define what successful performance would look like, you can't define a coherent training programme at all, let alone measure it efficiently or effectively' (p. 20). Reference has been made in previous chapters to what constitutes communication skills and the behavioural repertoires and underlying cognitions that go together to make up effective performance. These provide the basis of what is to be measured.

11.2 THE NATURE AND PROCESS OF EVALUATION

Various definitions have been offered to describe the nature of evaluation. Guilbert (1981) defined it as a continuous process, based upon criteria that have been co-operatively developed and concerned with measurement of the performance of learners, the effectiveness of teachers and the quality of the programme. It is continuous in that it may lead to a revision of educational objectives, or continuous in a formative sense by providing the learner with information on progress. The criteria refer to the acceptable levels of performance that have been established, while the co-operative aspect of evaluation involves a team approach from teachers and collaboration between teachers and students in implementing the evaluation programme. Training evaluation has also been viewed as the 'systematic application of principles of measurement at each stage of the training programme, to the depth and degree required to produce data in a meaningful form and which will assist the trainer in assessing the changes needed in any aspect of the training' (Foxon, 1986, p. 133). Evaluation is therefore the process of gathering information as well as the process of making decisions based upon this information.

Gallego (1987) further suggested that the definitions of evaluation fall into two main categories, qualitative and quantitative. The former largely reflects subjective judgements while the latter is best understood in terms of objective measurement. In making such a distinction it is perhaps better to think in terms of an evaluation continuum spanning these two pole positions.

In general, evaluative judgements are used to contribute to planning, improve present practices or products, or justify a practice or programme. Walsh and Green (1982) have defined various types of evaluation. Evaluations that contribute to planning are termed 'needs assessments'. Those that are performed to improve present practice or products are called 'formative evaluations'. This latter term is also used to describe continuous assessment of students, where information is systematically provided on an individual's progress during a course of study or training. This is distinct from certifying evaluation, which is used traditionally to position students in order of merit or qualify for some form of accreditation. Essentially, it is designed to protect society by preventing incompetent personnel from practising. 'Impact evaluations' refer to those processes that are carried out to justify a practice or programme.

In evaluation terms it is generally well accepted that there are four levels at which the quality or impact of a training course can be judged. Level 1 concerns the reaction of trainees to the programme. Level 2 relates to learning (i.e. what the participants knew after the course that they didn't know before). Level 3 focuses upon behaviour following the training with respect to on-the-job performance. Finally, Level 4 evaluation is concerned with outcomes (i.e. did the programme produce the results desired?). In the health-care field these may be viewed as ascending rungs of a ladder, of which patient outcomes and health status are the most important.

Outcomes, however, need first to be defined. This is achieved by clarifying and identifying the desired or possible results that could emanate from training application. Secondly, they require to be monitored in order to measure the extent to which they are being achieved. Thirdly, they must be assessed by exploring if the end result can be attributed to the training initiative. Thus, because of the multiplicity of variables affecting improvement in medical care and the complexity of outcome evaluation, it is important to attempt to assess the impact of training on practitioner satisfaction, knowledge and performance in order to document their links to patient health status.

In relation to student evaluation the assessment process should follow four main stages. These concern:

- the criteria or the acceptable levels of performance that the student must attain;
- the development of measuring instruments;
- the interpretation of the measurement data;
- the formulation of judgements as a basis for future decisions or actions.

Reference has already been made to the fact that any evaluative test procedure must be directly related to educational objectives. Moreover, any testing system must be realistic and practical and concentrate on those issues which are both important and relevant. In addition, it should be comprehensive, brief, precise, accurate and clear.

To underscore the importance of having clear objectives with tangible outcomes, Exercise 11.1 has been designed to assist trainers to begin to analyse and define their objectives in planning and implementing CST.

Exercise 11.1 Establishing the basis of a test instrument

Consider the CST programme that you are about to introduce. Against the background of the objectives you have established, list: (1) the contents of the course that you expect trainees to know and understand; (2) a set of behaviours that you expect trainees to recognize and accurately interpret; and (3) a set of behaviours that you expect trainees to adopt and integrate into their interpersonal communication performance. These may be set out under the following headings:

- Knowledge and understanding
- Recognition and interpretation
- Application and assimilation

Based on what the trainer's expectations of trainees are following such a course, it will be possible to begin to develop test instruments which are relevant to the training process and which have the capacity to fulfil the qualities of tests discussed later in this chapter.

11.3 SOME PROBLEMS IN EVALUATION

There is a myriad of problems that surround the evaluation of CST of which the following are both important and frequently encountered. Firstly, there is the problem of deciding what is to be evaluated. Education evaluation has a twofold purpose. One is concerned with the operational objectives of evaluation which include such features as the programme planning process, structure, decision-making procedures, personnel, physical facilities, finances, recruitment, training, public relations and administrative management. The other is concerned with the educational objectives dealing with aspects such as programme objectives, trainees, methods and techniques, materials and quality of learning outcomes (Knowles, 1980).

Secondly, there is the cost of undertaking assessment procedures, both in terms of finance and time. Both these factors can mean that severe restrictions are placed upon the type of evaluation that can be carried out and its essential worth. Thirdly, there is a possible lack of expertise on the part of course tutors in designing evaluative systems allied to CST that go beyond measuring mere intellectual skills to assess professional performance and patient outcomes. Fourthly, and linked to the previous factor, is the degree of difficulty in actually measuring practitioner performance in the work situation or patient health outcomes. Fifthly, there is the problem of designing test instruments which fulfil the criteria of validity, reliability, objectivity and practicability.

Such factors play an important part in the evaluation process at all levels of education. However, at the continuing education (CE) level other issues emerge linked to assessment. The fact that there is a lack of objective evaluation of CE courses may reflect the thinking that the provision of CE opportunities is a service to the profession and that as long as there is uptake of such courses that is sufficient evidence of their usefulness and effectiveness. There is also the concern that practitioners who voluntarily participate in CE programmes might consider formal evaluation an infringement of their professional rights and freedom, and might either refuse to take part in evaluation procedures or withdraw from participating in CE.

In the overall context of CE, Knowles (1980) highlighted four universal problems related to evaluation:

- The complexity of human behaviour and the myriad of variables affecting it make it impossible for us ever to be able to prove that it is 'our programme' alone that has produced the desired changes.
- To date the social sciences have not developed the rigorous research procedures and measurement instruments for producing the hard data required for evaluating many of the subtle and more important outcomes of a CE programme. (Considerable gains have, however, been made in this area in recent years.)
- Intensive evaluation procedures require substantial time and financial resources, which are not prepared to be committed by planners and participants, simply to document the value of training which they already see.
- CE is, unlike youth education, an open system in which participation is voluntary so that the worth of a programme is more readily tested by the degree of persistence and satisfaction of its participants.

These observations only serve to illustrate the complexity of the task facing a trainer at whatever level of training in respect of initiating evaluation. However, it is to the methodological strategies that we now turn in an attempt to provide practical advice on how testing can be implemented even in situations where the constraints are considerable.

11.4 QUALITIES OF THE ASSESSMENT PROCEDURE

As has been alluded to, the two main desirable qualities of any test are those of validity and reliability. A brief outline of these concepts is presented, firstly to alert trainers of the issues that require to be considered in the design of any evaluative test procedure in respect of CST, and secondly to provide some background information that will foster a better understanding and critical assessment of evaluative reports on the outcomes of training programmes. In addition, factors that can confound the evaluation process are highlighted and alternative actions are proposed.

11.4.1 Validity

Validity is concerned with the question: To what extent does the test instrument measure what it is intended to measure? Unfortunately, in designing tests the emphasis is often on answering factually orientated questions, despite teaching objectives including the application of principles coupled with the trainee's ability to develop problem-solving skills. Thus for tests to be valid they must be designed to cover all aspects of instruction including behavioural dimensions as well as factual knowledge.

Consider the example where a clinical nurse tutor wishes to design a test to determine if a student can effectively educate a patient on the use of stoma care products. In writing the test items the tutor only includes questions about the types of product, their unique features and the clinical situations where they are indicated. Here then is a situation where the test measures knowledge about stoma care products but does not measure what the tutor intended (i.e. it is not a valid measure of the advisory/explaining skills of the student).

It is perhaps obvious that a test may be valid for one purpose but not for another. However, the same test can have degrees of validity depending on its construction, so that the notion of validity is in fact a very relative one. It must also be remembered that the concept of validity is multidimensional. There are different types of validity, including content, criterion-related and construct validity. Content validity is of primary concern to tutors who wish to develop knowledge-based tests of a particular subject data. Criterion-related validity is concerned with comparing test scores to some external variable or variables (criteria) that measure the same trait. With criterion-referenced tests trainees are expected to reach a certain level of mastery (criterion level) of the material being studied before proceeding further. Tutors may use criterion-referenced pre-tests to predict which students will master the training or indeed where the mastery level should be set. In order to support both these decisions such pre-tests will require some estimate of criterion-related validity.

Criterion-referenced measurement has been used to judge practitioners' ability to interact with their patients. For example, elements such as avoidance of jargon, active listening, sensitively dealing with emotions and using open questions could be rated on a 0–4 scale where 0 equals total omission of the element and 4 represents exemplary use of the element. In addition, using this approach, evaluation pre- and post-scores can be measured to determine any changes in performance following training.

Finally, construct validity is designed to assess how well a test measures more abstract concepts such as 'problem-solving ability', 'awareness of patient needs', 'perceptions', 'anxiety', etc. Gronlund (1976) defined a construct as:

psychological quality which we assume exists in order to explain some aspect of behaviour. Reasoning ability is a construct. When we interpret test scores as measures of reasoning ability we are implying that there is a quality that can be properly called reasoning ability and that it can account to some degree for performance in the test. Verifying such implications is the task of construct validity. (p. 81)

11.4.2 Reliability

Reliability may be defined as the consistency with which a given test measures a specific variable. Thus it is concerned with the reproducibility of test scores on different occasions given the same testing conditions. It must, however, be recognized that valid results are by necessity reliable, but reliable results are not necessarily valid. While validity is a relative term, reliability is a strictly statistical concept and is expressed in terms of a reliability coefficient or through the standard error of the measurements made. (For further consideration of the statistical aspects of this feature see Speedie, 1985 and Page and Fielding, 1985.)

In considering reliability as a fundamental quality within a test it must also be recognized that the concept of reliability extends to those who administer the test, in the sense that observation-type tests require the observer to be reliable. Thus, while it is possible to construct a specific categorization system of behaviours or actions to be assessed, the rater must be consistent in terms of attention to, and interpretation of, the specific facets of these behaviours. This will mean that in any form of interaction analysis the propensity to be unstructured, ill-defined or highly subjective will be minimized by clearly defining the criterion to be assessed and providing precise instructions on the methods of scoring to be adopted. Evans *et al.* (1991) described the use of a criterion-referenced history rating scale to assess students' diagnostic efficiency following CST, its application being matched with high levels of inter-rater reliability.

11.4.3 Other characteristics of tests

In addition to validity and reliability, several other qualities are important to the test instrument. Firstly, it should be objective, in that independent examiners should agree on what constitutes a 'good' response to a particular question or task. Secondly, it should be practical, in that it can be carried out with limited expense and within a reasonable time frame. Ideally it should be easy to administer, yet the complexity of evaluating communication skills often militates against achieving this goal. Thirdly, against the background of the objectives set for training, the assessment procedure should reflect the weight of teaching in any particular area. Thus, assessment of trainees following a course on patient interviewing skills should seek to provide the correct balance in the evaluation procedure in terms of measurement of questioning skills, listening skills, explaining skills, etc. Fourthly, any test procedure should also be discriminatory, in that it should be possible to distinguish between good performance and poor performance of trainees in relation to a given variable. For example, in the health field such assessments have led to the recognition that practitioners have a tendency to avoid dealing with psychosocial aspects of patient care, concentrating on the physical aspects of disease.

11.4.4 Skewing of results

Within the evaluative process, or in developing an evaluation strategy, it is important to be aware of three factors that can confound the results. Firstly, the so-called Hawthorne effect concerns the degree to which the evaluative process itself may change the trainee's behaviour. Secondly, the halo effect involves overpositive rating by trainers or supervisors of their protégés. The third factor is that of separation of variables, i.e. the identification and elimination of the influence of non-training variables that exert a particular influence on the training results. This is particularly relevant to long-term evaluation, where it is realistically impossible to remove all factors that could contribute to a false-positive result.

11.4.5 An alternative paradigm

It has been suggested that evaluation of interpersonal skills training cannot be conducted in the same way as other types of training. Indeed Phillips and Fraser (1982) have spoken of the frustration of knowing the value of a learning experience and yet being unable to express it in a way meaningful to those who had participated in it. These workers argued that, because of problems of variability of course content to reflect individual needs, the reaction of participants to assessment and the differing evaluative requirements of cognitive, technical and behavioural skills, quantitative evaluation becomes almost impossible.

Such a position has led to the suggestion of a new research paradigm where co-operative inquiry is involved between a researcher and members of the training group (Heron, 1989). Talbot (1992) pointed out that such research 'contributes to the functional knowledge of how processes take place and what happens but is very weak on how to evaluate these data and make them verifiable or generalizable' (p. 28).

What has been advocated is a 'triangulation' approach, whereby a variety of methods are used to obtain different perspectives on the object of study (Cohen and Manion, 1985). This approach has two main advantages. Firstly, by illuminating different aspects of the training outcome a more holistic or multidimensional view can be obtained. Secondly, the degree of congruence of the results obtained from different methods provides a useful cross-check on the reliability and validity of each individual approach. Table 11.1 sets out an evaluation matrix which offers the opportunity of deciding upon the different elements which could be assessed and how that assessment could be approached.

Table 11.1 An evaluation matrix (Source: developed from Birnbrauer, 1987)

	Data accumulation, analysis and application						
Levels of evaluation	What could be measured?	What are the sources of data?	How should data be collected?	What analytical methods will be used?	What are the potential problems?	What solutions could be proposed?	How will the results be used?
Trainee reactions to course							
Training learning – knowledge – skills – attitudes							
Trainee behaviour/ performance on the job							
Organizational/ consumer outcomes							

11.5 METHODS OF EVALUATION

A wide range of methods has been employed to evaluate education and training programmes. Interviews with participants, programme advisory councils, questionnaires and instructional group feedback are all examples of methods that have been used to measure the operational objectives of a programme. Substantially, these reflect the degree of satisfaction of participants with the programme, but also provide some insight into processes, attitudes or behavioural changes.

The competency of practitioners relates to their knowledge, skills, attitudes and behaviours following a training programme and their ability to apply these in the patient-care setting. Examples of the methods used to evaluate these criteria include real or simulated practical tests, execution of a project, observational rating scales and tests, short open-answer questions, multiple choice questions and programmed examination (Guilbert, 1981). Some of these primarily relate to assessment of cognitively-based skills. However, real or simulated tests and observational recording go much further to chart actual performance. The use of 'patient simulators' (trained patient instructors) to teach and evaluate diagnostic, clinical and interpersonal skills is a good example of a performance indicator. In addition, the use of video to record and subsequently analyse performance is an increasingly used evaluative tool. Figure 11.1 sets out the types of methodologies that may be used to evaluate the competency of practitioners.

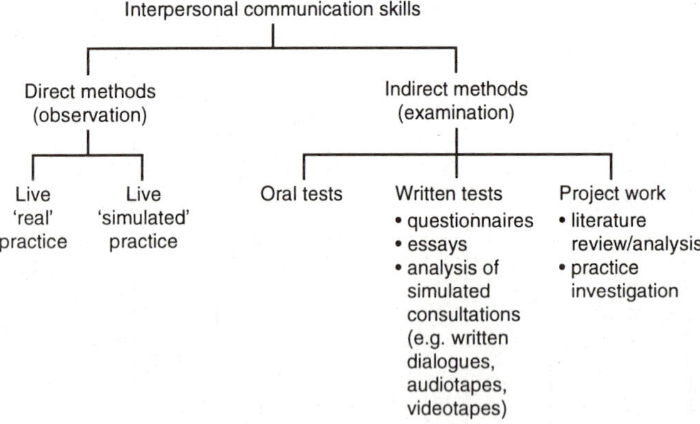

Figure 11.1 Evaluative methodologies to assess the outcome of CST.

As far as evaluation of patient health as a training outcome is concerned, this, as would be expected, is much more difficult. Here the criteria for evaluation focus upon monitoring, for example, compliance with drug therapy, disease control, death rates, discharge times from hospital, referral rates, surgery rates and the like.

11.5.1 Advantages and disadvantages of test procedures

Obviously in conducting CST there is the underlying assumption that communication skill can be learned and developed. Thus it is at the performance level that the trainer needs to direct evaluative efforts in order to assess the trainee's communicative ability, accepting of course that patient outcome measures are the ultimate test of effective communication. Against this background, indirect methods such as multiple-choice questionnaires, essay examinations and written analyses of patient–practitioner dialogues only serve to measure the cognitive abilities of the trainee along with, to some extent, writing skills. Oral examinations again tend to measure cognitive ability but do offer some insight into trainees' capacity to express themselves clearly. However, the degree to which this could be generalized to the work situation is clearly dubious. Furthermore, oral examinations often lack standardization, objectivity and reproducibility of results.

Direct evaluations do offer distinct advantages in the assessment of interpersonal skills. At the outset they permit examination of the candidate in a real or simulated situation through observation and analysis of performance. Secondly, they provide an opportunity to confront the trainee with specific situations that have not been illustrated during training, thereby assessing problem-solving and adaptive or applicative abilities. Furthermore, they indicate the degree to which generalization has occurred over tasks and persons. In this respect, as indicated in Chapter 2, Maguire, Fairbairn and Fletcher (1986) showed that, within the medical discipline, interviewing skills trained in a psychiatric setting were successfully applied to interviews with physically ill patients.

Thirdly, and connected to the previous issue, they also allow for attitudes to be observed and tested, as well as assessment of, and responsiveness to, a situation where there is a high degree of complexity. In considering practitioner attitudes it is important to point out that these can and do have an important bearing on the outcomes of performance. For example, Morrow and Hargie (1987b) indicated that the more positive a trainee's attitude to training the greater will be the degree of positive influence in communication behaviour. In relation to involvement by community pharmacists in patient counselling, Mason and Svarstad (1984) demonstrated that those pharmacists who had the most positive attitude to providing patient advice and education were also more involved in those activities. That attitudes frequently appear strong determinants of practice behaviour means that it is important in any training strategy to seek to develop constructive attitudes as well as verbal and non-verbal skills. Furthermore, McManus *et al.* (1993) reported attitudinal changes in students towards communication, after having being exposed to CST, as demonstrated by requests from trainees for further training in specific areas (e.g. breaking bad news, dealing with embarrassing subjects or with difficult patients).

Fourthly, direct evaluations allow for the assessment of communicative ability when under pressure. They also serve to distinguish between the important and trivial aspects of the encounter.

The disadvantages of such direct tests tend to centre on the difficulties in standardizing the conditions in the same way as is possible with a bench experiment. With actual patients, their responses cannot be controlled to obtain exactly the same behaviour with each trainee being assessed. Furthermore, such situations may suffer from intrusions of one kind or another and they may lack true observer objectivity. One way of overcoming the problem of reproducibility of patient responses is to use patient simulators who have been trained to act in specific but standardized ways from one trainee to another. However, this poses difficulties in terms of the time and expense involved in training simulations, and where a range of patient situations is emulated, ensuring equivalency of difficulty between them. One further disadvantage of direct tests is that they pose more logistical problems, especially when dealing with a large number of trainees.

11.6 APPLICATION OF EVALUATIVE METHODS

A distinction has already been made between direct and indirect evaluations that serve to identify or measure the outcomes of CST, and evaluations made by students or others of the actual programme of training, the tutors and the training techniques employed. It is important to give some consideration to these latter issues at the outset, the results of which will be of considerable value to the course designer in implementing future training.

11.6.1 CST process evaluation

Guilbert (1981) stated that ‘many psychometric studies have revealed the validity and the accuracy of student opinions as well as their close correlation with objective measurements of the instructor’s effectiveness’ (p. 415). Given this finding it is therefore both convenient and meaningful for the trainer to receive feedback from trainees. Unfortunately, some trainers see this as a threatening procedure damaging to their confidence and status as a teacher. Yet anyone who genuinely wants to develop and improve personal teaching performance will seek the opinions of students.

There are two main ways of conducting this form of evaluation feedback – verbal and written. Verbal feedback can either be carried out in a group context or at an individual level. It can range from being completely open, in which case participants are encouraged to make any comments on any aspects of the training, to being more structured, in that comments are invited on specific aspects of the course. One simple technique that provides very valuable feedback is to ask the group individually to state what was for them the most positive aspect of the training and also what was the most negative.

Written feedback may or may not accompany verbal feedback. In this situation various forms of questionnaire technique are used to gather information that will ultimately lead to the improvement of the training process. With simple evaluation questionnaires the purpose is to elicit a response to a statement. Here the statements should consist of a single component thought and specify clearly what is required to be measured. The statement should be presented in such terms that the trainee is required to express a favourable, neutral or unfavourable opinion. Ideally, equal numbers of the statements should be phrased positively and negatively to eliminate any suggestion of overall bias in the questionnaire. As far as provision of alternative responses is concerned 'Yes'/'No' answers serve only to give limited information. Instead a scaled answer is preferable and allows a greater appreciation of the students' opinions. Exercise 11.2 illustrates an example of part of a simple questionnaire of this type designed to gather feedback from a trainee group following completion of a CST course.

Exercise 11.2 Designing an evaluative questionnaire for trainee assessment of a CST course

Below are three examples of statements designed to obtain feedback from trainees in respect of their responses to a CST course. With your own training programme in mind, design a questionnaire to permit trainee evaluation of the programme, the tutor and the training techniques used.

In each of the following statements circle only **one** of the choices, using the following code: VSA = Very strongly agree; SA = Strongly agree; A = Agree; N = Neither agree nor disagree; D= Disagree; SD = Strongly disagree; VSD = Very strongly disagree.

1. This CST course has helped me to identify my own strengths and weaknesses in interacting with patients: VSA SA A N D SD VSD.
2. The analysis of my own performance on the video-replays was counterproductive: VSA SA A N D SD VSD.
3. This CST course did not really stimulate my interest in the processes involved in patient interactions: VSA SA A N D SD VSD.

For tabulation purposes the answers may be accorded a numerical value (e.g. 1–7). A further point in assigning numerical values to the range of answers is that the phraseology of the questions, either positive or negative, will dictate whether the continuum is ordered 1–7 or 7–1. It is also worth pointing out that a good evaluation instrument of this kind will have an equal number of positive and negative statements, for balance. Furthermore, the timing of the questionnaire will have a bearing on results, in that questionnaires administered immediately after training produce different results from those administered some time later (Morrow and Hargie, 1987b).

More complex questionnaires may be devised to identify not only the students' perceptions of reality in respect of the course of training but also their levels of expectation. In this type of question the item to be measured is clearly specified and a scale of answers is offered with a qualitative expression of each degree. Two questions are then asked, one dealing with trainee perception of the course, the other with trainee expectations of the course (Table 11.2). In analysing and interpreting this type of questionnaire the deviance between the means of the responses to question A and B gives a measure of the degree of dissatisfaction or satisfaction of the students in relation to that item. It should be remembered that dissatisfaction may be expressed in terms of lack or excess. Also, by adding the deviation scores across the whole range of items in the questionnaire it is possible to get an overall measure of satisfaction or dissatisfaction among trainees.

Table 11.2 Complex questionnaire: test item

Item: Relevance of videotaped exemplars
What is required to be measured is the degree of relevance of the exemplar material shown on the course by way of illustration of the skills in action.

Never relevant exemplars	1
Rarely relevant exemplars	2
Occasionally relevant exemplars	3
Frequently relevant exemplars	4
Always relevant exemplars	5

Question A. Where would you place this CST course on this evaluation scale?
Question B. Where would it be in order to satisfy you?

11.6.2 Evaluation of teaching techniques and tutors

It is not possible within the scope of this chapter to offer a comprehensive review of the research that has focused on the evaluation of the training techniques used to teach interpersonal communication. However, it is of value to consider some of the findings related to their implications for training practice, since such findings are formative in producing changes in teaching strategies.

Teaching techniques

While some of this research has already been mentioned in preceding chapters, there are four major aspects of teaching that are worth highlighting. The first is that of experiential learning where trainees are subject to practice. Indeed there are numerous examples of controlled studies demonstrating the superiority of students exposed to practice-based training over those who were not. For example, Kendrick and Freeling (1993) have evaluated the effects of a communication skills course for preclinical students. In this study the students initially received lecture-based instruction on doctor–patient communication and were subsequently divided up into small groups for more experiential style teaching. The group study schedule was so organized as to include an evaluation element at a time when two of the groups had received practice in interviewing general practice patients and two had not. The evaluation involved students identifying communication behaviours from a preprepared video of four extracts from doctor–patient consultations. What the results demonstrated was that, while all students were able to consistently identify specific behaviours relative to a preordained checklist, those students who had undergone the experiential interviewing training were significantly better than their 'untrained' counterparts in the areas of defining patient meanings and clarifying inconsistencies.

In a study of the use of a videotape programme to teach pharmacists communication skills comparative evaluation against a control group of learners not exposed to the video showed a statistically significant gain in knowledge within the experiential group (Campagna and Berger, 1990). However, another significant factor to emerge was that the videotape teaching technique used produced lower cognitive scores than expected, suggesting that this mode on its own is inadequate to achieve the desired outcomes. The passive video approach, for example, did not allow for involvement or role-play practice factors which are important for adult learners if skill is to be learned and assimilated (Grosswald, 1984).

Secondly, and linked to the former, is the issue of feedback. This has been comprehensively covered in Chapter 10, but it is worth reiterating that it is not practice which makes perfect but practice with appropriate feedback that makes for perfection.

Thirdly, the use of modelling techniques is formative, particularly using both positive and negative video exemplar material, allied to skill discrimination, communicative performance and behavioural generalization. Carroll and Monroe (1980), in a comprehensive review of the teaching of medical interviewing, identified a fourth factor, the specificity of instruction on particular skills. Programmes where individual skills were identified, demonstrated, practised and evaluated tended to be more effective than less structured programmes.

Tutors

Surveys of communication skills teaching in various health domains have clearly demonstrated the wide range of individuals involved in CST. Moreover, teachers range from those who are clearly experts in the theory and practice of this form of instruction to those who are merely 'interested staff'. Hargie and Morrow (1987b) argued for an interdisciplinary approach to skills training. Ideally, a behavioural scientist should be involved in the design, implementation and evaluation of CST in conjunction with a tutor representing the professional background of trainees. This type of work necessitates the marriage of two separate bodies of knowledge and if either is not adequately represented then the training experience may be impaired. The behavioural scientist will ensure that training focuses upon the communication issues without an over-emphasis upon professional content, while the practitioner–tutor can ensure that any discussion of communication takes place within the realities of the actual practice situation. Thus, a fine balance between 'process' and 'product' can be obtained. Evidence of trainee endorsement of this approach has been reported (Morrow and Hargie, 1986).

In addition, the feedback regarding the efficacy of tutors in CST would suggest that, as mentioned in the preceding chapter, there is a valuable role to be played by adjunct instructors, e.g. patients, student preceptors and patient simulators (Swanson and Stillman, 1990). This issue will be considered more fully later in relation to observation tests of trainee communication performance.

11.6.3 Trainee self-evaluation of outcomes

Trainee self-evaluation of outcomes is one step removed from observer-based practical tests. It is an attempt to obtain feedback from trainees regarding their behaviours following training, especially in situations where time and financial constraints make it impossible to go beyond this type of assessment. It must of course be recognized that this is an inherent limitation within this methodology, in that the reflections of the individuals concerned will be highly subjective. However, Hanson (1981) has pointed out that 'the limits of a self-reporting methodology must be weighed against the potential costs of a methodology using onsite observations' (p. 58).

Morrow and Hargie (1987b, 1995) have used a trainee-report technique to evaluate continuing education courses for pharmacists on developing communication skills. In each, participants were asked to complete a questionnaire stating the degree of influence the course had on them across a range of itemized behaviours consistent with the content of the course. The continuum of available responses for each item ranged from –3 to +3, minus values indicating a negative influence and plus values a positive influence, with 0 equalling no influence. In the first course (Morrow and Hargie, 1987b), the questionnaire was administered immediately following the training and 3 months after training. At both stages of evaluation pharmacists rated the influence of the course as being highly positive. Nevertheless, comparison of individual responses to this questionnaire showed a significant difference between the degree of influence at the end of the course and at the follow-up stage. This was predicted on the basis that the effects of continuing education and training decrease with time.

This finding, however, does have several important implications, not only with respect to the type of training employed but for the understanding and interpretation of this type of evaluative approach. Firstly, the fact that some courses may be of relatively short duration means that, if more time had been available to deal with each course component, more lasting impressions might have been made. Secondly, the decreased level of influence reported may also be attributed to the difference in levels of sensitivity and awareness provided in a training environment where behavioural consciousness was continually being stimulated, as opposed to the actual practice situation, where the same structured stimulation is not available. Thirdly, practitioners who incorporate new behaviours into their performance, to the extent that they become habituated or automated, may underestimate the contribution of previous influential factors. Fourthly, practitioners, subsequent to training, may experience particularly difficult interpersonal situations that call for skills outside the scope of a given course. Because such interactions may have had unsatisfactory outcomes, the course of training may be judged to be less effective. Allied to this is the fact that a short course cannot hope to cover all possible practice situations, and trainees may not be able to generalize the skills to other kinds of patient consultation. A final factor concerns the possibility that some desired behavioural changes may not be easily achieved. One good example of this identified by Morrow and Hargie (1987b) is the inability to provide a private area for patient counselling in a community pharmacy, despite the fact that within the course of training it was seen as a highly important factor in contributing to effective communication.

This latter factor does begin to raise the issue of the internal consistency of the test items in the questionnaire. To what degree are these items a product or a consequence of the course, or of influences entirely outside the training itself? Statistically it is possible to measure the internal consistency or correlation between items in a questionnaire from the results obtained from the surveyed group. By so doing items of dubious relevance can be omitted from the questionnaire. Oppenheim (1992) has discussed these issues and the reader is referred to this seminal text for detailed information on questionnaire design and analysis.

11.6.4 Indirect methods of trainee evaluation

Indirect methods of CST evaluation are largely pencil-and-paper-type tests, although they do vary considerably, ranging from straightforward traditional examination questions to written analysis of simulations or responses to videotaped vignettes. Firstly, the modified essay question (MEQ) which is a set of short, open-answer questions preceded by a case history, has been used to test the cognitive skills of trainees following CST (Weinman, 1984; Knox and Bouchier, 1985). Using both pre- and post-test results, or control *versus* test group results, these studies demonstrated clear gains in student knowledge following training. Moreover, they also tended to indicate increased student awareness and acceptance of the psychosocial dimensions of the case presentations, a feature that may underline the behavioural and affective changes found in other studies.

Secondly, Lezberg and Fedo (1980) described the use of:

- weekly written exercises requiring the demonstration by students of a knowledge of the practical application of specific communication principles;
- evaluation summaries of assigned articles dealing with practice-orientated communication situations and issues;
- participation in interviews;
- final examinations made up of multiple-choice questions and essay questions. Within this last written assessment, students were expected to create and analyse a dialogue between a patient and a pharmacist relevant to the practice situation.

Thirdly, an extension and refinement of this latter procedure has perhaps been the basis of the most meaningful forms of written or oral assessments, i.e. the response to videotaped scenarios of practitioner–patient consultations and audiotaped or written transcriptions of interviews (CINE, 1986). Such techniques are in essence similar to the discrimination phase of CST described in Chapter 8. They largely assess the cognitive and problem-solving skills of trainees and allow some indication as to their attitudes to any given situation. While such evaluations may be predictive of what happens in the practice context this is by no means guaranteed. Observation of trainees in practice is the only clear indicator of the performance effects of training.

Olson and Iwasiw (1987) have used the Behavioural Test of Interpersonal Skills for Health Professionals (BTIS) to evaluate the effects of training on listening skills with a group of registered nurses. This test consists of 28 videotaped vignettes of common patient–practitioner situations to each of which trainees are required to respond. In this programme, pre-training testing of nurses was carried out with the first 14 situations of the BTIS. Here the nurses recorded their responses on audiotape. Following training they were similarly tested with the other 14 situations. A control group of nurses, who received no training, was also evaluated using the 28-item BTIS instrument to ensure that the second half of the BTIS did not in itself elicit higher scores than the first half of the test. The audiotaped responses were subsequently scored by trained raters to measure any differences in listening behaviour. The results of the study demonstrated clear gains in nurses' listening skills following training.

Within the dental setting, Ter Horst, Leeds and Loogstraten (1984) used the videotaped vignette approach to evaluate the effects of CST with dental students. Here students were divided into a control group who did not receive training and an experimental group receiving CST. Following the course, students in both groups were asked to write down their reactions to a series of videotaped excerpts of dentist–patient interactions. These written responses were analysed independently by two raters against a pre-defined communication category checklist. Although there was some evidence of enhancement of performance of the training group over the non-training group on some of the categories assessed, the poor inter-rater reliability levels found in this evaluation meant that the validity of the findings was questionable. Such a study serves to demonstrate the complexity of tests to produce valid and reliable results.

Campagna and Berger (1990) used a particular educational model, that of Bloom's taxonomy, to develop an instrument to measure the overall cognitive gain of practitioners on a CST programme. In this study, of a continuing education course for community pharmacists, an experimental group exposed to a video teaching programme on communication skills was compared to a control group that viewed a similar-length video on a non-related subject. Both groups were pre-tested before being shown their respective videotapes and then post-tested following viewing. The experimental group scored significantly better than the control group. However, the authors have drawn attention to the fact of the influence of the testing procedure in that both groups showed a significant increase in their scores at post-testing.

In consideration of these indirect methods of assessment various advantages can be identified:

- In general terms these tests are relatively easy to prepare and pose few logistical problems in organization.
- Prepared materials, unlike real practice, can also be uniquely constructed to test key abilities on the part of the trainee.
- Indirect evaluations are usually both convenient to administer in relation to time and applicable where large numbers of trainees are involved.
- Because they are largely cognitive evaluations, judgement of the responses is made easier by virtue of being right or wrong, appropriate or inappropriate.
- Such tests are comparatively cheap to administer.

As far as disadvantages are concerned these focus on the fact that such evaluations often measure largely cognitive skills rather than communication skills *per se* (i.e. they indicate a trainee's knowledge and problem-solving abilities but they don't say how these are applied or what behaviours actually result in the work situation). Further, by virtue of the convenience of these methods and their other advantages, trainers may be reluctant to initiate more rigorous evaluation procedures. Reluctance to undertake more direct evaluation may also stem from the fact that within such a system standards for competent communication performance in practice, which cannot be compromised no matter how good a trainee is in other areas of patient care, need to be decided.

At a more specific level, in addition to the above there are a number of other considerations. These mainly concern the use of videotaped triggers or vignettes. Here, the very nature of these recorded incidents is such as to only reflect parts of an interaction. They therefore suffer from the disadvantage that their interpretation and any responses to them are isolated and not set within the context of the overall encounter. Video recordings, audiotapes and written dialogues of complete consultations overcome this difficulty, although the latter two largely omit non-verbal communication. However, video recordings are more costly to prepare and this cost may be recurrent if different situations are required from one assessment to another. The other value of complete consultations is that they can be structured to provide a programmed form of evaluation by conducting the trainee through the interaction and posing questions at strategic points in the process. Obviously by using this form of evaluation some of the above advantages are diminished in that it can be, for example, much more time-consuming to undertake.

Related to the above, reference has already been made in Chapter 8 to the use of interactive video. Such technology allows for trainees to be presented with a number of challenges to which they must give responses. For example, they could be asked to identify examples of self-disclosure, the types of emphasis used in a patient instruction context or the use of reinforcement techniques. Their responses can then be saved and stored, and subsequently marked by the tutor.

Project work

In the above section reference has been made to what could be described as more 'controlled' methods of trainee evaluation. Project work, while still an indirect approach, is perhaps more flexible in its operation and opens up the opportunity for students to demonstrate more adequately their understanding of communication behaviour and the processes involved. Here the emphasis tends to focus upon the dynamic problem-solving or analytical skills of the student rather than merely the recall of facts or pencil-and-paper tests.

In such situations, for example, students may be required, by way of investigation, to record and analyse professional interactions and prepare a thesis as part of an accredited programme of study. Thus, students are enabled to learn and be assessed using a practice-research-type approach. Not only do such activities aid learning and assessment but they can also contribute to a profession's knowledge of itself and how practitioners may need to modify their behaviours. For example, the report by Morrow *et al.* (1993) was a consequence of a final-year pharmacy student project designed to examine the questioning behaviour of pharmacists in community practice.

Although projects do offer wider evaluative opportunities, it must be pointed out that they suffer from the disadvantage that their marking by a tutor or supervisor may be more subjective than objective. Furthermore, any assessment may reflect wider criteria such as methodological design as distinct from aspects of communicative competence.

11.6.5 Direct methods of trainee evaluation

Since interpersonal skill is manifested by overt behaviours, observation of these actions is the most logical evaluation strategy. As indicated in Figure 11.1, two direct methods of observation have been used to assess interpersonal skills: live 'real' practice and live 'simulated' practice. Real practice evaluation refers to those situations where trainees are assessed during actual patient consultations. Simulated situations describe interactions where the consultation is staged either by employing trained patient simulators or through role-play. Because the former is difficult to implement, simulated encounters are most frequently used for assessment procedures. It should also be realized that direct methods of evaluation are potentially most threatening to trainees, so that this form of assessment tends to be used for students prior to qualification rather than qualified practitioners.

Simulated practice assessment

As previously indicated, patient simulators are individuals who are carefully trained to consistently present a patient problem to the trainee, with the encounter being carried out in a carefully controlled situation, such that meaningful evaluation of student performance is possible.

The advantages of simulations as an assessment technique are as follows.

- They can identify specific patient health-care issues or behavioural problems, emphasizing the skill areas to be evaluated.
- Patient simulators can describe symptoms and behavioural problems in specific ways.
- Patient simulators can provide structured feedback to trainers and also to trainees in respect of the learner's performance.
- Different trainees can be exposed to the same patient stimuli and comparative assessment can be carried out using the same criteria.
- The trainee is not committed to the actual care of the patient, so that the problems of eliciting and dealing with true presentations, if these were real patients being observed, are obviated.

The main disadvantage of this technique is that the physical conditions of a health problem cannot always be easily simulated (apart, of course, from using individuals who also actually suffer from the particular complaints). Also, training these individuals can be a costly and time-consuming procedure. The reader is again referred to the comprehensive review by Swanson and Stillman (1990) on the use of standardized patients for teaching and assessing clinical skills.

In an interesting study by Thompson (1992), candidates for membership of the Royal New Zealand College of General Practitioners were examined for their communication performance in two simulated patient interviews. To overcome any confounding effect of knowledge, candidates were briefed as to the patient's medical problem and its management. Scoring of performance was made by three raters and the results showed that there was no significant correlation between a candidate's performance in one situation and performance in a dissimilar situation. Thus performance was seen to be context-specific. Against this background, Thompson argued that it is necessary to (1) specify the domain of competence at the outset and define critical competencies; (2) test critical issues in a variety of ways since it is not possible to completely divorce context from skill; and (3) recognize that resource limitations will mean that evaluations test only a sample of the critical competencies.

An alternative to the use of trained patient simulators is the employment of role-play situations to evaluate interpersonal skills. Here either other trainees or trainers play the patient role and the individuals being assessed are observed in relation to their communication behaviour and scored using behavioural rating scales. The evidence to date clearly points in favour of the value of this technique to discriminate and measure communicative performance in trained and untrained personnel (CINE, 1986; Crute, 1986).

As indicated above, observation evaluation methodologies largely depend upon established behavioural checklists from which raters can, in a structured, standardized form, appraise the performance of the trainee. It must be remembered that with a single rater the objectivity of the assessment is questionable, so that a multiplicity of raters is preferable. However, for the results to be meaningful, inter-rater reliability must be demonstrated. In Exercise 11.3 an assessment schedule allied to interpersonal performance is illustrated. A wide variety of such checklists have been reported, for example, Kraan *et al.*, 1989, Maguire, Fairbairn and Fletcher, 1989 and Kendrick and Freeling, 1993.

Exercise 11.3 Direct assessment of trainee communication performance

Instructions

Videotape a real or simulated trainee-patient encounter. Replay the interaction and score it across the fourteen items listed according to the following nine-point scale: 8 = Excellent; 7 = Very good; 6 = Good; 5 = Satisfactory; 4 = Average; 3 = Unsatisfactory; 2 = Bad; 1 = Very bad; 0 = Appalling; N = Not applicable.

Communication skills

	Score: 0	1	2	3	4	5	6	7	8	N
1. Skill in establishing rapport										
2. Listening ability										
3. Self-presentation										
4. Skill in obtaining information										
5. Relevancy of information										
6. Adequacy of information										
7. Allows sufficient time for response										
8. Appropriate use of reinforcement										
9. Ability to monitor situation										

10. Use of appropriate speech
11. Use of appropriate language
12. Skill in explaining material/information
13. Adaptability
14. Skill in terminating session

Total score:
% score:

More extensive forms of skills checklist can be prepared that seek to itemize more precisely how an individual performs. For example, Kraan *et al.* (1989) developed a 68-item checklist to evaluate students', residents' and primary-care practitioners' interviewing skills. This inventory, the Maastricht History-Taking and Advice Checklist, has been extensively validated and covers six segments or subscales of communicative behaviour. The first three – reasons for the encounter, history taking and presenting solutions – substantially cover the content issues to be addressed, while the latter three – structuring the interview, interpersonal skills and communication skills – represent the practitioner's process skills in performing the consultation. This particular inventory provides a good example of the distinction between the 'what' and the 'how' of communication.

Exercise 11.4 is designed to illustrate how trainers can devise more complex evaluation procedures to assess interpersonal skill. Moreover, the design of this checklist gives more specific guidelines for raters and in that respect has the potential for greater consistency and reproducibility of results.

Exercise 11.4 Devising a behavioural checklist for interpersonal performance

Instructions

Firstly, the trainer should decide what are the target behaviours to be assessed in the communication skills evaluation. Secondly, choose an actual practitioner–patient situation where these target behaviours apply. Thirdly, outline a continuum of actions along each target behaviour. An example is given below for the trainer to practise with before devising his/her own scale. The trainer should fill in the blank squares appropriately.

Task

To instruct a newly diagnosed diabetic patient on her use of insulin therapy.

Sample target behaviours	**Continuum of actions**				
	−2	**−1**	**0**	**1**	**2**
When speaking with the patient the language used	often includes medical terms without explaining their meaning	often includes medical terms and sometimes explains their meaning	seldom includes medical terms but does not always explain their meaning	seldom includes medical terms but always explains their meaning	only uses terms that the patient understands
When questioned by the patient about psychosocial matters	always avoids any involvement	frequently avoids involvement but acknowledges existence of such problems			
In trying to promote understanding	never resorts to the use of illustrations or analogies				
When explaining administration technique					

Real practice assessment

This is the most difficult form of evaluation to carry out, particularly because of the organizational and ethical problems it presents, together with possible clinical effects of subjecting patients to such encounters. These latter two issues have been discussed previously in Chapter 7. Although it poses such difficulties, several reports have been made regarding the use of this technique. Within the medical field these evaluations have included both undergraduate students and qualified doctors. The observation techniques involved were primarily videotaped trainee–patient encounters rated against predetermined behavioural criteria. For example, in a unique follow-up study of the communication skills of young doctors who had received CST during their undergraduate education, Maguire, Fairbairn and Fletcher (1986) demonstrated the sustained effects of training where video feedback was employed. In this investigation 36 young doctors who as medical students had been randomly allocated to either video feedback training or conventional teaching in interviewing skills during a psychiatry clerkship were reassessed 5 years later. Of these 36, half had received feedback training and half had received conventional teaching on interviewing. The groups were matched for their pretraining interviewing skills and time after training. Each doctor was asked to obtain a history of the problems of three patients, two of whom were simulated patients and one real, representing psychiatric, life threatening and chronic disabling categories of illness. Each interview was video recorded and subsequently assessed by a trained psychologist against a predetermined interview rating scale. The results demonstrated that while both groups had improved their interviewing skills score after initial training the superiority of the feedback training group at that stage was maintained over the subsequent 4–6 years. This was consistent across the range of skills examined, with the exception of avoidance of jargon where both groups performed equally well. The control group scored particularly poorly on clarification, open questioning and covering psychosocial problems. Both groups scored poorly on opening and closing interactions but overall the trained group was viewed as being more competent, empathic, warmer and self-assured than the control group. The results also indicated that the effects of training in a psychiatric setting were generalized to other types of patient.

More recent work has demonstrated the benefit of skills training to patient satisfaction outcomes. In a controlled study of students' communicative performance and patients' satisfaction, Evans, Stanley and Burrows (1992) showed by patient interview tests carried out during a CST module (after the lecture phase but before a workshop phase) and then subsequent to the workshop training, that students exposed to the experiential training scored significantly better than their 'untrained' counterparts. Specifically, they received higher ratings for opening interviews, willingness and ability to discuss patients' psychosocial concerns, their effective use of silence, questioning style and clarity of questions, and their ability in closure routines.

When compared with patient satisfaction profiles, the patients of the trained student group reported higher satisfaction with all aspects of their interview than those subjected to the control group of students. In a number of the satisfaction variables (help given by the student, patients' perceptions of students' caring, student detection of anxiety and student transfer of information) the ratings rose from pre-training interviews through post-lecture interviews to peak after the skills workshops. What this work showed was the positive contribution of training to communication performance and patient awareness of these improved communication skills, reflected in their increased levels of reported satisfaction.

In a similarly organized study, Evans *et al.* (1991) carried out a structured analysis of the content of 30 history-taking consultations, 15 drawn randomly from each of two student groups, one subjected to CST and a control group. In each of five categories, interview introduction, problem diagnosis, patient instruction, summary and overall rating, the trained group performed significantly better than the control group. A finer-grained analysis of the diagnostic aspects of the interview showed the trained students to be more proficient than their control counterparts in several areas. Also it should be noted that the interview times for both groups were broadly similar, again demonstrating that their greater diagnostic efficiency was not a function of more time spent in the interview procedure.

In a review of the effects of counselling and communication in health care, Davis and Fallowfield (1991) predicted that there would be a number of measurable outcomes from the application of interpersonal skills in practice. These included professional satisfaction, diagnostic adequacy, patient satisfaction, treatment adherence, psychological benefits, improvement of patient understanding, memory and skills improved physical outcomes and prevention of disease. They go on to provide an analytical review of the research literature to support their assertions. What they demonstrated was the realistic potential (albeit given the difficulty of limiting the confounding variables) of linking skills training to health-care outcomes, the fourth level of evaluation identified at the outset.

Such findings certainly justify the implementation of CST to enhance the effectiveness of practitioner–patient consultations. Furthermore, they can also serve to highlight the areas of performance that are weakest, which are by implication prime targets for skills training intervention.

11.7 OVERVIEW

Evaluation of CST presents a formidable range of challenges to the trainer. Notwithstanding, evaluation cannot be considered an optional extra following training but must be viewed as an integral part within it. This chapter has therefore sought to identify and discuss a number of the central issues pertaining to assessment procedures. These included the nature and process of evaluation, the problems inherent in evaluation, the qualities of tests and the variety of methods of evaluation applied within the context of health professional training. Practical guidance has also been offered by way of facilitating meaningful implementation of these procedures within the resources available to the trainer.

PART FOUR

Towards Formulating a CST Programme

In this final part, a more integrated perspective will be brought to bear upon features of CST that were introduced separately in previous parts of the book. As stressed throughout, our intention is not to prescribe some 'standard' communication training programme for health workers. Rather we have adopted the philosophy of 'rather a fishing rod than a fish'. By presenting a broad conceptual framework and identifying key considerations that must be acknowledge in formulating training interventions, the intention is to encourage tutors to create their own programmes tailor made for their unique circumstances. To this end, Chapter 12 is devoted to a detailed exposition of the major factors that a tutor must take into account in designing a particular programme.

For any CST programme to be ultimately successful changes in thinking, feeling and behaving must be transferred, or carried over, to the ward, clinic, patient's home, or wherever health care is normally provided by the participants. It is not enough that such changes be confined to the training setting. Trainers must be aware, however, that such transfer does not necessarily occur automatically. Chapter 13, therefore, considers steps that can be taken to maximize the impact of training where it matters most – in the workplace.

Chapter 14 brings the book to a close. Here a broader look is taken at CST and its role in improving the quality of communication entered into by health professionals during the course of their duties. While improvements in training are necessary, it is argued that in isolation they may be insufficient to radically alter current standards of practice. Other influencing factors that need to be addressed are identified.

Designing and implementing the programme

12

12.1 INTRODUCTION

Communication skills training has characteristically been adapted in its application to meet the specific needs and diverse circumstances of a great variety of groups, resulting in the emergence of a plethora of specific programmes. Consequently, the approach in this chapter is not to attempt to develop some sort of generic 'archetypal' programme but rather to concentrate on the process of planning and designing as distinct from the end product. As a result the prospective trainer will, hopefully, be better prepared to tackle the job of formulating an instructional sequence best suited to a specific situation. Throughout, the emphasis will be placed upon practical issues and consequences. Planning issues to do with transfer of training, however, will be taken up in the following chapter.

When it comes to answering many of the procedural questions that a likely tutor would probably want to be addressed, such as when best to introduce CST or the most effective sequencing of content, one will search in vain for categorical empirical evidence upon which to base a reply. Frequently decisions have to be taken on other grounds, drawing upon, for example, formal theories and principles of curriculum planning and instruction as well as intuitions distilled from personal experiences with this method of training. There will be occasions in this chapter when we will draw unashamedly upon the many years of experience which we have now accumulated in CST work with a variety of health-professional groups.

12.2 FACTORS INFLUENCING PROGRAMME DESIGN

The form and substance of any programme are ultimately shaped by decisions taken in relation to a number of key considerations (see Figure 12.1 in Section

12.3). Each decision is determined by one or more of a number of constraining influences, including the needs and characteristics of the group, the objectives of the programme, resources available, the size of the group and the time available for training. In addition, what the trainer elects to do in one respect (e.g. practical activities) can have a limiting effect upon the options available in another (e.g. duration of course). To add a further dimension of complexity, influencing factors are to varying degrees interdependent, so that the impact of one may modify the significance of another in the decision-making process. Group size, for instance, can have a considerable impact upon the salience of the resources available. Group needs and characteristics should relate very obviously and directly to identified training objectives, etc.

12.2.1 Needs and characteristics of the group

As discussed in Chapter 7, a crucial starting point in the planning of any educational intervention is with the needs and characteristics of the group for which it is intended (Galbraith, 1990). Different categories of need can be thought of including normative, felt, expressed and comparative (Orr, 1992). Normative needs are defined in relation to some notional standard. Comparative needs are imputed on the basis of comparability with another group in receipt of training. In both cases the necessity of training will have been recognized by some third party, be it manager, administrator, educationalist or researcher. But the felt and expressed needs of participants themselves should not be overlooked in the process of curriculum design. Anastasi (1987) recommended that, as trainers, we 'Talk to potential participants . . . to see if they perceive any needs for increased communication skills' (p. 742). According to Tannenbaum and Yukl (1992), having members voluntarily participate in training rather than forcing compliance by making attendance mandatory is associated with higher motivation to learn, increased learning and more positive reactions to the instructional sequence. These are some of the advantages of having a highly motivated and committed group of trainees who acknowledge that further training is required and accept that the procedures being advocated will meet those objectives. Apart from influencing the specific instructional objectives, there are design implications for the content of training. With an already committed group, the amount of time devoted at the beginning to convincing the participants of the important effects of quality communication on patient outcomes, for example, can be reduced.

Those undertaking CST can be, both individually and collectively, enormously varied. Differences in academic ability, motivation, personality, gender, maturity, existing communicative competence, professional experience, to name but a few characteristics, may exist and influence the structure and operation of the intervention. Associations between certain trainee personality traits and attitude to this type of instruction have been reviewed (Crute, Hargie and Ellis, 1989; Irving, 1995). Significant negative relationships with participant 'anxiety' have been found, while 'extroverted', 'stable', and 'socially precise' trainees seem to be more favourably disposed to CST. The latter discovery is consistent with the conclusion drawn by Morrow (1986) that introverted students react less positively to instructional procedures incorporating elements of CCTV recording and feedback.

The relationship between personality of trainee and performance during training has also been explored. Crute, Hargie and Ellis (1989) reported that 'venturesome' student health visitors improved more as a consequence of training than those who were 'shy', and that the 'self-assured' improved more than those who were 'apprehensive', as measured by Cattell's 16 PF Inventory. While it isn't proposed that prospective trainees undertake a battery of personality tests prior to commencing CST, it is important for tutors to be aware of the influence that personality differences can exert on attitudes to and performance during training. Where possible, modifications to the instructional process should be made to accommodate them.

Gender may also be a further factor associated with reactions to elements of this form of training. Thus Norris (1986) produced evidence to suggest that male students may find role-play a more effective learning method than traditional lecture-based instruction, while the opposite is true for females.

As far as professional experience is concerned, students could be, on the one hand, just embarking upon training with little or no practical experience of the nature of the work. Indeed their appreciation of the significance of communication and the relevance of instruction in this sphere may be quite limited. On the other hand they may be practising professionals of many years standing, taking part in CST within the context of on-going career development. The requirements of these contrasting groups will evidently differ and must be acknowledged in their respective programmes. In-service trainees, unlike their inexperienced counterparts, can be expected to have decided views on such matters as professional practice. They typically arrive with already established interpersonal styles and strategies for dealing with different work situations. These presumably, as far as they are concerned, have served them more or less well in the past. Accordingly, they may not be readily predisposed to openly examine and modify what they do and ultimately they have potentially much more to lose in the process. Training will consequently represent more of a threat if it is construed as a situation where the instructor has 'all the answers' – if it is handled in what Knowles (1987) terms an overly 'pedagogical' way. Alternatively the group may resist this as an attempt at self-aggrandisement on the part of the instructor and become alienated. But this negativity need not happen if the trainer is sensitive to the particular characteristics of the group and organizes training to utilize the wealth of practical experience possessed by members.

12.2.2 The objectives of the programme

Following on from the general needs of the group, the focused attention given to meeting particular objectives has a strong influence upon decisions taken during programme planning. What takes place, and the experiences to which trainees are subjected, will be deemed to best achieve these outcomes. In keeping with what has already been said about the importance of taking the felt needs of students into account, the possibility of having training objectives emerge from a process of joint negotiation between tutor and trainees should be considered, especially with a more mature and experienced group. This collaborative approach has much to commend it under these circumstances. Faulkner (1993) outlined steps that can be taken from developing an agenda with the group at the outset encompassing not only participants' concerns but areas that the tutor feels are in the group's interests to include, through prioritizing issues, to agreeing upon content and the teaching and learning methods that will be followed in the delivery of the workshop sequence. There may also be room for negotiating methods of evaluating the intervention. While many trainers may feel apprehension about the prospects of surrendering some control over what takes place in this way, Faulkner (1993) reassuringly reflects that 'what is surprising is that the agenda generated by participants over many years of workshops has always included the majority of the material that the tutors wish to teach' (p. 127). The importance of this collaborative strategy for promoting consequent transfer of training will be addressed in the next chapter.

Within the over-riding aim of improving communicative competence, the primary objective that has traditionally typified the sort of training process featured in this book has been essentially performance-based. The intention has been to directly change what trainees do, how they behave and when they communicate. But, as has been stressed in this book, the roles that internal phenomena such as knowledge, beliefs, attitudes and values, together with situational parameters, have to play in the communicative process must be acknowledged and taken into account. Training objectives should be correspondingly catholic, incorporating:

- knowledge (e.g. knowledge of self, others, roles, situations and routines, etc.);
- cognitions (e.g. thought processes involved in social problem-solving and decision-making);
- perceptions (e.g. sensitivity to relevant social cues);
- attitudes (e.g. respect for the patient as a person, being non-judgemental, caring, etc.);
- beliefs and values (e.g. irrationality of beliefs such as that one must always 'grin and bear it', be liked by everyone, etc.);
- feelings (e.g. confidence, warmth, empathy, relaxation, etc.).

The relative emphasis placed upon these differing types of outcome has quite profound implications for designing the programme. If bringing about changes in knowledge and cognitive processes are prioritized then it is likely that more attention will be devoted to the sorts of instructional activity discussed in relation to the sensitization phase of training. As mentioned by Analoui (1993), 'for acquiring knowledge and gaining understanding, whether in connection with the task or social aspects of the job, methods such as a lecture, problem solving exercise, using documented real life case studies, workshops and classroom structured learning activities are all suitable means for . . . training' (p. 76). On the other hand, attitudes and feelings may be more successfully shaped through greater involvement in experiential activity involving simulation or some real-life encounter. Again, the incorporation of practical exercises must be based upon what the trainer is striving to achieve. Simulation exercises and games are often better suited to increasing familiarity with a procedure or system. Method-centred role-play lends itself better to training fairly simple skills, while less structured development role-plays are a more useful vehicle for coming to terms with complex processes, including counselling, and examining the feelings and personal issues which emerge. The content of training must also, of course, be in keeping with the goals of the module.

12.2.3 Resources available for training

The CST programme presented is frequently a compromise between what the trainer would ideally like to do and what can, in fact, be realistically accomplished. The resources that can be used must be taken into account. Some of these will already be recognized from earlier chapters. They include staffing, accommodation, equipment, materials and finance.

Staffing

As mentioned in the preceding chapter, we have found that having a tutor with a background in the behavioural sciences work alongside a colleague from the specific health profession is an ideal arrangement for carrying out CST. Others would seem to corroborate our views (Kagan, 1985; Whitehouse, 1991). Both tutors should be involved in planning as well as teaching. It may also be necessary, especially with large groups of students, to enlist the help of additional tutors to assist with practicals. Suitable staffing is probably the single most important resource that trainers can have at their disposal. The likely success or failure of the enterprise will rely heavily upon this factor. Unfortunately, there seems to be a dearth of suitable tutors in certain areas, such as nursing (MacLeod Clark and Faulkner, 1987) and medicine (Davis and Fallowfield, 1991). If need be, though, it is preferable to operate with fewer staff than accept tutors who are ill-suited to this form of training.

Tutors should:

- **have a knowledge of CST procedures**. If not, students will invariably sense their uncertainty and become de-motivated. Again such tutors, through force of circumstance, tend to 'do their own thing'. This commonly means seeking out familiar terrain and surreptitiously refocusing the exercise by concentrating, during feedback, on trainees' professional knowledge rather than interpersonal skill *per se*. Students find this both confusing and frustrating. It may therefore be necessary, and is indeed desirable, for tutors expressing interest to be provided with initial training by the CST member of the team.

- **be familiar with the experiential approach to teaching**. Many teachers feel uncomfortable with this approach and deficient in respect of it.
- **possess the skills being trained**. CST trainers often don't practise what they teach (Analoui, 1993). This is relevant for three reasons. Firstly, good practice lends credence to the programme. Secondly, tutors inevitably serve as models and, thirdly, such skills, together with corresponding personal attributes like sensitivity, openness, respect and genuineness, help create the supportive climate within which trainees can feel secure enough to take risks. For these reasons, Faulkner (1993) is adamant that 'before anyone is taught how to develop their ability to teach communication skills they must have a top-up on their own ability to interact effectively with patients and their families' (p. 114).
- **be committed to this form of communication skills training**. Assumptions and values held about education should be consonant with this approach. If students sense that the tutor is less than committed the high levels of motivation that they require to undertake this frequently demanding venture will be difficult to generate and sustain.
- **be knowledgeable of the profession**. The behavioural scientist in the partnership should have a sufficient working knowledge of the professional service provided to enable comment to be made about the skills in context.

Accommodation

Obtaining suitable accommodation for the practical parts of the programme is often the most difficult physical resource need to satisfy. The most desirable accommodation is that which is custom-built for work of this nature and a number of institutions in the UK can now boast interpersonal skills training centres. The one at the University of Ulster will be described for illustrative purposes. It presently comprises six CCTV labs. There is also access to a studio equipped to professional standards for recording and editing model tapes. Units are completely autonomous and consist of a recording room (28 m^2) and a playback room (14 m^2) where feedback tutorials are held. Playback rooms each contain a U-matic video cassette recorder, a colour TV monitor, an intercom, a system of cue lights which are used for relaying messages to the adjacent recording room and a wall-mounted remotely controlled video camera, together with control panel. This camera records through a window in the adjoining wall. Each recording room has two suspended omnidirectional microphones and various pieces of furniture which can be used to create a variety of settings, from a lounge to a consulting room. The tremendous advantage of this type of accommodation is that it enables a large number of students, working in separate subgroups, to undertake practicals, including video feedback provision, at the same time.

But CST can be attempted under more spartan conditions. These may, nevertheless, make the task of creating a facilitative group environment more or less difficult. This should not be discounted. Initial attitudes towards the perceived value of training are often founded upon such subtle cues as inadequate resources (Board and Newstrom, 1992).

The minimum requirement is probably a room large enough to give subgroups sufficient space to take part in practical activities without distracting each other. It should, of course, be warm, well ventilated, pleasant, comfortable and in a location that minimizes the likelihood of external noise or disturbance. Fixed furniture causes problems so chairs, desks, etc., should be movable.

Equipment

Here one tends to think primarily of CCTV and video recording equipment, comprising video recorder, video camera, microphone, TV/monitor. While not essential, as already stressed, it does offer a powerful instructional tool in the hands of a knowledgeable trainer. Many of the positive features that it affords in relation to modelling (Chapter 8) and as a feedback modality (Chapter 10) have already been discussed. These and others are discussed by, for example, Cartwright (1986) and Dowrick (1991).

Video recording equipment is now widely available in institutions engaged in the education and training of health professionals and is frequently used in CST work, as shown by the survey of medical schools undertaken by Frederikson and Bull (1992). While there are several competing systems from which to choose, the most common are Beta, U-matic (both developed by Sony) and VHS (by JVC) (Cartwright, 1986). The large format of U-matic, which uses ¾ in tapes and hence an increased recording surface, initially gave it an edge over its small-format rivals on the quality of the recorded image produced. However, technological developments have meant that, since the late 1980s, this advantage has been eroded. Indeed some of the latest generation of small-format Beta and VHS equipment offers better-than-broadcast quality pictures and has moved ahead. This, coupled with relative price, size and convenience has boosted their attractiveness, with VHS in particular becoming an extremely popular choice of system in the UK.

When it comes to deciding upon a videoing set-up, choices range from a simple camcorder at one end to a purpose-built centre, such as that described in the preceding subsection, at the other. The camcorder has been one of the most significant developments in video technology in the past few years. It combines a camera, microphone, video recorder and monitor in a single, highly portable unit. It is therefore technically possible to record a piece of interaction, including the sound, with a camcorder, and have one or two view the outcome. While this could be thought of as a basic set-up for CST work, it does have limitations.

Relying upon the built-in microphone means that sound sources close to the camcorder are more readily picked up than those further away, which may well include the participants involved in skill practice. Again, if it is intended to play back the recording in a group setting, the camcorder on its own is inadequate.

We would therefore recommend, as a basic system, something along the lines of the following:

- Video camera (or camcorder)
- Video recorder (even with a camcorder, this can be useful for rudimentary editing)
- External microphone
- Tripod
- Colour monitor or TV.

This elementary arrangement will enable the trainer to add a useful dimension to the training procedure at no great cost. Modern cameras are extremely light-sensitive, enabling them to operate quite successfully in normal room lighting, so this need not be a concern. Indeed some can function in as little light as 1 lux! Having a camera with a zoom lens is an extremely useful facility in CST, making it possible for the operator to zoom in on one of the participants, or isolate a particular piece of behaviour during recording, without having to physically move the camera about. There are also benefits to be gained from incorporating a remote control unit enabling the camera to be positioned inconspicuously and operated from a distance, thereby reducing reactivity.

Recording good quality sound can often pose more problems than vision and generally requires one or more extension microphones. These may either be stationary or of the levalier (or 'lapel') variety. The latter, being attached to the lapel or tie of the interactor, permits high-quality recordings to be made but may be intrusive. The attached cables can also get in the way and cause difficulties, although replacing these with portable transmitters is a common solution. There are different types of stationary microphone, each with distinct characteristics. Some are unidirectional and designed for recording a single speaker, while others are omnidirectional and cope better with group situations. Given the complexity of the area, it is often well worth while seeking specialized technical advice on sound to get best results.

The final component of the video set-up is the monitor or TV. Here little need be said apart from the fact that it should be technically compatible with the recorder. A remote control facility is also a big advantage.

If at all possible, and given suitable accommodation, the trainer should try to commission several video-recording set-ups so that subgroups can practise simultaneously. This enables larger numbers of trainees to engage in a practical session at the same time.

The potential of the audiotape medium as a cheap and readily available alternative, or complement, to video in providing feedback was mentioned in Chapter 10. It is also a means of modelling skills that are fundamentally verbal in nature. Audio recorders can be a useful resource when video facilities are limited, student numbers are large, or for students to record extra-classroom encounters, perhaps as a homework exercise.

More mundane, but still useful pieces of equipment include an OHP (overhead projector), black- or whiteboard, and flip-chart. The last can serve a useful purpose during the playback tutorial.

Materials

Items that can be listed under this subheading include books, handouts or manuals, skill assessment schedules, taped material on communication and communication skills, and blank video/audiotapes. There is an ever-increasing publication of books on communication skills and communication skills training, a considerable number of which are of relevance to the health professions. Some of these have already been extensively referred to. These books prove an invaluable source of lecture content, if lectures are intended to be used as part of the process of skill sensitization. They may also be drawn upon if skill handouts or manuals are put together by the trainer for distribution to trainees. Furthermore, students can be referred to them for further reading.

An alternative to compiling manuals and workbooks, although one which reduces the flexibility of training, is to adopt those that have been prepared on a commercial basis. These often incorporate skill assessment schedules. However, such schedules can quite easily be constructed by the trainer and, since this option takes into account the nuances of the particular programme, are frequently accepted as being more directly relevant and beneficial.

Commercially produced audio- and videotapes, often part of instructional packages on various aspects of the communicative process, are available to be used either instead of or together with model tapes that the trainer may make (see Chapter 8). Details of some of these, which are germane to health-care delivery, are given by Faulkner (1993).

As well as prerecorded tapes, blank tapes for recording skill practice are needed. This is usually one of the more easily met resource demands, especially in the case of the cheaper VHS variety. For the most part a single tape will be used and re-used, following feedback, during the next practical. There may be advantages, though, in keeping recordings (with students' permission) until the end of the programme so that students can replay and discuss them in their own time between sessions. By comparing later with earlier attempts, levels of improvement can (as a rule) be readily appreciated, thereby increasing motivation.

Finance

Most of the training resources already mentioned ultimately depend upon the size of the budget that can be drawn upon. With sufficient funding, adequate equipment and materials can readily be made available, suitable accommodation obtained and optimal levels of staffing countenanced! Indeed it is possible to improve the quality of staffing given sufficient finances to operate training for tutors in CST procedures.

12.2.4 Group size

Given adequate space, staff and video-recording facilities, large groups can be quite comfortably handled. Real practical difficulties arise when, with limited resources, programme objectives require every trainee to practise during each practical session devoted to a separate skill. While these problems may begin to manifest themselves during sensitization, if students are engaged in experiential exercises, it is principally at the stages of practice and discussion that they become chronic. Here they are exacerbated by the necessity for this part of training, if it is to be meaningful, to be conducted in small groups of ideally fewer than 10 students. Hobbs (1992) suggested that with more than this number, a co-worker is really required. The resolution of this dilemma will require decisions to be taken about the use of resources, constitution of subgroups and allocation of time to different training components, each of which will be discussed later in the chapter.

12.2.5 Time

The final constraining influence upon programme design is the amount of time that has been allocated to it. The feeling of never having quite enough time to incorporate all the facets of the communication process that seem relevant is a common complaint. It is perhaps exacerbated by the quintessentially experiential nature of CST. While this approach to teaching has much to commend it, it does tend to be time-consuming. One is sometimes faced with the decision of covering only core features thoroughly or incorporating additional material by, for instance, focusing upon several skills per session or reducing the amount of time devoted to practice and feedback.

If CST is added to an already crowded curriculum, as is sometimes the case, the time that can be given to it is often meagre, being squeezed into the few hours grudgingly relinquished by someone else or culled from students' private study. The depressingly low percentages of formal curriculum time in medicine, nursing and dentistry typically given over to communication skills work has already been mentioned. However, revisions of the nursing curriculum in the form of Project 2000 (UKCC, 1986) and undergraduate medical education (General Medical Council, 1993), give this area a greater prominence.

12.3 PROGRAMME CHARACTERISTICS

The practical consequences which the various sources of influence just reviewed have for decisions that shape the programme and give it identity will now be considered. These are outlined in Figure 12.1.

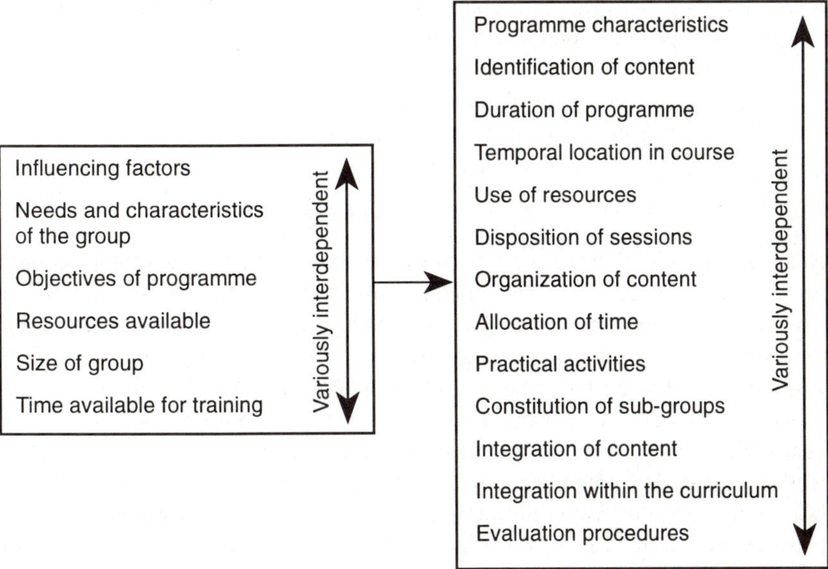

Figure 12.1 A decision-making framework.

12.3.1 Duration of programme

There is no definitive answer to the question of how long the CST programme should last. The most obvious determining factor is of course the amount of time available. Group size and available resources can also play a part. If subgroups have to practise consecutively rather than concurrently the total hours devoted to training (although not necessarily to each student) will be increased accordingly.

Programme objectives are additionally relevant. Dickson, Tittmar and Hargie (1984) distinguished between time- and competency-based programmes. The former take place within a fixed temporal framework, with a predetermined number of sessions being devoted to different content areas. With competency-based programmes the overall length and speed of progression through the sequence is determined by the systematic satisfaction of preordained criterion levels governing performance. While this individualized learning format is probably the more effective instructional approach, allowing for personal pacing and competency attainment as a basis for progression to more complex communicative processes or situations, its flexibility can create massive logistical problems. This is undoubtedly one of the reasons why CST in the health professions is invariably group-centred and time-based.

The length of programmes differs enormously. As a rough guide, in the health professions the average length is probably somewhere around 20 hours. It has been our experience that little can be accomplished in less than about 15 hours, unless it is intended to concentrate upon a single skill area or situation with minimal practice and feedback. It must be remembered that, in most cases, trainees have to be introduced to experiential techniques such as role-play and video recording, and that sufficient practice opportunities must be provided to encourage the transfer of training, as we shall see later.

12.3.2 Temporal location of programme in course

Remarkably little agreement exists as to the stage of training at which students profit most from CST. This is evidenced by the fact that, in the basic training curriculum of most professions, programmes of this type can be found from first through to final year (Hargie and Morrow, 1986a). The survey of medical schools in the UK on their teaching of communication skills, referred to previously, revealed that more than a third of this work took place in the first clinical year (Whitehouse, 1991). On other health-professional courses, much of it would seem to be located in first year and prior to any substantial clinical experience. As such, this form of training facilitates the bridging of theory and practice, thus providing a more systematic preparation for practical involvement in the clinical setting.

There may be disadvantages, though, identified by Dickson and Maxwell (1987), in placing CST too early in the course. Certainly undergraduate physiotherapy students surveyed by Maxwell, Dickson and Saunders (1991) reacted much more positively to CST in the final year of the course than those encountering it in the second year. Students at the beginning of their training typically embark upon CST without any real appreciation of what the job they are training for entails. Not only do they lack practical experiences to draw upon during the programme but they may even fail to appreciate the relevance of this input to their course. Compared with the natural science-based elements and technical skills of the profession, communication may appear, at first sight, familiar and unproblematic. Under these circumstances the trainer is well advised, perhaps through some experiential exercise, to begin by impressing the need for effective communication and the many problems of this type that can beset the neophyte when dealing with patients, staff and the public.

An additional pitfall in scheduling the programme at the beginning of training is that students, through lack of professional knowledge and experience, may feel ill-prepared to take part in professionally oriented practical activities. If, on the other hand, the programme isn't explicitly oriented towards their profession it often loses face validity. Students cannot see the relevance of what they are doing, even if prepared to accept that communication plays a part in their chosen profession.

Difficulties that can arise through only instituting CST towards the end of a course may be just as testing. Foremost among these is a possible lack of integration with other aspects of professional training. Additionally, students, having most likely taken part in lengthy periods of placement, can feel that there is little to be gained from a college-based procedure of this nature, which could be seen as artificial. To overcome such resistance it may be necessary to adopt the sort of approach that seems to work best with practising professionals. Thus experience (albeit limited) is acknowledged and built into training; felt needs are taken into account; content of training can target more complex skills, strategies or problematic situations; emphasis may be on *in vivo* practice or developmental role-plays; and a purposefully less directive style implemented during feedback than with the first-year counterpart.

An alternative to having CST at some particular juncture, and one which has enormous potential, is to organize it on a recurring basis throughout the duration of the course. This allows for basic concepts and simple skills to be built upon and developed in line with ongoing clinical knowledge, skills and professional expertise as training progresses year on year. There is a danger, nevertheless, that with relatively short, isolated sequences, the total CST programme may become extremely fragmented.

12.3.3 Disposition of sessions

This has to do with two central considerations. The first is the issue of whether sessions should be concentrated in time or spaced out with intervening periods when trainees are doing other things; the second, the extent to which separate sessions should be given over to isolated constituent elements of performance.

Massed versus *spaced practice*

By tradition, CST has been structured in keeping with the principles of spaced practice. The period of time between sessions is typically a week, in accordance, no doubt, with common timetabling habits. With the massed alternative, instruction is condensed so that skills and opportunities to practise them are introduced in quick succession. The rapid build-up of fatigue and decline in motivation which can result are weaknesses of massed practice, which may become particularly evident with the less mature, experienced and committed student. Again there is little opportunity for students to supplement class activities through readings or homework assignments.

The consensus of opinion, therefore, would appear to favour spaced practice but instances of programmes where sessions are scheduled in a decidedly more massed fashion can be found. These tend to be of the all-day workshop variety, often involving practitioners, and the organizing principle is invariably logistical rather than andragogical. A considerable amount of material can be covered in a short period with trainees who would find it inconvenient to attend on a number of occasions. While learning does undoubtedly take place, questions have been raised about the extent to which it is retained or transferred to the place of work.

Spaced practice has also hidden dangers, which should be recognized. If the interval of time between sessions is too long forgetting can occur to the detriment of cumulative learning effects. The optimum length of interval is not known and most probably varies depending upon such features as the group, homework assignments, concurrent placement experiences, etc. In some cases it could even be that a week, while convenient from a timetabling point of view, is too long!

Whole *versus* part practice

The founding of CST upon a reductionist philosophy permitting the analysis of complex interactive processes into simpler elements, has already been established. Practising these constituent elements separately is the hallmark of the 'part' approach. The 'whole' method of learning involves, in comparison, going through the complete activity on each practice session until mastery is achieved. But 'part' and 'whole' are relative terms. While it would be unimaginably cumbersome to accept 'health professional communication' as the undifferentiated content of training, programmes can be found that operate at a more holistic level than that of basic skills such as questioning, listening, etc. Participants may be required simply to practise taking a complete medical history (for example, Maguire, 1984b).

Several factors are relevant when deciding upon which approach to employ. Perhaps the most important is the nature of the task. Those that are highly complex, yet capable of being broken down into a number of simpler but meaningful constituent parts, lend themselves to part practice (Magill, 1993). Characteristics of the trainees, including ability, motivation, experience and learning style, are also salient. The less able student with little prior experience, who already possesses few of the skills, may be easily discouraged and should therefore benefit from concentrating initially upon molecular aspects rather than advanced processes such as interviewing or counselling. It is important, though, that they don't lose sight of the relationship between the element being practised and the holistic performance (e.g. between reflecting and counselling), otherwise the exercise may become meaningless for them. Being accustomed to learning in accordance with the part strategy will also be an advantage.

A further determining factor in choosing which method to implement is the total time available for training. Focusing upon single skills per session is time-consuming. With more able students it is often possible to combine two or even three skills that complement each other and can readily be practised in the same practical (e.g. paraphrasing and reflection of feeling). However, being too ambitious in this respect should be cautioned against.

A compromise between the 'whole' and 'part' options, which Magill (1993) maintains takes advantage of the benefits afforded by both, is the progressive-part technique. This involves concentrating initially upon the first and second content elements in isolation before practising both together. In the context of interviewing, questioning might be practised, then attending, then both together. The third component is likewise introduced on its own and then combined with the first two, and so on. The sequence reported by Tittmar, Hargie and Dickson (1978) for use with health visiting students was organized along these lines. Scheduling sessions in this manner is also a highly effective way of achieving the integration of training content.

12.3.4 Integration of content

If CST operates on the principle that skilled communication is capable of being analysed to reveal a number of simpler elements each of which can, in isolation, be targeted during instruction, then, at some point, thought must be given to issues of synthesis. One of the potential shortcomings of the 'part' method of training is that students, at the end of the sequence, may be highly accomplished in the performance of isolated components but unable to integrate them in carrying out the complete task. To claim success the CST procedure must incorporate mechanisms whereby the original communicative process can be reconstituted. In many instances the final session of the programme is set aside for this purpose as is the case, for example, in the short programme outlined by Hobbs (1992). The rationale would appear to be that the various bits and pieces can be readily and properly combined as the culmination to the sequence. But this may prove inadequate; integration of content should be an ongoing activity throughout the length of the programme.

A variant of the CST protocol was developed by Hargie, Dickson and Tittmar (1978) with this in mind and termed 'mini-teaching'. It incorporates a progressive-part format together with a systematic lengthening of skill practice episodes as training continues (see Table 12.1 for an illustration of this mode). This principle of progressively and systematically approximating the realities of the work setting has important consequences, it would seem, when it comes to promoting greater levels of skill retention and transfer, as we will see in Chapter 13.

Aspects of the integration of content to do with organization and choice of practical activity will be mentioned under these respective subheadings.

12.3.5 Identification of content

A variety of techniques for determining the aspects of communication forming the content of training was presented in Chapter 7. Options fall under three main headings; the intuitive, the analytical and the empirical. The procedure followed by any particular trainer faced with the task of designing a programme and identifying the most relevant facets of communication for a specific group to consider will largely be determined by the objectives of the programme, the time available and the resources that can be utilized. While empirical procedures are more 'scientifically' respectable and arguably furnish a more valid set of skills specifically tailored to the needs of a certain group, they are time-consuming and draw heavily upon the resources available, including equipment and materials, but particularly finance and personnel. Many of the techniques require a certain level of expertise to operate successfully.

Table 12.1 Outline of the practical element of a mini-teaching programme

Session	*Activity*	*Length of practice*
1	Introduction and familiarization	—
2	Introduction to video	5 min
3	Non-verbal communication	5 min
4	Questioning	5 min
5	Integration of NVC + Questioning	10 min
6	Reflecting	10 min
7	Integration of NVC + Questioning + Reflecting	15 min
8	Explaining	15 min
9	Integration of NVC + Questioning + Reflecting + Explaining	20 min
10	Opening	20 min
11	Closing	20 min
12	Integration of all skills	25 min
13	In-depth history interview	30 min

It is true to say that, in the majority of reported CST programmes, the skills featured have been established on the basis of intuition and analysis. A trainer with a straitened budget may not feel unduly disadvantaged if forced to adopt these approaches when planning modules on generic communication skills for basic level trainees. There may be less complacency, though, at the prospect of preparing, in the same way, to offer a CST programme in some more specialized area of the clinician's job. In this case there is a greater need to make use of some of the more sophisticated empirical procedures in order to identify the nuances of effective performance. Adams *et al.* (1994), for instance, unearthed subtle differences in physiotherapists' perceptions of skilled instrumental and affective behaviour when working with different patients including those categorized as outpatients, gynaecology and neurology.

12.3.6 Organization of content

Having identified material legitimately forming the content of training, decisions have to be taken in respect of its sequential organization over the length of the programme. Contrasting models for structuring the content of curricula in the health professions in a coherent and meaningful way are available (see, for example, Cork, 1987; Greaves, 1987; Burrell, 1988). Chronological, structural logic, problem-centred, spiral and inductive are types of sequence that would seem to be most evidently represented in the construction of different CST modules.

Chronological sequence

Here skills are presented in the temporal order in which they naturally occur in the commission of the interactive task. As discussed in Chapter 3, many social encounters follow a predictable course. According to the seminal study by Byrne and Long (1976), the typical GP–patient consultation comprises six episodes: relating to patient, discussing reasons for attendance, examining, considering patient's condition, detailing treatment or further investigation and finally terminating the interaction. This progression suggests that skills should be introduced in the order of opening skills, questioning (and perhaps reflecting), explaining and closure. Although this is an uncommon approach to design it was implemented in an early programme, described by Gibson *et al.* (1981), to teach social work students interviewing techniques.

Structural logic

Without doubt, the vast majority of CST programmes have been planned in accordance with this method. Here the determining factor is conceptual relationship and level of complexity. If one facet of a subject depends upon the prior understanding of another, the latter should precede the former in the instructional sequence. Such programmes often begin with a consideration of the key features of skilled interaction as presented in Figure 3.2.

It will be appreciated that the skills introduced in Chapters 4 and 5 differ in complexity. Some can be readily thought of as subskills of others (e.g. listening subsumes reflecting). Processes such as interviewing and counselling are located at a still higher level. Thus effective counselling involves successful listening together with a variety of other skills. The potential afforded by this differentiation in the arrangement of training was recognized by French (1994) as follows: 'By identifying skill levels according to increasing complexity and the interrelationships between skills, one can generate a hierarchy of social skills that can serve as a heuristic tool or "rule of thumb guide" to social skill learning in nursing practice' (p. 272). Similarly, both Newman and Fuqua (1990) and Faulkner (1993) discuss the advantages of beginning interpersonal training by providing a grounding in the simpler microskills of counselling such as eye contact, posture, open questions, summarizing, etc. before progressing participants to more advanced strategic issues, which govern interactive performance in situations with patients/clients and their families. An example of this approach to communication in nurse education is presented in Table 12.2.

Constructing a programme in keeping with the philosophy of structural logic has a number of advantages. Since earlier inputs are systematically extended and elaborated as instruction continues it inevitably promotes the integration of content. Cork (1987) indicated that it is particularly suited to groups having little background knowledge of the subject to draw upon. We would concur with this view. This approach works particularly well with students who have just commenced their professional training, with little or no knowledge of the discipline of communication or practical professional experience. Presenting material in this way also establishes a firm base on which to build further inputs, if required, at some subsequent stage.

Table 12.2 A programme organized according to the principles of structural logic (Source: example drawn from CINE, 1986)

Session	*Activity*
1	Communication in nursing
2	Elements of communication
3	Questioning skills
4	Listening and attending skills
5	Reinforcing and encouraging skills
6	Information-giving skills
7	Initiating and terminating interactions
8	Comfort and reassurance
9	Combining micro skills: the nursing process
10	Communicating with other members of the health-care team
11	Cancer and dying
12	Preparing a patient for discharge
13	Communicating with geriatric and stroke patients
14	Communicating with patients before and after surgery

Problem-centred sequence

Here the key organizing feature is a problem with which students are confronted. It may be generated by the trainer or drawn from students' own experiences, perhaps by means of a critical incidents procedure. The substance of training is introduced in an attempt to illuminate this concern and formulate solutions to it. In the case of the communication skills sequence for fourth and fifth year medical students outlined by Sanson-Fisher *et al.* (1991), on the theme of information transfer, the problem situations addressed centred on patient adherence, childhood behavioural difficulties, potentially threatening medical interventions, eating problems, sexual problems, alcohol-related problems and breaking bad news.

Morton and Kurtz (1982) argued strongly in support of the problem-centred approach in CST on the basis that:

> Adult learner commitment and involvement is heightened when learners perceive its relevance to their work concerns. For example, a family assistance worker may not be especially interested in the skill of immediacy, but if the skill is taught in the context of how to deal with a hostile client, the worker may be more likely to perceive its value and concentrate on learning it.
>
> *Morton and Kurtz, 1982, p. 413*

We have found the problem-centred approach an especially apt way of establishing a framework for training mature, sophisticated and professionally experienced groups. The situations selected should reflect the experienced needs of members. As a result they can readily relate, from the beginning of the programme, to what takes place and accept its relevance.

The spiral curriculum

This concept will be familiar to those with a background in curriculum design. It has been discussed by Burrell (1988), among others, as an approach to structuring the education and training of nurses. As far as CST is concerned, the thinking is to introduce core concepts and skills in their simplest form early in the course. As students progress, and as the curriculum 'spirals' upwards, this material is systematically reintroduced, with increasing layers of complexity added. For example, a CST sequence might commence with basic features of skilled interaction, such as those outlined in Chapter 3. This could be subsequently built upon by including core skills such as questioning, explaining, opening and closing, mentioned in Chapter 5. At the next turn of the spiral, this work could be further embellished by focusing upon the interviewing process, bringing in some of the material covered in Chapter 6.

The inductive approach

The particular circumstances of practising professionals who may have accumulated substantial clinical experience, and how this must be taken into account by the trainer, has been mentioned on several occasions. Under these circumstances a more inductive approach to structuring the training sequence can usefully be considered. Here the emphasis is very much upon the negotiated curriculum, which, as it happens, is quite often problem-centred. But rather than working through the three phases of the training process – sensitization, practice and feedback – a more thoroughgoing experiential framework can be set in place. Participants are accordingly given the opportunity to become involved in interaction at the outset. This may be with other participants, a patient simulator or indeed recordings of interactions with actual patients may be requested to be brought along. General principles guiding practice are then abstracted, following analysis and evaluation, in the context of discussion with peers and tutor. Thus trainees deal with a problem situation without prior sensitization to any specific tactics or strategies for coping. It is during feedback that these are established, together with more general principles relating to the nature of skilled interaction.

The inductive approach to structuring CST inputs can work well, especially with more mature, experienced trainees.

12.3.7 Practical activities

Procedures for offering skill practice opportunities were outlined in Chapter 9, including covert rehearsal; behaviour rehearsal; structured, semistructured and unstructured role-play (together with multiple role-play, fish-bowl, role-rotation and role-reversal variants); simulation exercises and games; and *in vivo* practice. Those selected for use in a particular programme inevitably depend upon one or more of the constraining factors mentioned in the first part of this chapter. Decisions taken with regard to temporal location of the input in the course, together with the organization and integration of content, also play a part. Perhaps the most central considerations, though, concern the characteristics of the group and the objectives established for the programme.

While there are few hard and fast rules, we have found that less mature, confident or experienced trainees do not cope as well with techniques such as covert rehearsal, unstructured or developmental role-play and, of course, *in vivo* practice. The relationship between group characteristics, needs and programme objectives has already been established. If the trainer is principally intent upon developing proficiency in the performance of relatively basic skills, structured or method-centred role-play and, perhaps, simulation exercises are suitable. Behaviour rehearsal may also be considered, depending partly upon the skill content. It is also an effective way of providing initial practice of more complex skills.

At more advanced levels, though, incorporating interactive strategies and situations, developmental role-play is often the preferred alternative. When the objective is essentially to increase awareness of certain difficult issues or to gain insights into the operation of some procedure, the fish-bowl variant of developmental role-play, as well as simulation exercises and games, is typically implemented. A particularly useful approach to changing attitudes and increasing self-awareness and sensitivity, on the other hand, is through procedures such as role-reversal.

The appropriateness of these techniques will also depend upon the stage of the programme at which they are introduced. With less sophisticated and confident students it may be best to begin with simulation games and exercises, which are usually viewed as less threatening, before moving on to role-play. Indeed, under these circumstances, Miles (1987) advocated concentrating largely upon didactic instruction at the start before gradually including experiential exercises as the programme unfolds.

The point at which particular practical activities are utilized becomes more significant when the sequence is organized in keeping with the principles of structural logic. In this case, after the introductory exercises, it is common to progress from the method-centred role-play of simpler skills to developmental role-play and, finally, perhaps *in vivo* practice. The latter two also promote the integration of earlier content and serve an important function in this respect.

12.3.8 Constitution of subgroups

The practice and feedback stages of training are, in most cases, undertaken in subgroups. If at all possible these should contain no more than ten members, with six being a figure to aim for. While teaching groups of this size is andragogically sound, it can pose considerable resource problems.

Two further points about the constitution of subgroups are worth making. One has to do with whether or nor to maintain the same subgroups for the duration of training. Keeping to original subgroupings enables members to become familiar and comfortable with each other so that greater levels of trust can be attained, thus promoting increased openness. Members should be dissuaded, though, from constantly practising with the same partner, since this may serve to limit the generalizability of training outcomes. One advantage of changing subgroups, on the other hand, is that each trainee can be offered a broader range of practice experiences and feedback opportunities.

The second issue concerns the homogeneity of subgroup composition. We tend to favour having a broad cross-section of the overall group represented in each subgroup. Differences in age, sex, experience, etc. often lead to a richer flux of views and opinions during feedback. If however, members differ in some important respect that has implications for how skills content would normally be implemented, or the types of situation encountered, then more selective groupings can be made.

12.3.9 Use of resources

Resources available frequently place a frustrating restriction upon the form which the programme takes. Here video recording equipment and staffing considerations immediately come to the fore. Being confronted with a large group of students and having only a single video unit to call upon can pose obvious problems. These are compounded if the trainer is adamant that the central objective of the module is essentially performance-oriented, requiring students to participate in practical activities designed to improve some aspect of their communicative repertoire. Nevertheless, much can be accomplished even under these circumstances.

Strategies to be considered include one or more of the following.

- Timetable subsections of the cohort for practicals at different times, perhaps on a rota basis.
- Have participants record 'in their own time' so that they come along to feedback sessions with recordings already made. This is obviously more convenient for them when working with audiotapes.
- Operate slightly larger subgroups of, say, ten members.
- Have only half the larger subgroup practise per session, with the rest having their turn on the next occasion. Those not actually practising can take part as role-play partners and contribute fully during feedback.

When staffing is the essential resource problem, it may not be possible to allocate a tutor to each subgroup. While trainees prefer to have their group led by a tutor (Martin, Jones and Hearn, 1994) it is uncertain if this is associated with improved training outcomes. The effects of tutor presence are likely to be mediated by what the tutor does, together with other features of the programme. Operating a flexible system whereby one tutor oversees several subgroups can, therefore, be contemplated. This can work particularly successfully with the more mature trainee. It is desirable, though, that:

- subgroups be thoroughly briefed prior to practice;
- one member of the subgroup be appointed as coordinator;
- a specific and clearly defined task be set;
- subgroups come together for a plenary session.

12.3.10 Allocation of time

The allocation of the total hours available to the different phases of the training process, and to different content, is a feature of many of the constraining influences already mentioned. As such it is extremely difficult to be other than tentative as to how to best distribute the time period given over to training. Nevertheless, the notion of 3–6 hours per week is a useful starting point. For the most part, with inexperienced groups, this should be spent on a single skill. More complex strategies or situations typically require longer, perhaps taking place over several weekly sessions.

Assuming that programme objectives are to directly improve performance in addition to increasing knowledge, sensitivity, self-awareness, etc., about a quarter of this time should be given over to skill sensitization, roughly the same to practice and the remainder to feedback. These proportions may vary, of course. As noted, an inductively organized programme does not have a sensitization phase as such, with more time devoted to reflection and discussion of practical experiences. More generally, and regardless of how training is structured, it is imperative that sufficient time be allowed for full and detailed feedback to be given.

12.3.11 Integration within the curriculum

Integrating the content of CST has already been discussed. When it forms part of a broader curriculum, the relationship of CST to other course elements must, in addition, be addressed. It would seem that, in practice, trainers are often negligent in this respect. This is borne out by the results of the survey by Hargie and Morrow (1986a) which identified three models of CST implementation. The **interspersed model** characterized training that was distributed throughout the curriculum. It was often poorly coordinated and arranged on an *ad hoc* basis. The **isolated model** was so called for several reasons. Communication studies tended to be taught by a social or behavioural scientist as an academic subject in a separate, self-contained unit. With no explicit attempt made to relate these concepts to health-care practice this, in as much as it did take place, was left entirely to the perspicuity of individual students.

The **integrated model** rectified many of these shortcomings. Here the organizing principle was identified as the application of communication issues to the interpersonal dimension of the health professions. The successful operationalization of this resolve was accomplished through a team-teaching strategy involving a behavioural scientist (usually a psychologist) together with a health-practitioner tutor. The unfortunate fact that in pharmacy much instruction appeared to reflect the first two, rather than the third model, led Hargie and Morrow (1986a, p. 174) to conclude 'that there was a need for more guidance and direction about how to organize and implement CST'. The need for greater attention to the fuller integration of communication skills into the broader medical (Whitehouse, 1991) and nursing (Faulkner, 1993) curriculum has also been voiced.

The relationship between elements of the curriculum that are college-based and those that are field-based deserves careful thought. If properly sequenced to complement each other, students can gain an invaluable learning opportunity. Having a period of placement following on from a CST programme organized in keeping with the principles of structural logic, for instance, provides opportunities for the integration of earlier content to take place through *in vivo* practice. Subsequent college-based work can, in turn, incorporate and build upon these experiences. In any case, when CST is taught as part of a course, it must link with the other elements to form a coherent and unified whole if a worthwhile outcome is to be achieved. Ellis and Whittington (1981, p. 176) encapsulated the sentiment admirably in the following succinct statement: 'At best [CST] is an integral part of an organism of which it is a microcosm: at worst it is a cosmetic graft soon rejected or isolated by the host.'

12.3.12 Evaluation

Establishing the most suitable strategies for evaluating the instructional intervention should also feature as part of the process of programme planning. Such evaluation may be conducted with different purposes in mind, as was indicated in Chapter 11. The major aim, in certain cases, is to assess students' levels of performance to enable judgements to be made about their competence as they proceed through training. Upon its completion, decisions have to be taken as to whether professional accreditation is merited. The procedure may alternatively be conducted with the primary intention of improving the quality of the programme itself. Subsequent inputs can be modified in accordance with feedback obtained in this way.

A variety of evaluation techniques from which choices can be made was outlined in the preceding chapter and categorized as direct or indirect. In deciding which to adopt the trainer should reflect upon several questions. What is the purpose of evaluation? What exactly is to be evaluated? What resources are available to facilitate evaluation? Depending upon the resolution of these issues, the techniques elected might range from a questionnaire designed to assess participants' reaction to the programme to the direct observation of practice with a patient in order to gauge personal competence as a basis for professional accreditation.

In terms of programme planning, evaluation enables subsequent interventions to be fine-tuned in order to maximize effectiveness, as represented in the model of CST outlined in the introduction to Part Three.

The essential considerations in designing and implementing a CST course are summarized in Table 12.3 and form the basis of Exercise 12.1.

Table 12.3 CST planning checklist

1. **Needs of a group**
   - felt
   - expressed
   - normative
   - comparative

2. **Characteristics of participants**
   - professional experience
   - motivation
   - personality
   - learning style
   - group size

3. **Objectives of programme**
   - knowledge
   - cognitions
   - perceptual awareness
   - attitudes
   - beliefs
   - feelings
   - behaviour

4. **Resources available**
   - staff
   - accommodation
   - equipment
   - materials
   - finance

5. **Time allocated for training**

6. **Programme options**
   - duration
   - temporal location in course
   - skills content
   - organization of content
     – chronological sequence
     – structural logic
     – problem-solving sequence
     – spiral curriculum
     – inductive approach
   - disposition of sessions
     – massed vs spaced
     – whole vs part
   - integration of sessions content
   - practical activities
     – simulation
     – *in vivo*
   - constitution of subgroups
   - allocation of time to different aspects of training

7. **Integration of programme within the curriculum**

8. **Evaluation**
   - direct techniques
   - indirect techniques

Exercise 12.1 Designing CST programmes

This exercise is intended to help the reader begin to apply the essential learning points of the chapter to the CST training which they provide. Having read Table 12.3, reflect back on the last CST course you conducted. Go down the checklist, noting those points that featured in your planning and running of it. Are there any other considerations which, with hindsight, would have improved the quality of the learning experience which you offered?

Alternatively, the reader may wish to think about a pending CST input. Once again, use the contents of Table 12.3 to check those aspects of planning and implementation to which you have given some thought. What about the others? Do decisions that would enhance the course need to be taken in respect of them?

12.4 OVERVIEW

This chapter has addressed a range of organizational and logistical issues pertinent to the planning and implementation of CST programmes. In so doing it extends the cross-sectional focus on the training procedure taken in preceding chapters.

Trainers must formulate programmes to meet the requirements of particular groups and within the realities of specific settings and sets of circumstances. CST is most effective when approached in this way. There is no template of 'the model programme' which can be immutably worked through on each and every occasion. In consequence, the focus in this chapter has very much been upon the process of devising a training sequence. This was discussed within a framework of decisions taken with regard to a range of features of the programme. These are determined by a set of immediate influencing factors including the needs and characteristics of the group, the objectives of the programme, resources available, size of group and the time that can be set aside for training. The fact that the formulation of certain programme characteristics can place constraints on choices available in respect of others was also acknowledged. Features discussed included the duration of the programme, temporal location in course, utilization of resources, disposition of sessions, organization of content, allocation of time, choice of practical activities, constitution of subgroups, integration of content and of the programme within the curriculum, and the selection of evaluation procedures.

13 Promoting transfer of training

13.1 INTRODUCTION

It will be recalled from the earlier discussion of the evaluation stage of the CST sequence that the ultimate criterion against which the worth of any training programme can be assessed is the extent to which positive changes are brought about in patient outcome measures (such as heightened satisfaction with care, increased compliance/cooperation with treatment and shorter recovery periods) and consequently, improvements in the quality and efficiency of institutionalized health-care delivery.

For the effects of training to work their way through and impact upon outcome measures of patients subsequently dealt with by trained personnel and hence be reflected in organizational indices of quality of care provision, several circumstances are necessary. Assuming that the content of training is appropriate, that the skills acquired are relevant to trainee needs and can bring about the desired changes in patient outcomes (i.e. that the skills content of training has social validity), it is further necessary for trainees to carry over their deployment from the training setting to the ward, clinic or patient's home. This statement may seem rather obvious and yet it raises a concern that is one of the most perplexing facing trainers. Participants may evince acceptable standards of skilled performance, in accordance with the objectives of the programme, in the training context but not when back in their work situation. In other words there can be little transfer of training.

Successful transfer of training, at its most basic, depends upon several conditions being satisfactorily met. The first has to do with learning and retention. Unless trainees, upon completion of their programme, have mastered its content and those learned changes in knowledge, attitudes, feelings, sensitivity or behaviour are relatively enduring, little impact upon actual practice with patients/clients can be expected. But while knowing what to do and when and how to do it is a necessary precondition for transfer to take place, it is not sufficient. The second requirement is that participants must be adequately motivated to behave accordingly. At the in-service level, this may mean changing established work routines. They must not only see advantage in modifying their customary practice in accordance with the objectives of training but be made to recognize that these altered ways of doing things are accepted and supported within the organizational setting. Thirdly, they must be given opportunities, when back on the ward, to implement what they have learned and retained from training, as they would want to.

Transfer of training should, therefore, be a matter of central concern to any instructor considering running a CST programme. This chapter will identify and discuss some of the major factors that seem to have an influence upon the carry-over of training effects from training to work contexts. Recommendations will also be made throughout for maximizing the transfer process. While many of these have to do with the process and content of the instructional sequence itself, and will take us back to the topic of programme design, the promotion of transfer has a much more wide-ranging remit. It is not only dependent upon the quality of instruction received (Campbell, 1988). The issue of transfer must be acknowledged and catered for at the very outset during the initial planning of the intervention. Board and Newstrom (1992) have argued strongly that it ultimately hinges upon a collaborative arrangement between the trainer, trainees and management (the latter in situations where participants are either in employment or have a work-based component to their course). Each party has areas of responsibility in the ultimate success of the training venture. Factors that have a bearing upon transfer have been located by Tannenbaum and Yukl (1992) in the pre-training and post-training environments as well as during programme delivery. This is the framework that will be used to structure the main body of the chapter. Before moving on to tackle these matters, however, some further attention must be given to more general issues to do with transfer.

13.2 THE PROBLEM OF TRANSFER

According to Analoui (1993), 'transfer ought to be seen as one of the single most important determining factors in the effectiveness of training programmes' (p. 6). It is perhaps something of a surprise, therefore, to learn that until comparatively recently it was an aspect of instruction that was largely ignored by trainers in general. It was not seen as being particularly problematic, the general assumption being that once participants were able to satisfactorily demonstrate learning outcomes in the training setting this would, as a matter of course, carry over to the job and be reflected in new work practices. From a more enlightened perspective, this optimistic way of thinking has been labelled 'train and hope' and has been roundly condemned as a wholly inadequate strategy for ensuring the ultimate success of the training venture (Marx and Ivey, 1988).

One of the consistencies noted by Kendall (1989) to emerge from research into the generalization of behavioural change interventions in a range of settings, with children as well as adults, is that such generalization 'does not routinely occur on its own' (p. 360). In human resource development terms, this has been an expensive lesson. According to figures cited by Garavaglia (1993) organizations in the USA invested more than $45 billion in formal employee training in 1992. Accepting the estimate by Board and Newstrom (1992), which they acknowledge to be generous, that only 50% of all training content is consistently applied to the job, the inevitable conclusion is that some $22.5 billions spent on human resource development is largely wasted.

But what about CST specifically? Are training outcomes subject to the same transfer vagaries? While a number of research evaluation studies and reviews attest to the effectiveness of this systematic, structured approach to communication skills instruction (Crute, Hargie and Ellis, 1989; Baker and Daniels, 1989; Anderson and Sharpe, 1991; Hargie, Morrow and Woodman, 1993; Thompson, 1994; Dickson and Bamford, 1995), it must be recognized that much of this work has relied upon training-based criteria rather than taking the further, but much more difficult step of following through the effects of instruction on performance in the workplace and consequently on patient/client outcome measures. Nevertheless some such research has been done. In an already cited study, Evans, Stanley and Burrows (1992) reported that medical students who undertook CST to improve their history-taking interviewing performance not only manifested superior skill in this regard when compared with a control group of students, but were associated with patients who expressed higher levels of satisfaction with all aspects of the interviews which these trained students conducted.

In sum, the problem of transfer is essentially twofold. One aspect is that much of the evaluative research carried out on CST has neglected to assess effectiveness at this level. The other is that, from the evidence which we do have, it seems as though, as with training in general, generalization from the training setting may be neither automatic nor guaranteed unless steps are taken to promote it.

13.3 A PERSPECTIVE ON TRANSFER

The terms 'transfer of training' and 'generalization' have been used interchangeably in the previous section. While referring to the same basic event, they do however derive from markedly different traditions of psychological enquiry and represent contrasting explanations of this general phenomenon, as explained by Dickson and Bamford (1995). Tannenbaum and Yukl (1992, p. 420) simply regard transfer of training as 'the extent to which trainees effectively apply the knowledge, skills and attitudes gained in a training context back to the job'. The further concept of 'transfer distance' has to do with the carry-over of training to work settings quite similar to the circumstances of training (near transfer) or significantly different (far transfer) (Laker, 1990). The latter of course represents a greater challenge to the trainer. The terms 'transfer of training' and 'generalization' will be used interchangeably in this chapter.

Basic thinking on transfer of training, which tended to accentuate the mere learning and retention of material, has been more recently extended in a promising way by those interested in human resource development. Accordingly, a much more holistic approach has been proposed. Ford and Fisher (1994, p. 242) advocated a systems perspective arguing that 'the training program cannot be viewed in isolation from the organizational system of which it is a part'. They go on to develop a model of the transfer process which specifies transfer outcomes not only (1) as the direct result of the learned knowledge, skills and attitudes brought about by the training programme, but also (2) as affected by the effects of a range of trainee characteristics and (3) as affected by features of the job context. Both (2) and (3) influence transfer outcomes directly and indirectly, the latter through impact on initial learning outcomes (Figure 13.1).

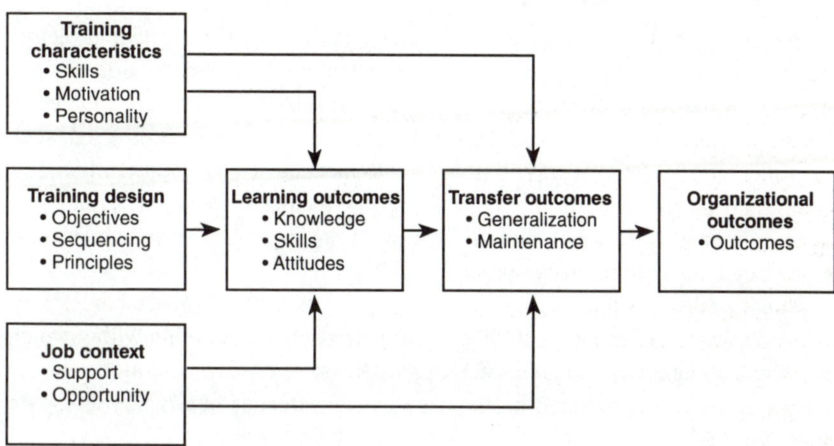

Figure 13.1 The transfer process. (Source: reproduced from Ford and Fisher, 1994, with the permission of the publishers of *Occupational Medicine: State of the Art Reviews*, Hanley & Belfis, Philadelphia, PA)

Along similar lines, Board and Newstrom (1992) developed the notion of the 'transfer partnership' as central to the effective representation of training in work. As such, a matrix of factors reflecting all parties in the training endeavour, trainers, trainees and management, is recognized. Furthermore, circumstances both before training commences and after it has finished should not be overlooked through a blinkered focus on the instructional programme alone (Tannenbaum and Yukl, 1992). Perhaps Analoui (1993) best encapsulated the essence of this more holistic outlook in the following statement:

> [The] concern for transfer should not be limited to remembering and retaining certain abstract material or knowledge and skills *per se*. When it comes to training situations, transfer encompasses a wide spectrum of activities, skills, knowledge and complex processes which should also include consideration of the values, behaviours and expectations of the trainers and prospective employers both during the training and after it is completed
>
> *Analoui, 1993, p. 6*

The breadth of this conceptualization will be reflected in the sections to follow.

13.4 THE SKILL MODEL OF INTERPERSONAL COMMUNICATION REVISITED

Some of the above thinking, and particularly the role of organizational factors on individual performance, deserves further attention. It has implications for our account of the communicative process as skilled activity sketched in Chapter 3. There, it will be recalled, social performance was held to be goal-directed, such that interactors behave in ways best judged to meet those ends, constantly modifying their performance in the light of ongoing feedback. Personal variables of interactors and situational factors, it was argued, provide a framework for contextualizing the interactive process.

But it may be useful to give particular prominence to broader contexts of interpersonal engagement, including the organization or institution within which individuals engage in situated interaction (Dickson, 1995a). The model of the interactive process presented in Chapter 3 can be extended in this way as shown in Figure 13.2.

Such situated interaction (e.g. admitting a patient to the ward) may be handled markedly differently by the nurse from one hospital to another, indeed from one ward to another, on account not of personal qualities and dispositions but rather of the organizationally imposed constraints, together with expectations and acceptable, informal standards of conduct, that prevail. In reviewing a number of studies from the nursing literature which make this point, May (1990) observed that:

> Research which seeks to place NPI [nurse–patient interaction] and NPR [nurse–patient relationships] in context emphasizes the ways in which the social organization of nursing work exerts powerful forces on the forms which episodes of NPI take, and the effects of this upon the way in which nurses understand and define the social relationships in which they are implicated.
>
> *May, 1990, p. 309*

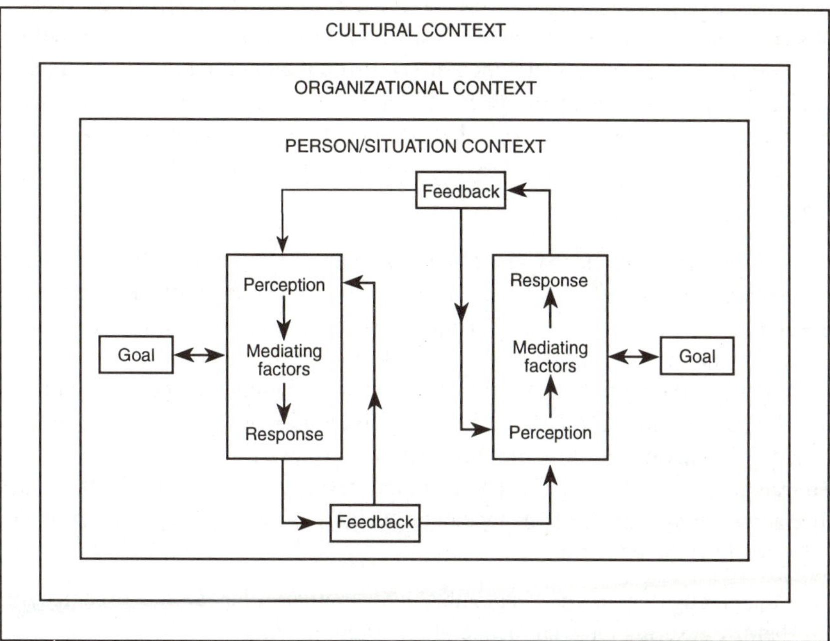

Figure 13.2 Contextualized model of interpersonal communication skill.

Furthermore, Fielding and Llewelyn (1987) claimed that the manifestation of what could be regarded as poor communication may actually have a number of benefits for staff, given the nature of the organization and that person's role in it!

The point is that the degree to which a health-care worker manifests skilled communication with a patient is a feature not only of personal characteristic and situational factors that pertain but is also embedded within and reflective of broader organizational/institutional concerns. As such, the organizational setting is one of the parameters of transfer of training given prominence, as we have seen, by those taking a holistic perspective of the topic. These matters will be included in the subsequent focused discussion of factors which determine transfer and corresponding recommendations on how to promote it. This work, as previously stated, cannot be left to be carried out during training, however. It must be begun in advance of it and continue after the programme has been completed. The remainder of the chapter will be structured in three sections addressing each of these phases.

13.5 PRETRAINING FACTORS AND STRATEGIES

Board and Newstrom (1992) are adamant that the extent to which training is implemented in work practices is ultimately a feature of the collaborative relationship created between the trainer, the trainee and the manager. Each has a distinct contribution to make which varies across the three phases from before training to during training and then afterwards, creating a matrix of challenges and opportunities. But unless there is complementarity and joint commitment the results of training in the work environment are likely to be impaired.

13.5.1 The manager

We will use the term 'manager' loosely to broadly refer to all in the health-care organization who are involved in organizing or supervising others, who have some authority to make decisions about work practices and be particularly influential in the cultivation of a certain work climate in the ward or clinic. The manager can therefore be located at different strata within the organization from ward sister to unit manager and beyond. Board and Newstrom (1992) believe that these individuals 'hold the most significant keys to resolving the problem of transfer of training' (p. 22). These authors reveal a range of contributions that the active involvement of management at this pre-training stage can provide. They include the following.

- Enunciating the mission statement and strategic plan of the organization thereby ensuring the congruence of the training initiative.
- Ensuring that the skills targets of training are reflected in recognized and accepted performance standards in the work setting.
- Being seen to be enthusiastically in support of the training initiative both in word and action. This endorsement can be given in a number of ways, formally and informally.
- Recognizing further training implications for the success of the programme among line managers. Transfer of training may have a knock-on effect, exposing training needs on the part of supervisors. It is important that they themselves have the skills in question, are able to recognize and monitor their use among staff and provide continued guidance and support as and when necessary. A working knowledge of the format and content of training will be an advantage.
- Serving as a role model by demonstrating the targeted attitudes, sensitivities, knowledge and behaviours in dealing with others in comparable situations. It may make little sense extolling the virtues of a training programme designed to improve staff's ability to listen to patients when senior colleagues are seen to exclusively pursue their own agendas in interactions.
- Reviewing training content and design before the programme is finalized. This can help ensure that the programme is valid in respect of meeting the identified needs of staff and is in keeping with the broad cultural values of the organization and its members.
- Selecting trainees to attend. It is important that participants be selected for the right reasons. These should have to do with who has the most pressing

need for new or improved skills to enable them to do their job more successfully, rather than who can most be done without for a day, or whose turn it is! (Trainee characteristics that affect the success of transfer are reviewed below.)

- Considering features of the organization, its operation, culture and climate than will most likely facilitate or inhibit the implementation of change, once participants return from training. The manager should be prepared to take steps to minimize the latter.
- Acknowledging and reinforcing training outcomes when they do show through on the ward or in the clinic.

13.5.2 The trainer

Traditionally trainers have concentrated upon improving the design of their inputs when giving thought to encouraging transfer (Garavaglia, 1993). In doing so the assumption has been that quality of training alone is sufficient. This is now generally accepted to be a rather narrow outlook. Several additional contributions are required from the trainer at this stage. These include the following.

- Sharing responsibility with both managers and trainees for ensuring that practices of health-care delivery actually change. Based upon survey data, Kotter (1988) reported that one of the most frequently cited causes of restricted training success was failure to include management in the behaviour change process. Another was failure to directly involve those to whom training was being offered, resulting in difficulties of acceptance of, and engagement with, the initiative. Setting in place and sustaining a facilitative working relationship encompassing trainer, trainee and management should, therefore, be considered as a useful point of departure for the process of identifying needs, deciding upon content and designing the programme. Trainees who have made a contribution to, or at least been consulted in, the process of putting the programme together are more likely to recognize it as a means of meeting their needs and be accepting of it (Wlodkowski, 1985). There is good reason to believe that those who recognize the benefits of training are more likely to make the effort to transfer what they get from it (Huczynski and Lewis, 1980).
- Developing 'trainee readiness' is a further strategy mentioned by Board and Newstrom (1992), of relevance at this pretraining stage. Those participants who had received advanced information about the programme, in a study by Baldwin and Magjuka (1991), expressed greater commitment to applying what they learned to the job.

A central tenet of adult education, espoused by Knowles (1987), is that the more mature learner has a need to know why they should learn what is being taught otherwise they are unlikely to willingly invest time and effort in it. He advocated that, 'one of the first tasks of the adult educator is to develop a "need to know" in the learners – to make a case for the value **in their life performance** of their learning what we have to offer' (Knowles, 1987, p. 170). This can be done in a number of ways. At the very least, and perhaps with preservice students, it may involve an experienced professional attesting to the relevance of the programme to those who would aspire to the profession. But the message can often be delivered much more impactfully by creating experiences, perhaps through simulation, that demonstrate how the quality of health-care delivery can often suffer through poor interpersonal communication (see Exercise 13.1).

Exercise 13.1 Relevance of CST

Aim

To heighten students' awareness, at the outset, of the need for effective interpersonal communication in quality health-care delivery.

Preparation

Prepare role-play scenario and two reasonably structured role briefs, one for Mrs Green (or could be Mr Green), the other for Dr Jones.

Scenario: The interaction takes place between Mrs Green and Dr Jones during a brief (about 3–4 minute) consultation in the busy Health Centre where Dr Jones practises.

Mrs Green: You are quite fit and active as you approach middle age. One of your loves is gardening and you spend as much time as possible in the garden. Some people see you as a lonely person but you don't mind your own company. People often make you nervous and uncertain. In the summer you take full advantage of the sun trap by the shed and sunbathe there at every opportunity. Recently you have noticed a little mark by the side of your nose. All this talk about the dangers of excessive sunbathing has got you really worried. You have had little need to contact Dr Jones as a rule. Talking to doctors isn't easy for you and for some time you have simply tried to put the matter out of your mind, hoping that the mark will go away. It hasn't and you have started to convince yourself that it could be serious. Finally, you pluck up the courage to make an appointment. Dr Jones seems rather unconcerned about your facial mark but begins asking you about your family, diet, exercise and such like. You can't seem to get him back to what you want to talk about.

Dr Jones: Mrs Green is one of your patients but you don't really know her very well. Upon arrival she seems quite a shy, timid lady, and is obviously concerned about a lesion on her face which you believe to be quite innocent. You do notice, however, some slightly raised yellowish nodules on her eyelids that suggest possible high blood cholesterol. This is worth pursuing, despite the fact that you are running behind and still have some house calls to do. You begin to enquire about family history, lifestyle, etc.

Organization

You can use either the fish-bowl approach by having two volunteers enact the scenario at the front of the class. Alternatively the group can be divided up into smaller groups of three to five, with the others acting as observers. It is important, of course, that participants see only their own role-play brief.

Discussion

The discussion should centre on how the consultation was experienced by Mrs Green. Probable feelings of frustration and confusion, and how these would probably affect subsequent follow-up, can be explored. The importance of dealing adequately with patent's concerns, issues of power and control, time-management, relationship between clinical and interpersonal competence, etc. can also be brought out in underscoring the centrality of effective interpersonal communication in health-care delivery.

Trainees who are or have been practising professionals have, of course, a background of direct experience that can be drawn upon. The potential threat that can be engendered by any attempt at personal assessment of practice, particularly of communicative practice it seems, must be recognized. If handled sensitively within a context of trust, however, this can be the most meaningful approach to establishing a state of readiness to learn. One of the findings to emerge from a piece of research conducted by Noe and Schmitt (1986) was that trainees' reactions to initial skill assessment was a significant predictor of their level of satisfaction with the programme. Perhaps this was a consequence of their greater recognition at the outset that the programme had something worthwhile to offer. Furthermore, Williams, Thayer and Pond (1991) reported a strong connection between satisfaction with the accuracy of assessment and motivation to transfer following training.

In addition to those ways of engineering receptivity already mentioned, trainee expectation of follow-up activity or assessment has been linked to declared intention to implement learning when back in the work setting (Baldwin and Magjuka, 1991).

While, strictly speaking, design matters are largely handled pretraining, we will hold over this topic and deal with it when we discuss factors during training that influence generalization of outcomes.

13.5.3 The trainee

Pretraining contributions made by trainees centre on applying their knowledge, abilities and motivation to planning, assessment and preparation. The resources which they bring to training are also important. We have already considered, in the preceding chapter, a range of participant characteristics which should be taken on board when designing the programme. Here we will extend this avenue by examining additional factors that seem particularly relevant to the transfer process. If we keep in mind the model of this process developed by Ford and Fisher (1994) and presented earlier (Figure 13.1), it will be appreciated that trainee differences in such areas as skills, motivation and personality can have direct effects on react to instruction and the benefits derived. These factors can also have a bearing on transfer outcomes, both directly and indirectly, the latter via influences on initial learning. The implication is that those trainee characteristics already mentioned in the last chapter also have a potential contribution to make, both directly and indirectly, to the transfer process. Likewise, additional characteristics about to be addressed at this point may well affect engagement with the learning experience *per se*. The variables to be considered now, however, have more commonly been mentioned in the literature, specifically in connection with issues of transfer, and have been included here on that basis.

Cognitive styles

People have different preferred strategies for handling learning tasks and assimilating information. Focusing upon one of these categorizations, the holism *versus* serialism dichotomy (Pask, 1976) has been implicated in the ease with which trainees are able to transfer (Harris, 1985; Jonassen and Grabowski, 1993). While some learners may have the versatility to acquire knowledge by means of either strategy, it seems that most prefer one or the other. Holists approach a body of material in a typically more thematic fashion, looking for broad relationships within it and quickly identifying underlying principles and generalities. By contrast, serialists tend to become absorbed in the narrow detail of specific aspects of the material rather than conceptualizing the global picture. As a result, the formation of abstractions and generalities based upon specific experiences may be much more difficult for them to accomplish. This is particularly pertinent since many feel that it is the creation, retention and subsequent application of such principles that lies at the heart of the transfer process (Gardiner, 1984). Interestingly, it may well be that CST, given its reductionist approach of identifying various elements of interpersonal processes, is well suited to the serialist learner (although there is some evidence that holists may be better equipped to benefit from simulation exercises – Rowland and Stuessy, 1987). Nevertheless, this serialist learning style that makes CST so compatible may ironically make it all the more difficult for the participant to operate at the level of abstraction necessary to derive the sorts of rules and generalizations required for subsequent regulation of performance in the workplace.

Trainers must therefore be sensitive to preferred approaches to learning and be prepared to accommodate individual needs when possible. It has been reported that mismatching cognitive style and mode of instruction can lead to poorer learning outcomes (Jonassen and Grabowski, 1993).

Self-efficacy

This is a belief in one's ability to carry out some designated task to an acceptable standard of performance and it has been proposed as a significant factor in accounting for transfer success (Noe, 1986). As expressed by Ford and Fisher (1994), 'employees who are confident that they can meet the objectives of a training programme (high levels of self-efficacy) will be more likely to not only learn the training material but to transfer that material to the worksite' (p. 244). In one of the few studies to investigate how self-efficacy affects the acquisition of skilled interaction, Gist, Stevens and Bavetta (1991) reported that those taking part in a programme of negotiation training who scored highest on this attribute were most successful in maintaining standards of performance over a 7-week period.

Belief in one's ability to succeed at certain tasks can be altered. Some of the ways in which such changes can be brought about have been outlined by Bandura (1989) and applied specifically to the improvement of training by, for example, Latham (1988). These have relevance for the design and delivery of CST. They include the following.

- **Enactive mastery**. The training experience should be such as to present participants with a sequence of tailored challenges that require their active involvement in meeting and overcoming, but which ultimately lead to a successful outcome. Expressed in the words of the old adage, 'nothing succeeds like success'. Tasks and exercises to which trainees are exposed must be carefully selected to ensure that they do not make unreasonable demands and inevitably condemn those taking part to failure.
- **Extrinsic reinforcement**. As mentioned in Chapter 10, it is good training practice to provide extrinsic feedback on performance especially in the early stages of the skill acquisition process. This feedback can serve as reinforcement, especially when it takes the form of tutor or peer praise.
- **Goal setting**. Clear goals and standards help people to make judgements about how well they are doing. As training progresses, increased involvement in the activity, together with improved levels of skill, is associated with the development of intrinsic sources of reinforcement. Knowing that one is 'doing well' carries its own rewards. Here trainees can benefit from being encouraged to set realistic goals and subgoals together with attainable standards of performance. Materials used, including model tapes, etc., should be selected with thought given to tacit messages about unrealistic performance standards that might unintentionally be conveyed to the training group.

Expectations

The expectations that trainees have of training tend to be related to how they engage with the sequence and the impact that ultimately the experience has on practice outcomes (Ford and Fisher, 1994). Two related sets of expectations have been noted by Noe (1986). The first have to do with the investment of time and effort in the programme leading to mastery of the content in accordance with the learning objectives established, the second with the likelihood of learned skills being applicable to the job. If it is felt that it is all very well spending time listening to patients within the specialized training environment but that there is little time for such practice in the real world of the busy ward or clinic, minimal transfer can be anticipated. We have already dealt with the contributions of the trainer and the manager in creating facilitative trainee expectations as they approach training.

Trainee attitudes

Trainee attitudes towards the job they do and their career development have been found by Noe and Schmitt (1986) to be predictive of training outcomes. Those reporting a higher degree of job involvement showed greater acquisition of key behaviours emphasized in the training programme. Similarly, participants who were more career conscious demonstrated greatest improvements in on-the-job performance. The authors speculated, 'Perhaps, individuals who have a career strategy are more willing to apply training content to their work because of an awareness of the relationship between behaviour improvement and career mobility' (Noe and Schmitt, 1986, p. 518).

To conclude this section, a range of contributions can variously be made by managers, trainers and trainees before the training programme is offered to maximize impact that carries through to the job.

13.6 TRAINING FACTORS AND STRATEGIES

Again, in accordance with the matrix of considerations determining transfer proposed by Board and Newstrom (1992), all three parties, management, trainers and trainees, have roles to play during training in ensuring ultimate success. The major focus of the section, however, will be on training design and delivery issues.

13.6.1 The manager

Once the programme gets under way, management commitments centre on the following.

- Communicating continued support for the initiative.
- Preventing interruptions by, for example, refusing to take participants away to deal with work matters unless absolutely necessary.
- Reallocating participants' work during training so that they are not constantly weighing their commitment to the programme against the backlog of work that their attendance will cause.

- Recognizing trainee participation and monitoring attendance.
- Anticipating the return to work. Thought should be given to what changes in personnel, facilities or procedures need to be made to facilitate the implementation of the learning to the workplace. Does a more private space need to be created in the community pharmacy, for example, where customers can be taken aside and counselled if necessary?
- Participating in transfer action planning. Board and Newstrom (1992) stressed that every training programme should incorporate a session devoted to helping participants identify ways in which learning can be applied to their job, anticipating influences facilitating and inhibiting these innovations and how they can be handled, and making a commitment to change. The drawing up and signing of a contract along these lines is one way of substantiating such a commitment.
- Deciding upon appraisal. What steps are necessary to monitor transfer during work, and are trainees made aware of these? This in itself can serve to enhance commitment to carry over and make use of skills and techniques acquired during training. Furthermore, are there plans to incorporate these into an appraisal scheme whereby employees will receive periodic evaluation and feedback on performance? Will this be reflected in tangible benefits for staff in terms of promotion prospects, pay increases, etc.? These are all relevant questions.

13.6.2 The trainer

The point has already been made that, traditionally, the source of poor transfer has been looked for in faulty programme design and implementation. As we have seen, a broader approach to the issue is now advocated. However, to avoid 'throwing the baby out with the bath water', the very real contribution of design and delivery issues to the wider application of training effects must not be neglected. While it should not be assumed that these matters are the trainer's sole responsibility, we would contend that the trainer is the party with particular expertise in, and primary responsibility for, such matters.

There are a number of useful sources offering advice on how to organize training with the maximizing of transfer in mind. The following guidelines are distilled primarily from the work of Stokes and Baer (1977), Stokes and Osnes (1988), Baldwin and Ford (1988) and Dickson and Bamford (1995).

Ensure the contextual validity of training content

A variety of approaches to identifying the interpersonal skills content of training was introduced in Chapter 7 and further considered, in the last chapter, in relation to constructing a programme. A principal cause of poor transfer is the teaching of skills that are, in the final analysis, largely irrelevant to doing the job (Bernstein, 1982; Newstrom, 1986). When a group of trainers was asked by Newstrom (1986) to rank a list of nine types of barrier to effective transfer, 'Trainees' perception of impractical training programme' was placed fourth, just in front of 'Trainees' perceptions of irrelevant training content'! Additionally, one of the reasons given by executives for failing to operationalize training outcomes was limited confidence in the utility of the training procedure in 'the real world' (Baldwin and Ford, 1988). For the skills content of training to be taken on board and implemented, Sailor *et al.* (1988) argued that it must be appropriate, desirable, useful, practical and adaptable.

By actively involving trainees and management in establishing training needs and identifying skills to be targeted in training, the chances that highly relevant skills content will be included are increased. It will be recalled that several of the methodologies of skill identification outlined in Chapter 7, such as constitutive ethnography and the Delphi technique, derived the skills content of the programme from the observations, experiences and judgements of, if not always the actual participants *per se*, at least their professional colleagues.

Maximize similarity between the training and work environments

The assumption here, and indeed the assumption that we have made throughout, is that training, or some part of it, will be offered 'off-site', i.e. that it will not take place as the participant does the job at the normal place of work. While drawbacks of 'on-site' training have been voiced by Analoui (1993), one of the advantages is that difficulties of transfer tend to be reduced. By organizing training in this way, what Laker (1990) referred to as 'transfer distance' is minimized. As a general rule of thumb, the greater the dissimilarity between the circumstances of training and those of the job, the greater the transfer distance and the less likely the effects of training are to emerge in the workplace. The implication is that training should recognize and incorporate conditions and circumstances of the workplace as much as possible. This is commonly referred to as the **principle of identical elements**.

Transfer between two settings is facilitated by the extent to which one resembles the other or, in learning theory terms, by the extent to which they share common stimulus and response elements (Thorndike and Woodworth, 1901). But some attributes of the training setting seem to be more crucial than others and these may differ according to the task being learned. Baldwin and Ford (1988) made a distinction between the physical and psychological fidelity of training and work settings and suggested that psychological fidelity may be more pivotal. In other words it is not necessary to attempt to create a **physically** accurate replication of the workplace for trainees to be able to subsequently apply what they have learned when they get back there.

In CST, it is therefore more important to try to create a psychological reality within which participants can recognize themselves doing their job than it is to have elaborate props and stage settings (Dickson and Bamford, 1995). This is not to deny that the latter can sometimes promote the former, but it is usually more productive to pay attention to the learning materials, exercises and instructional techniques employed with a particular group. Care must be taken to ensure that role-play and simulation exercises, as part of skill practice, not only incorporate the significant structural features of the work situation focused upon but that trainees are sensitively and progressively introduced to these, perhaps unfamiliar, learning methods along the lines suggested earlier in the book. As noted by Analoui (1993), 'The way in which an individual trainee subjectively perceives the simulator in use, affects his acceptance of the reality of the training situation in hand. It is the comparison between this perceived reality and the actual workplace situation which largely determines the success of the learning activity' (p. 68). If exercises seem inappropriate to participants so that they find it difficult to engage with them, it is unlikely that much carry-over, or indeed initial learning, will take place.

Train 'loosely'

The recommendation here is not to be too rigid and regimented in the planning and delivery of the instructional sequence. There is real danger that highly structured approaches to CST may become just that, so that each session follows exactly the same pattern, with exactly the same personnel, in exactly the same location, using exactly the same exercise and materials. Apart from the sheer tedium that can result, this ossification tends to militate against any performance changes that do take place, operating outside this narrow set of highly predictable training circumstances.

It is important to introduce variety by, for instance, presenting and giving trainees an opportunity to operationalize skills in a range of relevant practice scenarios, encouraging participants to work with different group members so that they learn how to modify skill usage to accommodate individual idiosyncrasies, even exploring alternative and personally more comfortable strategies and tactics for accomplishing goals. There should be no assumption that there is always only one correct way of dealing with most interpersonal encounters. Noe and Ford (1992) pointed to the advantages of behavioural variability (i.e. having alternative approaches to similar situations or problems). Training should not only be tolerant of such diversity but strive to promote it through encouraging members to generate and try different options, attempt variations upon a theme, etc., within the safety of the training setting.

Promote mediation

This training dimension has already been hinted at. After all, in much of CST, examples of performance are presented, not with the intention of promoting mindless behaviour replication, but rather the abstraction of broader principles governing action. Viewing a diversity of instances of skill deployment, including some examples of poor practice, can facilitate this process.

When learning occurs in the form of abstracted principles and heuristics governing responding under what might appear on the face of it to be quite diverse sets of circumstances, transfer of responding from one to the other is facilitated (Garavaglia, 1993). Individuals are not merely responding reflexively to environmental stimuli. If they were, they would probably only display ways of doing things acquired through training under demonstrably similar stimulus conditions to those that applied during instruction. This would obviously militate against the carry-over effect. Mediating schemata enable underlying situational commonalities to be recognized, enabling appropriate skilled performance to take place.

The potential of different types of mediator, including imagery, to aid transfer has been explored by Cartledge and Milburn (1995). Since, however, most cognitive processes rely upon verbal representations of objects and events, language-based mediation has more to offer than most of the alternatives. As such, Goldstein, Gershaw and Sprafkin (1986) recommended teaching trainees general principles governing successful performance. Encouraging learners to generate their own rule-oriented learning points in the form of principles underlying the performance of observed models was found by Decker (1980) to subsequently enhance generalization to a greater extent than having the learning points provided by the trainer.

The notion of mediation is further extended by Cornford (1991), who emphasized the importance of a supporting cognitive model of interpersonal activity according to which meaning can be attached to happenings and corresponding decisions can be taken as to what to do. This is one of the reasons why we feel it to be so important to present trainees with the skills model of interaction, outlined in Chapter 3 and further elaborated in the present chapter, in the early stages of the training programme. Without such a framework, Cornford (1991) claimed, microskills procedures often do little to help trainees integrate training content.

Reduce the distinctiveness of training

Programmes of skills training have quite distinctive features that set them apart in terms of how social intercourse is normally transacted. We can think of role-play and other forms of simulation, the presence of video equipment, etc., which add a certain uniqueness to the practice interaction. The use of augmented forms of feedback on performance through peer and tutor comments, video replays and so on additionally serve to set training apart. It is important that, as training progresses, increasing attention is placed on more naturally occurring feedback cues available within the interactive episode.

It is advantageous, as we have already seen, to structure the training sequence carefully so that demands never outstrip the group's evolving abilities to cope successfully. Self-efficacy can suffer otherwise. On the other hand, there is never any guarantee that the skills that in training seemed invariably to bring about the desired outcome will continue to do so in the real world of the ward or clinic. Such lack of instant and continued success when back at work can lead to a retreat to old ways and poor transfer. A further reduction of the distinctiveness of training, as the programme unfolds, should therefore be in respect of the diet of rewards that accrue from skilled performance. At the level of extrinsic reinforcement, praise from tutors, for example, should be scaled down so that it is no longer contingent upon every acceptable performance. Intrinsic reinforcement can also be made more sporadic, and more akin to what the trainee can hope to expect when doing the job, by including practice situations that present a greater degree of challenge. With role-play and simulation involving peers, this is seldom a problem in the closing stages of training when participants have developed relationships which tolerate giving each other 'a harder time' without causing offence.

Allow for overlearning

Overlearning, or continued practice beyond the point of initial acquisition, has been found to increase resistance to subsequent skill atrophy. Without the retention of skills, of course, there can be little hope of them being carried over to the job. Dickson and Mullan (1990) speculated that, since those skills in their programme that showed least evidence of generalization were included towards the end, minimal levels of acquisition might have accounted for limited transfer. This means that it is important to give participants the opportunity to practise skills on a number of occasions under a variety of circumstances so that new patterns of behaviour are integrated into more established ways of handling situations. Unfortunately for programme planners, there is no easy formulaic method of deciding just how much practice is necessary for each skill. Hagman (1980), however, advanced the idea of an optimum amount which will vary depending upon the type of skill and the circumstances of training.

Graded instructional sequence

One of the elements of training advocated by Roffers, Cooper and Sultanoff (1988), specifically designed with the maximization of transfer in mind, was the structuring of content so as to promote gradual integration both within the parameters of the programme and between the programme and the work setting. The training protocol that Hargie, Dickson and Tittmar (1978) called 'mini-teaching', which, as mentioned earlier, incorporated a progressive-part practice format together with a systematic lengthening of skill practice episodes as training progressed, was designed for a similar purpose. This principle of progressively and systematically approximating the realities of the interpersonal task, as typically conducted in the workplace, was further refined by Dickson (1981), who produced evidence that it might lead to greater levels of skill retention and generalization. Similarly, Cornford (1991) found that a sequenced practice programme of graded task difficulty, in conjunction with accompanying cognitive instructional procedures, led to effectively generalized skill acquisition and consolidation.

Progressively building in greater patient/client contact as the instructional sequence unfolds is a further application of this strategy with preservice students. Just when and at what rate it should be implemented will depend upon the level of sophistication of the group. Participants may be given tasks to carry out with patients/clients, stemming from and extending work in class. This can be built into a session or as 'homework' between sessions, depending upon the wider planning of the programme. It can involve the audio or indeed video recording of a piece of interaction, with the patient's permission of course, to be brought back to the next sessions for analysis and discussion. This is an excellent way of encouraging transfer, especially if supervisory staff can become increasingly involved as the programme proper comes to an end.

Extensions of standard skills programmes

Mention has been made of transfer action planning and the manager's contribution to it. The need to extend traditional skills training procedures in such ways by building in a specific focus on how training content can be successfully carried beyond training has been recognized relatively recently. Over the past few years a number of instances have been reported of trainers including additional structured techniques in standard training packages with the aim of producing more lasting and flexible outcomes.

Relapse prevention training (RPT) (Marx, 1982) is one such technique, based upon self-management procedures, which has attracted considerable attention in training circles generally (Wexley, 1984) and CST in particular (Marx and Ivey, 1988). An evaluation study of the impact of having a relapse prevention component as part of a supervisory skills training programme concluded that, 'even devoting a minimal amount of training time to a discussion of "slips" and relapse prevention strategies may help increase training effectiveness' (Noe, Sears and Fullenkamp, 1990, p. 326). Similar self-management-based techniques have also been found to promote the generalization of negotiating skills to a novel negotiating scenario not featured in the training sequence (Gist, Bavetta and Stevens, 1990).

As typically operated, RPT is part of the formal training programme, with usually the last session or sessions being devoted to it. Its inclusion seems to be particularly apt under circumstances where the work setting is less than conducive to changed practices. Briefly, RPT involves the following steps:

- restatement of the specific skill/s focused on in training;
- commitment to retaining and using the skill – this can be done with the help of a decision matrix which sets out the advantages and disadvantages of using and not using the skill as intended;
- recognition of the fact that lapses are possible, also distinguishing between lapse and relapses and accepting that one slip does not negate the benefits of training – emotional consequences such as disappointment or self-recrimination can also be recognized as unhelpful and more positive approaches talked through;

- identification of similarities and differences between training and job environments;
- prediction of problem areas where applying the new learning is anticipated to be particularly difficult – sources of such difficulty should be teased out;
- analysis of available resources and coping mechanisms – resources that can be mobilized (e.g. the emotional support of a fellow trainee can be valuable in a situation where a nurse has been acquiring listening skills as part of a more patient-centred approach), and coping mechanisms made available (e.g. better time management/reorganization of priorities to create more time to devote to the discussion of patients' psychosocial concerns), should be illuminated;
- planning and practice of application – participants should construct work-based scenarios derived from the problem areas and incorporating the difficulties derived from Stage 5; the strategies and tactics identified for overcoming these are then tried out with other members of the group, using role-play and simulation;
- monitoring the use of the target skill back on the job – participants may be encouraged to develop a viable assessment scheme for monitoring their use of the skill. There are several ways of doing this. One possibility is a structured diary, to be completed at times such as lunchtime or at the end of the day by noting when the skill was used, how and with what effect. Also, occasions when it could/should have been but wasn't can be included, together with a commitment to act differently under similar circumstances in the future. Ideally, management should be prepared to set aside the short period of time to complete this task each day. Self-reinforcement possibilities can also be discussed, so that trainees are aware of the need to recognize their achievements.

Fuller expositions of RPT are provided by Marx (1982), Marx and Ivey (1988) and Board and Newstrom (1992). A worksheet that can form the basis of an RPT-type session is provided in Figure 13.3.

13.6.3 The trainee

The trainee's main contribution to the task of promoting transfer during training is to, firstly, attend the programme as and when required and, secondly, participate in it fully and with an open mind. In the case of in-service training, the prospects of change to customary practices can engender insecurity and provoke an almost reflexive resistance. The upshot can be an unconducive attitude of sullen acquiescence or indeed active resistance. Learning, and particularly experiential learning, is minimal under these circumstances. While not recommending an unquestioning acceptance of everything presented, the trainee should be prepared to engage fully with the sequence, keeping an open mind as to possibilities for improving practices. 'Tried and tested' does not mean that established ways of doing things cannot be bettered.

1. The essentials of the skill are ______________________________

____

2. Work situations where it would be appropriate to use the skill ______________________________

____

3. Advantages of using the skill in each of these situations ______________________________

____

4. Disadvantages of using the skill in each of these situations ______________________________

____

5. Commitment of using the skill in each of these situations ______________________________

____

6. Differences between training and work settings ______________________________

____

7. Things at work which could help me in using the skill ______________________________

____

8. Ways of accessing this help ______________________________

____

9. Work situations where failure to use the skill is most likely ______________________________

____

10. Things which will make it difficult to use the skill ______________________________

____

11. Ways of overcoming these inhibitors ______________________________

____

12. What I would find most helpful now to enable me to counteract these inhibitors __________

____

Figure 13.3 Transfer training worksheet.

13.7 POST-TRAINING CONSIDERATIONS

Several related premises have been at the centre of our thinking on transfer throughout this chapter. One is that successful transfer is not solely a feature of the design and delivery of the training experience, although these features are of crucial importance, as we have seen in the last section. Carry-over is not due solely to increased knowledge, modified attitudes, enhanced sensitivity or newly honed skills. In addition, trainees must be sufficiently motivated to implement training outcomes and know when to do so. Furthermore, the organizational environment within which the trainee works must be accommodating to such change. Ford and Fisher (1994, p. 245) substantiated this view in their comment that 'training research has noted the importance of the immediate job context as critical to transfer. This context can either support or inhibit the transfer of training.' Some of these facilitating and inhibiting influences have been identified and discussed by Goldstein (1985).

Further and related premises are that management and trainees, as well as the trainer, have a part to play in making transfer happen and that their collaborative work commences before the training input and continues after it has finished. Here the post-training involvement of managers, trainers and trainees will be discussed.

13.7.1 The manager

The assumption to be made here is that management is the party best placed to effect organizational change that may be necessary to facilitate transfer. As such, a number of managerial contributions should be borne in mind.

Creating an organizational environment conducive to change

As put by Hayes (1990), 'training can only be effective within an organization framework which permits and promotes its efficiency' (p. 42). Referring explicitly to CST, Hargie and Tourish (1994, p. 1386–1387) expressed a similar viewpoint: 'Trainees are unlikely to find their attitudes changed at all unless the organization as a whole is moving in a similar direction. For this reason, many corporate training programs fail. The message of the training is not systematically reinforced throughout the organization, and hence the attitudinal changes which may have begun during a training programme atrophy upon return to the workplace.'

Three distinct but related aspects of the organizational environment have been mentioned by Ford and Fisher (1994). Firstly, there must be an appropriately dynamic climate, which embraces flexibility and innovative practice, where staff feel comfortable with change and sufficiently secure to try out new ways of doing things while accepting possible risks involved in abandoning old ways, and which ultimately derives from the same corporate values reflected in training.

Secondly, the support of fellow workers is crucial. Organizational climate is one thing but different departments and work groups can develop, to a certain extent, their own sets of routines and norms. Where these countermand training outcomes, it is highly unlikely that new practices will be sustained.

Finally, trainees must be given the opportunity to use new-found knowledge and skills. If their work is such that they seldom have a chance to apply what they have learned, generalization can scarcely be expected. Similarly, if the implementation of new practices necessitates certain additional equipment or other resources, it is the responsibility of management to ensure that these are provided. Of course trainees must not only have opportunities to make use of training but also to recognize those opportunities.

Monitoring performance

Participants should be encouraged to monitor their use of the new skill. Self-monitoring is an extremely potent technique for sustaining targeted activity. Supervisory monitoring can also create a basis for informed decision-making on current work practices and furnish valuable feedback on the worth of training. This can be further and usefully developed through a mentoring system of matching newly trained and more skilled staff.

Providing support and reinforcement

Managers and supervisory staff must be alert to instances of transfer and be ready to promote them when they do occur though recognition and praise. Unfortunately opportunities here are often missed, 'managers are often reluctant, unskilled, or unavailable to provide the feedback and reinforcement necessary to facilitate skill utilization' (Noe, Sears and Fullenkamp, 1990, p. 317).

Acting as a model

In an early piece of research, Fleishman, Harris and Burtt (1955) made the intriguing finding that only those trainees whose supervisors manifested behaviours targeted in training routinely showed evidence of carry-over.

Reducing initial job pressures

Making changes to set habits and routines may initially add to the pressures of work. Tasks may take longer, fewer patients may be seen, etc. These concerns have to be taken into account by management and accommodated. If they are not, regression to old ways may prove the convenient option.

Providing a system of aides-memoires

Having written and graphic material in the form of posters, cards, etc. strategically placed at the work site can help to keep training current and cue appropriate behaviour.

Including trained performance in formal staff appraisal procedures

This can send a powerful message about the value placed on this aspect of the job as well as providing a sound basis for reinforcing quality performance in a very tangible fashion.

13.7.2 The trainer

In addition to possible involvement in some of the activities listed immediately above, the trainer can make further contributions at this post-training stage.

Evaluate training

Some of the ways in which this can be done are covered in Chapter 11. The point here is that evaluation should include an assessment of transfer. Making trainees aware of the fact that such a follow-up will be conducted can promote a greater carry-over.

Hold 'booster sessions'

These are short training interventions held some time after the completion of the original programme, targeting the same content and designed to strengthen initial acquisition. It is claimed by Faulkner (1993) that the most successful workshops are those that have a 1- or 2-day follow-up session roughly 6 months after the original training. This can be particularly advantageous in situations where skills are important but not frequently deployed.

13.7.3 The trainee

There are several specific contributions that participants can make, following the completion of training, to the transfer process.

Exercising self-management techniques

Some reference has already been made to these both in relation to self-monitoring and relapse prevention training. By taking such steps as setting explicit goals, monitoring performance, and applying self-reinforcement, performance on targeted skills can be kept to the fore and sustained.

Operating a 'buddy' system

Here two learners pair up for the purposes of sustaining change through mutual commitment, advice and support. It may be a way of persisting with a commitment to change even in the face of other inhibiting aspects of the work environment.

13.8 OVERVIEW

Ultimately the success of training must be measured against improvements in health-care delivery and consequent increases in the quality of service offered. Unless the effects of training in improved interpersonal skills are reflected in changed work practice the venture will have been futile. In this chapter the importance of not leaving transfer to chance has been accentuated. The traditional approach of 'train and hope' is entirely inadequate. A further inadequacy is the belief that successful transfer will be guaranteed if the trainer makes a good job of designing and delivering the package. While this is a necessary condition for carry-over, it is not sufficient. The approach taken in this chapter has emphasized a more holistic approach to the task involving management, trainer and trainees in collaboration. Each has a contribution to make. Furthermore, these contributions are not confined to their respective roles during the running of the programme. What happens before and after the instructional sequence must not be neglected. These junctures offer significant opportunities for promoting transfer of training. A range of factors that influence carry-over together with strategies which can be used to this end were outlined.

Concluding comments 14

The ability to communicate effectively is now regarded as central to the provision of quality health care. Without it the establishment of facilitative relationships within which changes can take place in values, attitudes, feelings, knowledge, beliefs and ultimately habits and practices is impossible. There is evidence to suggest that patients who are related to by staff in an interpersonally skilled fashion can benefit not only psychologically and behaviourally but also physically (Ley, 1988; Ong *et al.*, 1995). Furthermore, it has been claimed by Ray (1993), among others, that recipients of health care place primary emphasis upon the communication skills of practitioners in making overall judgements on their professional competence. Attributions of competence produce feelings of confidence. Having confidence in a health practitioner, of course, has further implications for the likelihood of complying with therapeutic decisions. There is, unfortunately, also evidence that patients frequently express dissatisfaction with the extent of appropriate communication engaged in by health workers (Meredith, 1993; Buetow, 1995). The advent of consumerism within the NHS has, of course, given this reaction added import.

A premise of this book has been that one of the causes of poor communication is a lack of skill amongst health workers. There is evidence in substantiation. References to failings in this regard are common in the literature (Maguire and Faulkner, 1988; Davis and Fallowfield, 1991; Sellick, 1991; Audit Commission, 1993). A corollary is that training has been inadequate, either through insufficiency or inappropriateness.

It would seem that recommendations for innovation in this area of the curriculum have, in many instances, found those with an executive responsibility decidedly ill-prepared. While readily agreeing in principle with the legitimacy of such an endeavour, MacLeod Clark and Faulkner (1987) discovered that less than 5% of nurse tutors surveyed in schools and colleges of nursing throughout the UK felt that they were ready to offer such teaching. This disquiet was further reflected in the expressed need for suitable training in how to teach communication skills. This book has been written to meet the requirement by trainers for information on and guidance in apposite techniques for promoting students' interpersonal proficiency in professional contexts.

The CST process elaborated encompasses preparation, training and evaluation phases. The training phase, in turn, incorporates sensitization, practice and feedback components and is in keeping with our underlying concepts of communicative competence and skill. Throughout, however, we have been at pains to dispel the illusion of CST as a fixed and immutable regime that must be inflexibly adhered to in all circumstances. Rather we have striven to encourage tutors, within the resource constraints imposed upon them, to mould and adapt the basic model, in accordance with guidelines provided, to accommodate the needs of diverse student groups. Indeed, one of the advantages of the system is its tolerance of variability in terms of skill content, institutional setting, and trainee population. In addition to being flexible, there is merit in the tutor adopting an open approach to CST by monitoring the effectiveness of the programme, in accordance with the techniques discussed in Chapter 11, and being prepared to use such feedback to make further modifications and refinements in an attempt to ensure that the aims of training are fully met.

We have focused upon training as one method of enhancing the quality of the interpersonal dimension of the health worker's job. It would be naive, however, to assume that training alone will bring about the changes that we seek. Reflecting on the contextualized model of interpersonal communication outlined in Figure 13.2 and presented in the last chapter, it will be recalled that interaction takes place within a framework of organizational and cultural influences and is shaped accordingly. Cultural differences have been found to be at the root of some doctor–patient problems of relating (Bowes and Domokos, 1995). More generally, Fielding and Llewelyn (1987), discussing poor practice in nursing, suggested that our culture does not place a high value upon communication for its own sake. The ultimate effectiveness of CST must therefore depend upon broader structural changes associated not only with the education and training of health workers but with the conceptualization, organization and administration of health-care provision.

14.1 REPLACING THE BIOMEDICAL MODEL OF CARE

The traditional adherence to an essentially medical model of the patient, derived from the natural sciences, has led to a characterization of the patient as a purely biological entity comprising a complex of physical and chemical systems and subsystems, within which pathology can be defined and treated, rather than as a fellow human being with a personal dignity and needs that may be psychosocial as well as physical. Attitudes of medical staff, as a result, 'may be manifested as a tendency to see the patient as a thing or to concentrate upon the parts rather than the whole' (Tahka, 1984, p. 3). Under these circumstances the necessity for skilled communication is unlikely to be fully appreciated. A broader conceptualization of human well-being is required, incorporating contributions from the social and behavioural sciences, if improvements in standards of communication in health-care delivery are to be achieved (Hunt, 1988; Davis and Fallowfield, 1991; Epstein *et al.*, 1993).

14.2 SENIOR STAFF AS GOOD ROLE MODELS

Reference has already been made to the impact that broad cultural effects can have on the interchange between health-care provider and recipient. Microcosmically, the culture of care that pertains in an institution or part of it, such as a clinic or ward, is also highly significant. In a study of factors that influence how nurses communicate with cancer patients, Wilkinson (1991) found that the ward on which they worked was highly significant. On some wards nurses tended to avoid patients' concerns by using blocking tactics, while on others their psychosocial needs were facilitated. The contribution of the sisters to promoting facilitative ways of relating was highlighted 'as one factor which could influence how the other ward staff communicate with patients, as these sisters were observed acting as role models for the ward staff' (p. 686). Messages can be sent in many and sometimes subtle ways. Lillie (1985) drew attention to how the use of language by staff can serve to trivialize (e.g. talking 'baby talk' to the old or to the mentally handicapped adult) or dehumanize (e.g. labelling of patients as 'the hysterectomy in bed 2' or 'the asthmatic in 6').

If the general ethos of the ward is such that a low priority seems to be given to relating interpersonally to patients, students will no doubt behave accordingly. Greenwood (1993) reported that the reality which often confronted student nurses on the ward was an approach to patient care that was disease-oriented and essentially task-centred. It is improbable that college-based teaching in patient-centred communication will have a lasting influence on students' health-care practices if it is at variance with what is experienced by them in 'the world of work'. As we have seen in Chapter 13 when discussing how to promote the transfer of training, it is pointless making the effort to train if participants are to be placed in a work setting that neither values in real terms those ways of relating to patients/clients nor is prepared to facilitate them.

14.3 ORGANIZATIONAL AND ADMINISTRATIVE FACTORS

A variety of organizational and administrative factors, which reflect present-day realities of the health service, militates against good communication (May, 1990). Reductions in funding inevitably increase the pressures under which staff work. Clearly this has implications for the quality of interpersonal relationships formed not only with patients, but also with colleagues (McIntee and Firth, 1984). Faced with an ever-increasing case-load and the necessity to prioritize, it is likely that the physical rather than psychosocial needs of patients will be attended to. The time available to talk with and listen to patients is also likely to be curtailed. Indeed, health workers in several studies have expressed a desire to spend longer with patients and their families, particularly when a counselling/support role is called for (Bergen, 1991; Seale, 1992). A regression to old attitudes and ways of thinking, typified by accusations of 'skiving' levelled at nurses caught taking time to talk to patients, must be guarded against.

On the other hand, it has been argued that doctors often grossly overestimate the additional time taken to accommodate a more patient-centred communicative style. Epstein *et al.* (1993) reported findings that patient-centred consultations take, on average, only 1 minute longer than physician-centred alternatives. In actual fact, allowing patients to give their accounts of experienced problems and what caused them can facilitate a more accurate diagnosis. Patient feelings of having been understood can lead to greater confidence in that diagnosis. Patient understanding of, and indeed participation in, treatment decisions is likely to promote greater compliance with therapeutic recommendations. All in all, the total amount of time spent with a patient could actually be reduced in the long run, in circumstances where good communicative practice prevails (DiMatteo, 1994).

As a footnote, Davis and Fallowfield (1991) suspected that in many instances, health professionals use 'lack of time' as an excuse when they don't communicate properly with patients, really because of a lack of either confidence or skill. Furthermore, Thompson (1994) reviewed some evidence to suggest that there is little correlation between time spent with the patient *per se* and quality of communication entered into.

While accepting the difficulty of the task under present economic circumstances, policy makers, planners and administrators must acknowledge the value of effective interpersonal communication with patients (even if only on the hard economic basis of less stressed patients making quicker recoveries and being discharged from hospital sooner) and be prepared to take steps to promote it.

14.4 RELATIONSHIPS AMONGST THE HEALTH PROFESSIONS

A further organizational issue has to do with internal status hierarchies and the relationships amongst health professionals. The internal social structure of the NHS has a clearly identifiable status hierarchy extending from consultants down through doctors and paramedics to nurses and ancillary staff (Burton, 1985). The direction of power and influence follows. This structure militates against full and open discussion between strata taking place on the basis of equality, for the good of the patient. It also causes dilemmas for some who may avoid getting involved in conversations with patients about their diagnosis or prognosis lest they incur the wrath of a higher-status colleague whose policy is not to divulge such information. In the study by Wilkinson (1991) already mentioned, sisters of wards where facilitative communication with patients was practised had sought the agreement of doctors for any qualified member of staff to discuss issues of diagnosis and prognosis if asked by the patient. This resulted in '. . .an environment of openness, where nurses were not frightened to talk truthfully with the patients for fear of getting into trouble' (p. 687). Although changes are taking place, the transition for some health professions, from a subservient to a more collegiate relationship with others, still has some way to go.

14.5 GREATER SUPPORT FOR HEALTH WORKERS

Poor levels of communication may be self-serving for health professionals (Fielding and Llewelyn, 1987). We should not lose sight of the fact that, unfortunately, some health workers may feel that it is not in their best interests to engage with patients in the manner that patients have a right to expect them to. Abraham and Shanley (1992) suggested two possible reasons. One is a fear of having a lack of knowledge exposed if the sort of relationship is encouraged where patients feel at liberty to ask questions about their condition. The other has to do with an erosion of power and control. The traditional practitioner-centred style of interacting is one in which health workers retain power and control. There may be a number of immediate advantages in this arrangement for them. Unfortunately, it often leads to lack of patient satisfaction. What is more, lack of compliance may even be one of the few ways that patients have of asserting their autonomy, under these circumstances (Thompson, 1994). Evidently, better communication has to be accompanied by a revision of the nature of this relationship between patient and health-care provider in many cases.

Emotional self-protection has also been cited as a reason why staff maintain a distance from patients. The avoidance of all but the most superficial communication by nurses when dealing with patients may be a defensive strategy operating in the interests of preventing possible personal distress. This is most probable in areas of health care that are potentially more emotionally difficult, such as working with the terminally ill or the bereaved. Poor communication, using blocking tactics, etc., may therefore be a method for coping with occupational stress and avoiding 'burn-out' (May, 1990). One-fifth of the nurses sampled by Seale (1992), who dealt specifically with terminal illness, felt that they did not receive adequate emotional support in their work. Improved support systems for staff under these circumstances are obviously required if patients are to benefit from better communication. Faulkner (1993) outlined ways in which health professionals can be facilitated in this regard. Greater improvements in communication skills were found by Faulkner and Maguire (1984) among nurses working with mastectomy patients in ward contexts, where staff experienced group cohesion and support, compared to the community setting where nurses often had a strong feeling of working on their own.

Clearly these contextual realities of CST must be acknowledged. It would be naive to believe that CST can, single-handedly, reverse the impression, all too frequently formed, of health professionals as poor communicators. We are convinced, however, that it has an invaluable contribution to make as part of a wider movement that recognizes the centrality of this facet of professional competence and is pledged to improving it.

References

Abraham, C. and Shanley, E. (1992) *Social Psychology for Nurses*, Edward Arnold, London.

Adamek, M. (1994) Audio-cueing and immediate feedback to improve group leadership skills: a live supervision model. *Journal of Music Therapy*, **31**, 135–164.

Adams, J. (1987) Historical review and appraisal of research on the learning, retention, and transfer of human motor skills. *Psychological Bulletin*, **101**, 41–74.

Adams, N., Bell., J., Saunders, C. and Whittington, D. (1994) *Communication Skills in Physiotherapy-Patient Interactions*. Research Report, Centre for Health and Social Research, University of Ulster, Jordanstown.

Adelman, R. D., Greene, M. G., Charon, R. and Friedmann, E. (1992) The content of physician and elderly patient interaction in the medical primary care encounter. *Communication Research*, **19**, 370–380.

Aiken, L. R. (1994) *Aging: An Introduction to Gerontology*. Sage, Thousand Oaks, CA.

Ainsworth-Vaughan, N. (1992) Topic transitions in physician–patient interviews: power, gender and discourse change. *Language in Society*, **21**, 409–426.

Albert, S. and Kessler, S. (1976) Processes for ending social encounters. *Journal of the Theory of Social Behaviour*, **6**, 147–170.

Alexander, S., Whittingham, S. and Peppard, H. (1993) The development of an interactive videodisc to facilitate students' acquisition of interviewing skills in systems analysis courses. *IFIP Transactions A – Computer Science and Technology*, **35**, 107–115.

Alloy, L. and Lipman, A. (1992) Depression and selection of positive and negative social feedback: motivated preference and cognitive balance. *Journal of Abnormal Psychology*, **101**, 310–313.

Analoui, F. (1993) *Training and Transfer of Learning*, Avebury, Aldershot.

Anastasi, T. (1987) Communication training, in *Training and Development Handbook: A Guide to Human Resource Development*, (ed. R. Craig), McGraw-Hill, New York.

Anderson, L. and Sharpe, P. (1991) Improving patient and provider communication: a synthesis and review of communication interventions. *Patient Education and Counselling*, **17**, 99–134.

Annett, J. (1969) *Feedback and Human Behaviour*, Penguin, Harmondsworth.

Antaki, C. and Lewis, A. (eds) (1986) *Mental Mirrors: Metacognition in Social Knowledge and Communication*, Sage, London.

Archer, R. (1979) Role of personality and the social situation, in *Self-disclosure*, (ed. G. Chelune), Jossey-Bass, San Francisco, CA.

Argent, J., Faulkner, A., Jones, A. and O'Keefe, C. (1994) Communication skills in palliative care: development and modification of a rating scale. *Medical Education*, **28**, 559–565.

Argyle, M. (1972) *The Psychology of Interpersonal Behaviour*, 2nd edn, Penguin, Harmondsworth.

Argyle, M. (1988) *Bodily Communication*, 2nd edn, Methuen, London.

Argyle, M. (1994) *The Psychology of Interpersonal Behaviour*, 5th edn, Penguin, Harmondsworth.

Argyle, M., Furnham, A. and Graham, J. (1981) *Social Situations*, Cambridge University Press, Cambridge.

Argyle, M. and Kendon, A. (1967) The experimental analysis of social performance, in *Advances in Experimental Social Psychology*, vol. 3, (ed. L. Berkowitz), Academic Press, New York.

Arkowitz, H. (1981) The assessment of social skills, in *Behavioral Assessment. A Practical Handbook*, (eds M. Hersen and A. Bellack), Pergamon Press, New York.

Armstrong, P. (1982) The 'needs meeting' ideology in liberal adult education. *International Journal of Lifelong Education*, **1**, 330–334.

Armstrong, D. (1991) What do patients want? Someone who will answer their questions. *British Medical Journal*, **303**, 261–262.

Audit Commission (1993) *What Seems to be the Matter: Communication between Hospitals and Patients*, HMSO, London.

Aune, R. K. and Kikuchi, T. (1993) Effects of language intensity similarity on perceptions of credibility, relational attributions, and persuasion. *Journal of Language and Social Psychology*, **12**, 224–237.

Authier, J. (1986) Showing warmth and empathy, in *A Handbook of Communication Skills*, (ed. O. Hargie), Croom Helm, London.

Badenoch, J. (1986) Communication skills in medicine: the role of communication in medical practice. *Journal of the Royal Society of Medicine*, **79**, 565–567.

Bailey, C. and Butcher, D. (1983) Interpersonal skills training 11: the trainer's role. *Management Education and Development*, **14**, 106–112.

Baker, B. and Daniels, T. (1989) Integrating research on the microcounselling programme: a meta-analysis. *Journal of Counselling Psychology*, **36**, 213–222.

Baker, S., Daniels, T. and Greeley, A. (1990) Systematic training of graduate-level counsellors: narrative and meta-analytic reviews of three major reviews. *Counselling Psychologist*, **18**, 355–421.

Baker, S., Johnson, E., Kopala, M. and Strout, N. (1985) Test interpretation competence: a comparison of microskills and mental practice training, *Counsellor Education and Supervision*, **25**, 31–43.

Baker, S., Johnson, E., Strout, N. *et al.* (1986) Effects of separate and combined overt and covert practice modes on counselling trainee competence and motivation, *Journal of Counselling Psychology*, **33**, 469–470.

Baldwin, T. (1992) Effects of alternative modelling strategies on outcomes of interpersonal skills training. *Journal of Applied Psychology*, **77**, 147–154.

Baldwin, J. and Baldwin, J. (1981) *Behavior Principles in Everyday Life*, Prentice-Hall, Englewood Cliffs, NJ.

Baldwin, T. and Ford, K. (1988) Transfer of training: a review and directions for future research. *Personnel Psychology*, **41**, 63–105.

Baldwin, T. and Magjuka, R. (1991) Organisational training and signals of importance: effects of pre-training perceptions on intentions to transfer. *Human Resource Development*, **2**, 25–36.

Bandura, A. (1977) *Social Learning Theory*, Prentice-Hall, Englewood Cliffs, NJ.

Bandura, A. (1986) *Social Foundations of Thought and Action: A Social Cognitive Theory.* Prentice-Hall, Englewood Cliffs, NJ.

Bandura, A. (1989) Perceived self-efficacy in the exercise of personal agency. *Psychologist*, **2**, 411–424.

Barker, J. R. and Tompkins, P. A. (1994) Identification in the self-managing organization: characteristics of target and tenure. *Human Communication Research*, **21**, 223–240.

Barnlund, D. C. (1993) The mystification of meaning: doctor–patient encounters, in *Perspectives on Health Communication*, (eds B. Thornton and G. Kreps), Waveland Press, Illinois.

Baron, R. (1988) Negative effects of destructive criticism: impact on conflict, self-efficacy, and task preference. *Journal of Applied Psychology*, **73**, 199–207.

Bartlett, F. (1948) The measurement of human skill. *Occupational Psychology*, **22**, 83–91.

Batty, R., Barber, N., Moclair, A. and Shackle, D. (1993) Assertion skills for clinical pharmacists. *Pharmaceutical Journal*, **251**, 353–355.

Baum, B. E. and Gray J. J. (1992) Expert modeling, self-observation using videotape, and acquisition of basic therapy skills. *Professional Psychology: Research and Practice*, **23**, 220–225.

Becker, M. and Maiman, L. (1975) Sociobehavioral determinants of compliance with health and medical care recommendations. *Medical Care*, **13**, 10–24.

Becker, M. and Maiman, L. (1980) Strategies for enhancing patient compliance. *Journal of Community Health*, **6**, 113–135.

Becker, M. and Rosenstock, I. (1984) Compliance with medical advice, in *Health Care and Human Behaviour*, (eds A. Steptoe and A. Mathews), Academic Press, London.

Beisecker, A. E. (1990) Patient power in doctor–patient communication: what do we know? *Health Communication*, **1**, 105–122.

Beisecker, A. E. and Beisecker, T. D. (1990) Patient information-seeking behaviors when communicating with doctors. *Medical Care*, **28**, 19–28.

Bell, C. (1991) Using training aids, in *Gower Handbook of Training and Development*, (ed. J. Prior), Gower, Aldershot.

Bellack, A. and Hersen, M. (eds) (1988) *Behavioural Assessment*, Pergamon, New York.

Bensing, J. (1991) *Doctor–patient Communication and the Quality of Care*, NIVEL, Amsterdam.

Bensing, J. and Dronkers, J. (1992) Instrumental and affective aspects of physician behavior. *Medical Care*, **30**, 283–298.

Bergen, A. (1991) Nurses caring for the terminally ill: a review of the literature. *International Journal of Nursing Studies*, **28**, 89–101.

Berger, B. A. and Felkey, B. G. (1989) A conceptual framework for focusing the teaching of communication skills on compliance gaining strategies. *American Journal of Pharmaceutical Education*, **53**, 259–265.

Bermosk, L. S. and Mordan, M. J. (1964) *Interviewing in Nursing*, Macmillan, New York.

Bernstein, G. (1982) Training behaviour change agents: a conceptual view. *Behaviour Therapy*, **13**, 1–23.

Bernstein, L. and Bernstein, R. (1980) *Interviewing: A Guide for Health Professionals*, 3rd edn, Appleton-Century-Crofts, New York.

Bettinghaus, E. P. and Cody, M. J. (1994) *Persuasive Communication*, 5th edn, Harcourt Brace, Orlando, FL.

Biggs, S. J. (1991) Trigger tapes and training, in *Practical Guide to Using Video in the Behavioural Sciences*, (ed. P. Dowrick), John Wiley, New York.

Billow, J. A. (1990) The status of undergraduate instruction in communication skills in US Colleges of Pharmacy. *American Journal of Pharmaceutical Education*, **54**, 23–26.

Bilodeau, E. and Bilodeau, I. (1961) Motor-skills learning, *Annual Review of Psychology*, **12**, 243–280.

Bird, J., Hall, A., Maguire, P. and Heavey, A. (1993) Workshops for consultations on the teaching of clinical communication skills. *Medical Education*, **27**, 181–185.

Birnbrauer, H. (1987) Evaluation techniques that work. *Training and Development*, July, 53–55.

Blanck, P. D., Buck, R. and Rosenthal, R. (eds) (1986) *Nonverbal Communication in the Clinical Context*, Pennsylvania University Press, Philadelphia, PA.

Bland, M. and Jackson, P. (1990) *Effective Employee Communications*, Kogan Page, London.

Blenkinsopp, A., Robinson, E. and Panton, R. (1994) Do pharmacy customers remember the information given to them by the community pharmacist? in *Social Pharmacy: Innovation and Change*, (eds G. Harding, S. Nettleton and K. Taylor), Pharmaceutical Press, London.

Bligh, D. (1971) *What's the Use of Lectures*, D. A. and B. Bligh, Briar House, Exeter.

Block, M., Schaffner, K. and Coulehan, J. (1985) Ethical problems of recording physician–patient interactions in family practice settings. *Journal of Family Practice*, **21**, 467–472.

Blondis, M. and Jackson, B. (1982) *Nonverbal Communication with Patients*, John Wiley, New York.

Blumberg, H. H., Davies, M. F. and Kent, V. (1986) Interacting in groups, in *A Handbook of Communication Skills*, (ed. O. Hargie), Croom Helm, London.

Board, M. and Newstrom, J. (1992) *Transfer of Training*, Addison-Wesley, Reading, MA.

Boice, R. (1983) Observational skills. *Psychological Bulletin*, **93**, 3–29.

Borisoff, D. and Merrill, L. (1991) Gender issues and listening, in *Listening in Everyday Life*, (eds D. Borisoff and M. Purdy), University of America Press, Maryland.

Borisoff, D. and Purdy, M. (eds) (1991) *Listening in Everyday Life*, University of America Press, Maryland.

Boster, F. and Mongeau, P. (1984) Fear-arousing persuasive messages, in *Communication Yearbook 8*, (eds B. Bostrom and B. Westley), Sage, Beverly Hills, CA.

Bottero, W. (1994) The changing face of pharmacy: gender and explanations of women's entry to pharmacy, in *Social Pharmacy: Innovation and Development*, (eds G. Harding, S. Nettleton and K. Taylor), Pharmaceutical Press, London.

Bottomley, V. (1993) Department of Health Press Release. H93/65, 29th March.

Bowes, A. and Domokos, T. (1995) South Asian women and their GP's: some issues of communication. *Social Sciences and Health*, **1**, 22–34.

Bowman, F. M., Goldberg, D. P., Millar, T. *et al.* (1992) Improving the skills of established general practitioners: the long-term benefits of group teaching. *Medical Education*, **26**, 63–68.

Bradburn, N. and Sudman, S. (1980) *Improving Interview Method and Questionnaire Design: Response Effects to Threatening Questions in Survey Research*, Aldine Press, Chicago, IL.

Bradley, A. and Phillips, K. (1991) Interpersonal skills training, in *Gower Handbook of Training and Development*, (ed. J. Prior), Gower, Aldershot.

Bradshaw, P., Ley, P., Kincey, J. and Bradshaw, J. (1975) Recall of medical advice: comprehensibility and specificity. *British Journal of Social and Clinical Psychology*, **14**, 55–62.

Brandes, D. and Philips, H. (1978) *The Gamester's Handbook*, Hutchinson, London.

Brearley, S. (1990) *Patient Participation: The Literature*, Scutari Press, Middlesex.

Briggs, K. (1986) Assertiveness: speak your mind. *Nursing Times*, **82**, 24–26.

Brinko, K. (1993) The practice of giving feedback to improve teaching. *Journal of Higher Education*, **64**, 576–593.

Brook, C. (1985) Providing feedback: the research on effective oral and written feedback strategies. *Central States Speech Journal*, **36**, 14–23.

Brooks, W. and Heath, R. (1985) *Speech Communication*, W. C. Brown, Dubuque, I.A.

Brosius, H. and Bathelt, A. (1994) The utility of exemplars in persuasive communications. *Communication Research*, **21**, 48–78.

Brown, R. (1988) *Group Processes: Dynamics Within and Between Groups*, Basil Blackwell, Oxford.

Brown, G. (1997) Explaining, in *A Handbook of Communication* Skills, 2nd edn, (ed. O. Hargie), Routledge, London.

Brownell, J. (1993) Listening environment: a perspective, in *Perspectives on Listening*, (eds A. Wolvin and C. Coakley), Ablex, Norwood, NJ.

Bruneau, J. (1993) Empathy and Listening, in *Perspectives on Listening*, (eds A. Wolvin and C. Coakley), Ablex, Norwood, NJ.

Bruner, J. and Tagiuri, R. (1954) The perception of people, in *Handbook of Social Psychology*, (ed. G. Lindzey), Addison-Wesley, Reading, MA.

Bryman, A. (1986) *Leadership and Organizations*, Routledge & Kegan Paul, London.

Buckley, R. and Caple, J. (1990) *The Theory and Practice of Training*, Kogan Page, London.

Buckman, R. (1992) *How to Break Bad News: A Guide For Health-Care Professionals*, Macmillan, London.

Buetow, S. (1995) What do general practitioners and their patients want from general practice and are they receiving it? A framework. *Social Science and Medicine*, **40**, 213–221.

Buller, D. B. and Aune, R. K. (1992) The effects of vocalics and nonverbal sensitivity on compliance: further tests of the speech accomodation explanation, *Western Journal of Speech Communication*, **56**, 37–53.

Buller, D. B. and Street, R. L. (1992) Physician–patient relationships, in *Applications of Nonverbal Behavioral Theories and Research*, (ed. R. S. Feldman), Lawrence Erlbaum Associates, Hillsdale, NJ.

Burgoon, M., Birk, T. S. and Hall, J. R. (1991) Compliance and satisfaction in physician–patient communication. *Human Communication Research*, **18**, 177–208.

Burgoon, M., Callister, M. and Hunsaker, F. (1994) Patients who deceive: an investigation of patient–physician communication. *Journal of Language and Social Psychology*, **13**, 443–468.

Burgoon, M., Hunsaker, F. and Dawson, E. (1994) *Human Communication*, Sage, Thousand Oaks, CA.

Burley-Allen, M. (1995) *Listening: The Forgotten Skill*, John Wiley, New York.

Burnard, P. (1992) *Interpersonal Skills Training: A Sourcebook of Activities for Trainers*, Kogan Page, London.

Burrell, T. (1988) *Curriculum Design and Development: A Procedure Manual for Nurse Educators*, Prentice-Hall, Hemel Hempstead, Herts.

Burton, M. (1985) The environment, good interactions and interpersonal skills in nursing, in *Interpersonal Skills in Nursing: Research and Applications*, (ed. C. Kagan), Croom Helm, London.

Busby, A. and Gilchrist, B. (1992) The role of the nurse in the medical ward round. *Journal of Advanced Nursing*, **17**, 339–346.

Butterill, D., O'Hanlon, J. and Book, H. (1992) When the system is the problem don't blame the patient: problems inherent in the interdisciplinary inpatient team. *Canadian Journal of Psychiatry*, **37**, 168–172.

Byrne, P. and Long, B. (1976) *Doctors Talking to Patients*, HMSO, London.

Cairns, L. (1986) Reinforcement, in *A Handbook of Communication Skills*, (ed. O. Hargie), Croom Helm, London.

Campagna, M. A. and Berger, B. A. (1990) Using Bloom's taxonomy to assess pharmacists' learning as a result of viewing a program on communication skills. *American Journal of Pharmaceutical Education*, **54**, 7–14.

Campbell, J. (1988) Training design for performance improvement, in *Productivity in Organisations*, (eds J. Campbell, R. Campbell and associates), Jossey-Bass, San Francisco, CA.

Caney, D. (1983) The physiotherapist, in *The Study of Real Skills*, vol. 4 (ed. W. Singleton), MTP Press, Lancaster.

Caporael, L. and Culbertson, G. (1986) Verbal response modes of baby talk and other speech at institutions for the aged. *Language and Communication*, **6**, 99–112.

Carlson, R. (1984) *The Nurse's Guide to Better Communication*, Scott, Foresman & Co, Glenview, IL.

Carroll, J. and Monroe, J. (1979) Teaching medical interviewing: a critique of educational research and practice. *Journal of Medical Education*, **54**, 498–500.

Carroll, J. and Monroe, J. (1980) Teaching clinical interviewing in the health professions: a review of empirical research. *Evaluation and the Health Professions*, **3**, 21–45.

Cartledge, G. and Milburn, J. (1995) *Teaching Social Skills to Children and Youth: Innovative Approaches*, Allyn & Bacon, Boston, MA.

Cartwright, A. (1964) *Human Relations and Hospital Care*, Routledge & Kegan Paul, London.

Cartwright, S. (1986) *Training with Video*, Knowledge Industry Publications, White Plains, NY.

Cassata, D. (1978) Health communication theory and research an overview of the communication specialist interface, in *Communication Yearbook 2*, (ed. B. Ruben), International Communication Association, Transaction Books, New Jersey.

Cavalier, R. (1991) The multiple dimensions of interactive video, in *Practical Guide to Using Video in the Behavioural Sciences*, (ed. P. Dowrick), John Wiley, New York.

Caves, R. (1988) Consultative methods for extracting expert knowledge about professional competence, in *Professional Competence and Quality Assurance in the Caring Professions*, (ed. R. Ellis), Croom Helm, London.

Chalmers, R. (1983) Chair report of the study committee on preparation of students for the realities of contemporary pharmacy practice. *American Journal of Pharmaceutical Education*, **47**, 393–401.

Chalmers, K. and Luker, K. (1991) The development of the health visitor–client relationship. *Scandinavian Journal of Caring Science*, **5**, 33–41.

Chandler, M. H. H. (1989) Teaching interview techniques utilizing an instructional videotape. *Educational Gerontology*, **15**, 377–383.

Charlesworth, E. and Nathan, R. (1984) *Stress Management*, Corgi Books, London.

Chomsky, N. (1965) *Aspects of the Theory of Syntax*, MIT Press, Cambridge, MA.

Christensen, P. (1988) The nature of feedback student teachers receive in post-observation conferences with the university supervisor: a comparison with O'Neal's study of co-operative teacher feedback. *Teaching and Teacher Education*, **4**, 275–286.

Cialdini, R. (1988) *Influence: Science and* Practice, 2nd edn, Scott, Foresman & Co., Glenview, IL.

CINE (1986) *Report of the Communication in Nursing Education Curriculum Development Project (Phase 1)*, Health Education Council, London.

Clare, A. (1993) Communication in Health. *European Journal of Disorders of Communication*, **28**, 1–12.

Cohen, L. and Manion, L. (1985) *Research Methods in Education*, Routledge, London.

Cohen-Cole, S. (ed.) (1991) *The Medical Interview: The Three-Function Approach*, Mosby/Year Book, St Louis, MO.

Collins, J. and Collins M. (1992) *Social Skills Training and the Professional Helper*, John Wiley, Chichester.

Collins, W. J. N., Slater, M. and Smart, G. J. (1993) *Dental Hygienist Syllabus and Objectives*, School of Dental Hygiene, Guy's Hospital, London.

Condon J. T. (1992) Medical litigation. The aetiological role of psychological and interpersonal factors. *Medical Journal of Australia*, **157**, 768–770.

Cooke, P. (1987) Role-playing, in *Training and Development Handbook: A Guide to Human Resource Development*, (ed. R. Craig), McGraw-Hill, New York.

Cooley, E. (1994) Training an interdisciplinary team in communication and decision-making skills. *Small Group Research*, **25**, 5–25.

Cooley, R. and Roach, D. (1984) A conceptual framework, in *Competence in Communication: A Multidisciplinary Approach*, (ed. R. Bostrom), Sage, Beverly Hills, CA.

Corah, N. L., O'Shea, R. M. and Bissell, D. (1985). The dentist–patient relationship: perceptions by patients of dentist behaviour in relation to satisfaction and anxiety. *Journal of the American Dental Association*, **111**, 443–446.

Cork, N. (1987) Approaches to curriculum planning, in *Nursing Education: Research and Developments*, (ed. B. Davis), Croom Helm, London.

Cornford, I. (1991) Microteaching skill generalisation and transfer: training preservice teachers in introductory lesson skills. *Teaching and Teacher Education*, **7**, 25–56.

Cox, K., Bergen, A. and Norman, I. J. (1993) Exploring consumer views of care provided by the Macmillan nurse using the critical incident technique. *Journal of Advanced Nursing*, **18**, 408–415.

Crichton, E., Smith, D. and Demanuele, F. (1978) Patient recall of medication information. *Drug Intelligence and Clinical Pharmacy*, **12**, 591–599.

Crossman, E. (1960) *Automation and Skill. DSIR Problems of Progress in Industry, No. 9*, HMSO, London.

Crute, V. (1986) Microtraining in health visitor education: an intensive examination of training outcomes, feedback processes and individual differences. Unpublished PhD thesis, University of Ulster, Jordanstown.

Crute, V., Hargie, O. and Ellis, R. (1989) An evaluation of a communication skills course for health visitor students. *Journal of Advanced Nursing*, **14**, 546–552.

Cryer, P. (1988) Video feedback sessions for improving lecturing: participants' reactions to this method of academic staff development. *Programmed Learning and Educational Technology*, **25**, 112–118.

Cummings, J., Hansen, E. and Sillings, R. (1990) Teaching interviewing skills by interactive video: intertalk. *Journal of School Psychology*, **28**, 3–96.

Danish, S., D'Augelli, A. and Brock, G. (1976) An evaluation of helping skills training: effects of helper's verbal responses. *Journal of Counselling Psychology*, **23**, 259–266.

Davidhizor, R. (1992) Interpersonal communication: a review of eye contact. *Infection Control and Hospital Epidemiology*, **13**, 222–225.

Davis, H. and Fallowfield, L. (1991) *Counselling and Communication in Health Care*, John Wiley, Chichester.

Davis, B. and Ternuff-Nyhlin, K. (1982) Social skills training. The assessment of training in social skills in nursing, with particular reference to the patient profile interview. *Nursing Times*, **78**, 1765–1768.

Decker, P. (1980) Effects of symbolic coding and rehearsal in behaviour-modelling training. *Journal of Applied Psychology*, **65**, 627–634.

Decker, P. (1983) The effects of rehearsal group size and video feedback in behaviour modelling training. *Personnel Psychology*, **36**, 763–773.

Department of Health (1992a) *The Health of the Nation*. HMSO, London.

Department of Health (1992b) *The Patient's Charter*. HMSO, London.

Department of Health and Social Security (1986) *Primary Health Care: An Agenda for Discussion*, HMSO, London.

De Paulo, B. M. (1992) Nonverbal behavior and self-presentation. *Psychological Bulletin*, **111**, 203–243.

Derlega, V., Metts, S., Petronio, S. and Margulis, S. (1993) *Self-disclosure*, Sage, Newbury Park, CA.

DeVito, J. A. (1993) *Essentials of Human Communication*, Harper Collins, New York.

DeVito, J. A. (1995) *The Interpersonal Communication Book*, Harper Collins, New York.

Dichter Institute for Motivational Research, Inc. (1973) *Communicating the Value of Comprehensive Pharmaceutical Services to the Consumer*, American Pharmaceutical Association, Washington, DC.

Dickson, D. (1981) Microcounselling: an evaluative study of a programme. Unpublished PhD thesis, Ulster Polytechnic.

Dickson, D. (1995a) Communication and Interpersonal Skills, in *Community Health Care Nursing*, (ed. D. Sines), Blackwell Science, Oxford.

Dickson, D. (1995b) Learing av ferdigheter i kommunikasjon: rollespill som instruksjonsmetode, in *Kommunikasjon som Social og Tverrkulturell Kompetanse*, (eds F. Ask and O. Sletta), Tapir Forlag, Trondheim, Norway.

Dickson, D. (1997) Reflecting, in *A Handbook of Communication Skills*, 2nd edn, (ed. O. Hargie), Routledge, London.

Dickson, D. and Bamford, D. (1995) Improving the interpersonal skills of social work students: the problem of transfer and what to do about it. *British Journal of Social Work*, **25**, 85–105.

Dickson, D. and Maxwell, M. (1985) The interpersonal dimension of physiotherapy: implications for training. *Physiotherapy*, **71**, 306–310.

Dickson, D. and Maxwell, M. (1987) A comparative study of physiotherapy students' attitudes to social skills training undertaken before and after clinical placement. *Physiotherapy*, **73**, 60–64.

Dickson, D. and Mullan, T. (1990) An empirical investigation of the effects of a microcounselling programme with social work students: the acquisition and transfer of component skills. *Counselling Psychology Quarterly*, **3**, 267–263.

Dickson, D., Saunders, C. and Stringer, M. (1993) *Rewarding People*, Routledge, London.

Dickson, D., Tittmar, H. and Hargie, O. (1984) Social skills training in the preparation of the counsellor of the alcoholic, in *Advanced Concepts in Alcoholism*, (ed. H. Tittmar), Pergamon, Oxford.

Dillard, J. P. (1995) Rethinking the study of fear appeals: an emotional perspective. *Communication Theory*, **4**, 295–323.

Diller, L. (1990) Fostering the interdisciplinary team, fostering research in a society in transition. *Archives of Physical Medicine and Rehabilitation*, **71**, 275–278.

Dillon, J. (1986) Questioning, in *A Handbook of Communication Skills*, (ed. O. Hargie), Croom Helm, London.

Dillon, J. (1990) *The Practice of Questioning*, Routledge, London.

Dillon, J. (1997) Questioning, in *A Handbook of Communication Skills*, 2nd edn, (ed. O. Hargie), Routledge, London.

DiMatteo, M. (1994) The physician–patient relationship: effects on the quality of health care. *Clinical Obstetrics and Gynecology*, **37**, 149–161.

DiMatteo, M. and DiNicola, D. (1982) *Achieving Patient Compliance: The Psychology of the Medical Practitioner's Role*, Pergamon, New York.

DiMatteo, M. and Hays, R. (1980) The significance of patients' perceptions of physician conduct: a study of patient satisfaction in a family practice center. *Journal of Community Health*, **6**, 18–34.

DiMatteo, M., Hays, R. and Prince, L. (1986) Relationship of physicians' nonverbal communication skill to patient satisfaction, appointment compliance and physician workload. *Health Psychology*, **5**, 581–594.

DiMatteo, M., Taranta, A., Friedman, H. and Prince, L. (1980) Predicting patient satisfaction from physicians' nonverbal communication skills. *Medical Care*, **18**, 376–386.

Dimbleby, R. and Burton, G. (1985) *More Than Words: An Introduction to Communication*, Methuen, London.

Downs, C. W. (1988) *Communication Audits*, Scott, Foresman & Co., Glenview, IL.

Dowrick, P. (1991) *Practical Guide to Using Video in the Behavioural Sciences*, John Wiley, New York.

Dowrick, P. and Jesdale, D. C. (1991) Modeling, in *Practical Guide to Using Video in the Behavioural Sciences*, (ed. P. Dowrick), John Wiley, New York.

Drummond, H. (1992) *The Quality Movement*, Kogan Page, London.

Dryden, W. and Feltham, C. (1994) *Developing Counsellor Training*, Sage, London.

Duffield, C. (1993). The Delphi technique: a comparison of results obtained using two expert panels. *International Journal of Nursing Studies*, **30**, 227–237.

Dunn, W. and Hamilton, D. (1984) Continuing pharmaceutical education and the competence based approach – a discussion. *Journal of Social and Administrative Pharmacy*, **2**, 136–143.

Duryea, E. (1990) Doubling: enhancing the role play technique in schools. *Journal of School Health*, **60**, 106–107.

Eastwood, C. (1985) Nurse–patient communication skills in Northern Ireland – the educational problems. *International Journal of Nursing Studies*, **22**, 99–104.

Ebesu, A. S. and Miller, M. D. (1994) Verbal and nonverbal behaviors as a function of deception type. *Journal of Language and Social Psychology*, **13**, 418–442.

Eckes, T. (1994) Features of men, features of women: assessing stereotypic beliefs about gender subtypes. *British Journal of Social Psychology*, **33**, 107–123.

Edwards, H. and Noller, P. (1993) Perceptions of overaccomodation used by nurses in communication with the elderly. *Journal of Language and Social Psychology*, **12**, 207–223.

Eisler, R. and Frederiksen, L. (1980) *Perfecting Social Skills*, Plenum Press, New York.

Ekman, P. and Friesen, W. (1969) The repertoire of nonverbal behaviour: categories, origins, usage and code. *Semiotica*, **1**, 49–98.

Ekman, P. and Friesen, W. (1982) Measuring facial movement with the facial action coding system, in *Emotion in the Human Face*, (ed. P. Ekman), Cambridge University Press, Cambridge.

Ellis, A. and Beattie, G. (1986) *The Psychology of Language and Communication*, Weidenfeld & Nicolson, London.

Ellis, R. and Whittington, D. (1981) *A Guide to Social Skill Training*, Croom Helm, London.

Emmanuel, M. (1985) Auditing communication practices, in *Inside Organisational Communication*, (eds C. Reuss and R. DiSilvas), Longman, Harlow.

Enelow, A. J. and Swisher, S. C. (1986) *Interviewing and Patient Care*, 3rd edn, Oxford University Press, Oxford.

Epstein, R., Campbell, C., Cohen-Cole, S. *et al.* (1993) Perspectives on patient–doctor communication. *Journal of Family Practice*, **37**, 377–388.

Ericsson, K., Krampe, R. and Tesch-Romer, C. (1993) The role of deliberate practice in the acquisition of expert performance. *Psychological Review*, **100**, 363–406.

Evans, B. J., Stanley, R. O. and Burrows, G. D. (1992) Communication skills training and patients' satisfaction. *Health Communication*, **4**, 155–170.

Evans, B. J., Sweet, B. and Coman, G. J. (1993) Behavioural assessment of the effectiveness of a communication programme for medical students. *Medical Education*, **27**, 344–350.

Evans, B. J., Stanley, R. O., Mestrovic, R. and Rose, L. (1991). Effects of communication skills training in students' diagnostic efficiency. *Medical Education*, **25**, 517–526.

Ewles, L. and Simnett, I. (1992) *Promoting Health: A Practical Guide to Health Education*, 2nd edn, John Wiley, Chichester.

Falloon, I., Lindley, P., McDonald, R. and Marles, I. (1977) Social skills training of out-patient groups: a controlled study of rehearsal and homework. *British Journal of Psychology*, **131**, 599–609.

Faulkner, A. (1980) The student nurse's role in giving information to patients. Unpublished MLitt thesis, University of Aberdeen.

Faulkner, A. (1992) Communication skills in cancer and palliative care: the need to evaluate. *Medical Encounter*, **8**, 8–10.

Faulkner, A (1993) *Teaching Interactive Skills in Health Care*, Chapman & Hall, London.

Faulkner, A. and Maguire, P. (1984) Teaching assessment skills, in *Recent Advances in Nursing 7: Communication*, (ed. A. Faulkner), Churchill Livingstone, Edinburgh.

Fedor, D., Rensvold, R. and Adams, S. (1992) An investigation of factors expected to affect feedback seeking: a longitudinal field study. *Personnel Psychology*, **45**, 779–805.

Feldman, R. S. (1985) *Social Psychology: Theories, Research and Applications*, McGraw-Hill, New York.

Feldman, R. S. and Rime, B. (eds) (1991) *Fundamentals of Nonverbal Behaviour*, Cambridge University Press, Cambridge.

Feltham, C. and Dryden, W. (1994) *Developing Counsellor Supervision*, Sage, London.

Fichten, C. and Wright, J. (1983) Videotape and verbal feedback in behavioural couple therapy: a review. *Journal of Clinical Psychology*, **39**, 216–221.

Fielding, R. and Llewelyn, S. (1987) Communication training in nursing may damage your health and enthusiasm: some warnings. *Journal of Advanced Nursing*, **12**, 281–290.

Fillmore, C. (1979) On fluency, in *Individual Differences in Language Ability and Language Behaviour*, (eds C. Fillmore, D. Kemper and W. Wang), Academic Press, New York.

Fishbein, M. (1982) Social psychological analysis of smoking behaviors, in *Social Psychology and Behavioural Medicine*, (ed. J. Eiser), John Wiley, Chichester.

Fisher, R. C. (1992) Patient education and compliance: a pharmacist's perspective. *Patient Education and Counselling*, **19**, 261–271.

Fisher, C. M., Corrigan, O. I. and Henman, M. C. (1991) A study of community pharmacy practice. *Journal of Social and Administrative Pharmacy*, **8**, 15–23.

Fisher, S. and Groce, S. (1990) Accounting practices in medical interviews. *Language in Society*, **19**, 225–250.

Fitts, P. and Posner, M. (1973) *Human Performance*, Prentice-Hall, London.

Fleishman, E., Harris, E. and Burtt, H. (1955) *Leadership and Supervision in Industry*, Monograph no 33, Personnel Research Board, Ohio State University, Columbus, OH.

Fletcher, J. (1990) *Effectiveness and Cost of Interactive Videodisc Instruction in Defence Training and Education*, (IDA Paper P-2372), Institute for Defense Analyses, Alexandria, VA.

Fletcher, C. and Freeling, P. (1988) *Talking and Listening to Patients. A Modern Approach*, Nuffield Provincial Hospitals Trust, London.

Foot, H. (1986) Humour and laughter, in *A Handbook of Communication Skills*, (ed. O. Hargie), Croom Helm, London.

Ford, J. and Fisher, S. (1994) The transfer of safety training in work organisations: a systems perspective to continuous learning. *Occupational Medicine*, **9**, 241–259.

Forgas, J. P. (1983) What is social about social cognition?. *British Journal of Social Psychology*, **22**, 129–144.

Forgas, J. P. (1994) The role of emotion in social judgments: an introductory review and an Affect Infusion Model. *Journal of Social Psychology*, **24**, 1–24.

Foxon, M. (1986) Evaluation of training: the cost of the impossible. *Training Officer*, May, 133–137.

Frederikson, L. and Bull, P. (1992) An appraisal of the current status of communication skills training in British Medical Schools. *Social Science and Medicine*, **34**, 515–522.

French, P. (1994) *Social Skills for Nursing Practice*, 2nd edn, Chapman & Hall, London.

Friedman, H. S. (1979) The concept of skill in nonverbal communication: implications for understanding social interaction, in *Skill in Nonverbal Communication: Individual Differences*, (ed. R. Rosenthal), Oelgeschlager, Gunn & Hain, Cambridge, MA.

Fritz, P., Russell, C., Wilcox, E. and Shirk, F. (1984) *Interpersonal Communication in Nursing*, Appleton-Century-Crofts, Norwalk, CT.

Frost, R., Benton, N. and Dowrick, P. (1990) Self-evaluation, videotape review and dysphoria. *Journal of Social and Clinical Psychology*, **9**, 367–374.

Fuller, F. and Manning, B. (1973) Self-confrontation reviewed: a conceptualisation for video playback in teacher education, *Review of Educational Research*, **43**, 469–528.

Furnham, A. (1983a) Social skills and dentistry. *British Dental Journal*, **154**, 404–408.

Furnham, A. (1983b) Situational determinants of social skill, in *New Directions in Social Skill Training*, (eds R. Ellis and D. Whittington), Croom Helm, London.

Furnham, A., King, J. and Pendleton, D. (1980) Establishing rapport: interaction skills and occupational therapy. *British Journal of Occupational Therapy*, **43**, 322–325.

Gahagan, J. (1984) *Social Interaction and its Management*, Methuen, London.

Galbraith, M (ed.) (1990) *Adult Learning Methods: A Guide for Effective Instruction*, Krieger, Malabar, CA.

Gallant, J., Thyer, B. and Bailey, J. (1991) Using bug-in-the-ear feedback in clinical supervision: preliminary evaluations. *Research on Social Work Practice*, **1**, 175–187.

Gallego, A. (1987) Evaluation in nursing education, in *Nursing Education: Research and Developments*, (ed. B. Davis), Croom Helm, London.

Gallois, C. (1993) Prologue. *Journal of Language and Social Psychology*, **12**, 3–12.

Gamsu, D. S. and Bradley, C. (1987) Clinical staff's attributions about diabetes: scale developments and staff vs patient comparisons. *Current Psychological Research and Reviews*, **6**, 69–78.

Garavaglia, P. (1993) How to ensure transfer of training. *Training and Development*, **47**, 63–68.

Gardiner, D. (1984) Learning for transfer. *Issues in Social Work Education*, **4**, 95–105.

Garko, M. (1992) Physician executives' use of influence strategies: gaining compliance from superiors who communicate in attractive and unattractive styles. *Health Communication*, **4**, 137–154.

Garrud, P. (1990) Counselling needs and experience of junior hospital doctors. *British Medical Journal*, **300**, 445–447.

Garvin B. J. and Kennedy, C (1990) Interpersonal communication between nurses and patients. *Annual Review of Nursing Research*, **8**, 213–234.

Gask, L., Goldberg, D. and Boardman, A. (1991) Training general practitioners to teach psychiatric interviewing skills: an evaluation of group training. *Medical Education*, **25**, 444–451.

Geldard, D. (1993) *Basic Personal Counselling*, 2nd edn, Prentice-Hall, Sydney.

Gelso, C. and Fassinger, R. (1990) Counselling psychology: theory and research on interventions. *Annual Review of Psychology*, **41**, 355–386.

General Medical Council (1993) *Tomorrow's Doctor: Recommendations on Undergraduate Medical Education*, General Medical Council, London.

Gerry, M. E. (1989) An investigation into the assertive behaviour of trained nurses in general hospital settings. *Journal of Advanced Nursing*, **14**, 1002–1008.

Gershen, J. (1983) Use of experiential techniques in interpersonal skill training. *Journal of Dental Education*, **47**, 72–75.

Gibson, F., Lewis, J., Loughrey, J. and Lount, M. (1981) Developments in the teaching of social work skills. *Social Work Education*, **1**, 8–14.

Gill, C. (1973) Types of interview in general practice: the flash, in *Six Minutes for the Patient: Interactions in General Practice Consultation*, (eds E. Balint and J. Norell), Tavistock, London.

Gilley, J. (1990) Demonstration and simulation, in *Adult Learning Methods: A Guide for Effective Instruction*, (ed. M. Galbraith), Krieger, Malabar, CA.

Gist, M., Bavetta, A. and Stevens, C. (1990) Transfer training method: its influence on skill generalisation, skill repetition, and performance level. *Personnel Psychology*, **43**, 501–523.

Gist, M., Stevens, C. and Bavetta, A. (1991) The effects of self-efficacy and post-training intervention on the acquisition and maintenance of complex interpersonal skills. *Personnel Psychology*, **44**, 837–861.

Glueckauf, R. L. and Quittner, A. L. (1992) Assertiveness training for disabled adults in wheelchairs: self-report, role-play, and activity pattern outcomes. *Journal of Consulting and Clinical Psychology*, **60**, 419–425.

Goldberg, D., Smith, C., Steele, J. and Spivey, L. (1980) Training family doctors to recognise psychiatric illness with increased accuracy. *Lancet*, **ii**, 521–523.

Goldhaber, G. and Rogers, D. (1979) *Auditing Organizational Communication Systems*, Kendall Hunt, Texas.

Goldstein, I. (1985) Organisation analysis and evaluation models. Paper presented at the meeting of the American Psychological Association, Los Angeles, August.

Goldstein, A., Gershaw, N. and Sprafkin, R. (1986) Structured learning: research and practice in psychological skill training, in *Handbook of Social Skills Training and Research*, (eds L. L'Abate and M. Milan), John Wiley, New York.

Goldstein, A. and Sorcher, M. (1974) *Changing Supervisor Behavior*, Pergamon, New York.

Gorden, R. (1980) *Interviewing: Strategy, Techniques and Tactics*, 3rd edn, Dorsey Press, Homewood, IL.

Gordon, J. (1991) Measuring the 'goodness' of training. *Training*, August, 19–25.

Gray, D. (1988) Counselling in general practice. *Journal of the Royal College of General Practitioners*, **38**, 50–51.

Greaves, F. (1987) *The Nursing Curriculum: Theory and Practice*, Croom Helm, London.

Greenberg, M. A. and Stone, A. A. (1992) Emotional disclosure about traumas and its relation to health: effects of previous disclosure and trauma severity. *Journal of Personality and Social Psychology*, **63**, 75–84.

Greene, J. O. (1988) Cognititve processes: methods for probing the black box, in *A Handbook for the Study of Human Communication*, (ed. C. H. Tardy), Ablex, Norwood, NJ.

Greene, M. G., Adelman, R. D., Rizzo, C. and Friedmann, E. (1994) The patient's presentation of self in an initial medical encounter, in *Interpersonal Communication in Older Adulthood: Interdisciplinary Theory and Research*, (eds M. L. Hummert, J. W. Wiemann and J. F. Nussbaum), Sage, Thousand Oaks, CA.

Greenspoon, J. (1955) The reinforcing effect of two spoken sounds on the frequency of two responses. *American Journal of Psychology*, **68**, 409–416.

Greenwood, J. (1993) The apparent desensitisation of student nurses during their professional socialisation: a cognitive perspective. *Journal of Advanced Nursing*, **18**, 1471–1479.

Gregg, V. (1986) *Introduction to Human Memory*, Routledge & Kegan Paul, London.

Griffiths, R. (1974) The contribution of feedback to microteaching technique, in *Microteaching Conference Papers*, (ed. A. Trott), APLET Occasional Publications No. 3.

Gronlund, N. (1976) *Measurement and Evaluation in Teaching*, 3rd edn, Macmillan, New York.

Grosswald, S. J. (1984) Designing effective educational activities for groups, in *Continuing Education for Health Professions*, (eds J. S. Green, S. J. Grosswald, E. Suter and D. B. Walthall), Jossey-Bass, Washington, DC.

Guilbert, J. (1981) *Educational Handbook for Health Personnel*, World Health Organization, Geneva.

Gulley, H. (1968) *Discussion, Conference and Group Process*, Holt, Rinehart & Winston, New York.

Hadlow, J. and Pitts, M. (1991) The understanding of common health terms by doctors, nurses and patients. *Social Science and Medicine*, **32**, 193–196.

Hagman, J. (1980) *Effects of Training Task Repetition on Retention and Transfer of Maintenance Skill.* ARI Research Report 1271, Alexandria, VA.

Hamilton, M. A., Rouse, R. A. and Rouse, J. (1994) Dentist communication and patient utilization of dental services: anxiety inhibition and competence enhancement effects. *Health Communication*, **6**, 137–158.

Hammond, S. L. and Lambert, B. L. (1994) Communicating about medications: directions for research. *Health Communication*, **6**, 247–251.

Hanson, A. (1981) Use of standards of practice in the design and evaluation of a continuing education programme. *American Journal of Pharmaceutical Education*, **45**, 56–60.

Harding, G., Taylor, K. and Nettleton, S. (1994) Working for health: interprofessional relations in health centres, in *Social Pharmacy: Innovation and Change*, (eds G. Harding, S. Nettleton and K. Taylor), Pharmaceutical Press, London.

Hargie, C., Dickson, D. and Tourish, D. (1994) Communication skills training (CST) and the radiography profession: a paradigm for training and development. *Research in Radiography*, **3**, 6–19.

Hargie, O. (1994) Editorial introduction, in *Group Performance*, (eds H. A. M. Wilke and R. W. Meertens), Routledge, London.

Hargie, O. (1997a) Interpersonal communication: a theoretical framework, in *A Handbook of Communication Skills*, 2nd edn, (ed. O. Hargie), Routledge, London.

Hargie, O. (1997b) Communication as skilled performance, in *A Handbook of Communication Skills*, 2nd edn, (ed. O. Hargie), Routledge, London.

Hargie, O. and Bamford, D. (1993) *Interpersonal Helping Skills: Videotapes 1–3*, University of Ulster, Jordanstown.

Hargie, O., Dickson, D. and Hargie, C. (1995) The effects of religious affiliation in Northern Ireland upon levels of self-disclosure of undergraduates. *International Journal of Adolescence and Youth*, **5**, 173–187.

Hargie, O., Dickson, D. and Tittmar, H. (1978) Mini-teaching: an extension of the microteaching format. *British Journal of Teacher Education*, **4**, 1–6.

Hargie, O. and Gallagher, M. (1992) A comparison of the core conditions of client-centred counselling in real and role-play counselling episodes. *Counselling*, **3**, 153–157.

Hargie, O. and McCartan, P. (1986) *Social Skills Training and Psychiatric Nursing*, Croom Helm, London.

Hargie, O. and Marshall, P. (1986) Interpersonal comunication: a theoretical framework, in *A Handbook of Communication Skills*, (ed. O. Hargie), Croom Helm, London.

Hargie, O. and Morrow, N. (1986a) A survey of interpersonal skills teaching in pharmacy schools in the United Kingdom and Ireland. *American Journal of Pharmaceutical Education*, **50**, 172–174.

Hargie, O. and Morrow, N. (1986b) Analytical and practical considerations of illustrative model videotapes. *Journal of Audiovisual Media in Medicine*, **9**, 65–68.

Hargie, O. and Morrow, N. (1986c) Using videotape in communication skills training: a critical evaluation of the process of self-viewing. *Medical Teacher*, **8**, 359–364.

Hargie, O. and Morrow, N. (1987a) Interpersonal communication: the sales approach. *Pharmacy Update*, **3**, 320–324.

Hargie, O. and Morrow, N. (1987b) Introducing interpersonal skills training into the pharmaceutical curriculum. *International Pharmacy Journal*, **1**, 175–178.

Hargie, O. and Morrow, N. (1989) The effectiveness of microtraining in developing pharmacists' communication skills: a study of personality and attitudes. *Medical Teacher*, **11**, 195–203.

Hargie, O. and Morrow, N. (1991) The skill of self-disclosure, parts 1 and 2. *Chemist and Druggist*, **235**, 343–344 and 769–770.

Hargie, O. and Morrow, N. (1995) An evaluation of a presentation skills course for pharmacists. *International Journal of Pharmacy Practice*, **3**, 101–105.

Hargie, O., Morrow, N. and Woodman, C. (1992) Consumer perceptions of and attitudes to community pharmacy services. *Pharmaceutical Journal*, **249**, 688–691.

Hargie, O., Morrow, N. and Woodman, C. (1993) *Looking Into Community Pharmacy: Identifying Effective Communication Skills In Pharmacist–Patient Consultations*, University of Ulster, Jordanstown.

Hargie, O. and Saunders, C. (1983) Training professional skills, in *Using Video: Psychological and Social Applications*, (eds P. Dowrick and S. Biggs), John Wiley, Chichester.

Hargie, O., Saunders, C. and Dickson, D. (1994) *Social Skills in Interpersonal Communication*, 3rd edn, Routledge, London.

Hargie, O. and Tourish, D. (1993) Assessing the effectiveness of communication in organisations: the communication audit approach. *Health Services Management Research*, **6**, 276–285.

Hargie, O. and Tourish, D. (1994) Communication skills training: management manipulation or personal development. *Human Relations*, **47**, 1377–1389.

Harris, R. (1985) The transfer of learning in social work education, in *Educating Social Workers*, (eds R. Harris, M. Baker, P. Reading *et al.*), Association of Teachers in Social Work Education, Leicester.

Harris, M. (1994) *Magic in the Surgery: Counselling and the NHS: A Licensed State Friendship Service*, Research Report 20, Social Affairs Unit, London.

Hartley, P. (1993) *Interpersonal Communication*, Routledge, London.

Hassett, J. (1992) Simplifying ROI. *Training*, September, 53–57.

Hayes, J. (1990) Perceptions of the factors which influence the transfer of learning. *Journal of Public Sector Management*, **3**, 23–26.

Heath, C. (1986) *Body Movement and Speech in Medical Interaction*, Cambridge University Press, Cambridge.

Heath, R. L. and Bryant, J. (1992) *Human Communication Theory and Research: Concepts, Contexts and Challenges*, Lawrence Erlbaum Associates, Hillsdale, NJ.

Hein, E. (1973) *Communication in Nursing Practice*, Little, Brown & Co., Boston, MA.

Herman, C. P., Zanna M. P. and Higgins E. T. (1986) *Physical Appearance, Stigma and Social Behavior*, Lawrence Erlbaum Associates, Hillsdale, NJ.

Heron, J. (1989) *The Facilitator's Handbook*, Kogan Page, London.

Herzmark, G. (1985) Reactions of patients to video recording of consultations in general practice. *British Medical Journal*, **291**, 315–317.

Hewes, D. and Planalp, S. (1987) The individual's place in communication science, in *Handbook of Communication Science*, (eds C. Berger and S. Chaffee), Sage, London.

Hewitt, C. (1984) Training in social skills, in *Occupational Therapy in Short-Term Psychiatry*, (ed. M. Willson), Churchill Livingstone, Edinburgh.

Hirsh, H. L. (1986a) The physician's duty to stop, look, listen and communicate. *Medical Law*, **5**, 449–461.

Hirsh, H. L. (1986b) Physicians and nurses: partners in communication. *Medical Law*, **5**, 463–475.

HMSO (1993) *Health Services Commissioner for England, for Scotland and for Wales, Annual Report for 1992–93*. HMSO, London.

Hobbs, T. (1992) *Experiential Training: Practical Guidelines*, Routledge, London.

Hogstel, M. (1987) Teaching students observational skills. *Nursing Outlook*, **35**, 89–91.

Holli, B. and Calabrese, R. (1991) *Communication and Education Skills: The Dietician's Guide*, Lea & Febiger, Philadelphia, PA.

Hopson, B. (1981) Counselling and helping, in *Psychology and Medicine*, (ed. D. Griffiths), Macmillan, London.

Horn, R. and Cleaves, H. (1980) *The Guide to Simulation Games for Education and Training*, Sage, Beverly Hills, CA.

Huczynski, A and Lewis, J. (1980) An empirical study into the learning transfer process in management training. *Journal of Management Studies*, **17**, 227–240.

Hughes, K. (1994) An investigation into nonverbal behaviours associated with deception/concealment during a negotiation process. Unpublished DPhil thesis, University of Ulster, Jordanstown.

Hummert, M. L. (1994) Stereotypes of the elderly and patronizing speech, in *Interpersonal Communication in Older Adulthood: Interdisciplinary Theory and Research*, (eds M. L. Hummert, J. W. Wiemann, and J. F. Nussbaum), Sage, Thousand Oaks, CA.

Hummert, M. L., Wiemann, J. W. and Nussbaum, J. F. (eds) (1994) *Interpersonal Communication in Older Adulthood: Interdisciplinary Theory and Research*, Sage, Thousand Oaks, CA.

Hung, J. and Rosenthal, T. (1978) Therapeutic videotaped playback: a critical review. *Advances in Behavioural Research and Therapy*, **1**, 103–135.

Hunt, M. (1988) Talking to terminally ill patients at home. *Nursing Times*, **84**, 58–59.

International Medical Benefit/Risk Foundation (1993) *Improving Patient Information and Education on Medicines. Report from the Foundation's Committee on Patient Information*, International Medical Benefit/Risk Foundation, Geneva.

Irving, P. (1995) A reconceptualisation of Rogerian core conditions of facilitative communication: implications for training. Unpublished DPhil thesis, University of Ulster, Jordanstown.

Ivey, A. and Authier, J. (1978) *Microcounselling: Innovations in Interviewing. Counselling, Psychotherapy and Psychoeducation*, Charles C. Thomas, Springfield, IL.

Ivey, A., Ivey, M. and Simek-Dowling, L. (1987) *Counselling and Psychotherapy: Integrating Skills. Theory and Practice*, 2nd edn, Prentice-Hall, Englewood Cliffs, NJ.

Izard, C. (1977) *Human Emotions*, Plenum Press, New York.

Jacklin, C. N. (ed.) (1992) *The Psychology of Gender*, vols 1–4, Edward Elgar, Cheltenham.

Jackson, L. D. (1992) Information complexity and medical communication: the effects of technical language and amount of information in a medical message. *Health Communication*, **4**, 197–210.

Jackson, L. D. (1994) Maximizing treatment adherence among back-pain patients: an experimental study of the effects of physician-related cues in written medical messages. *Health Communication*, **6**, 173–191.

Jackson, E. and Katz, J. (1983) Implementation of interpersonal skill training in dental schools. *Journal of Dental Education*, **47**, 66–71.

Jarvis, P. (1983) *Professional Education*, Croom Helm, London.

Jarvis, P. and Gibson, S. (1985) *The Teacher Practitioner in Nursing, Midwifery and Health Visiting*, Croom Helm, London.

Johnson, D. W. (1990) *Reaching Out: Interpersonal Effectiveness and Self-Actualisation*, Prentice-Hall, Englewood Cliffs, NJ.

Johnson, D. W. and Johnson, F. (1987) *Joining Together: Group Theory and Group Skills*, 2nd edn, Prentice Hall, Englewood Cliffs, NJ.

Johnston, D. (1990) The prevention of cardiovascular disease by psychological methods, in *Proceedings of the Second Conference of the Health Psychology Section. Occasional Papers* 2, (eds P. Bennett and J. Weinman), British Psychological Society, Leicester.

Jonassen, D. and Grabowski, B. (1993) *Handbook of Individual Differences, Learning, and Instruction*, Lawrence Erlbaum Associates, Hillsdale, NJ.

Jones, C. (1984) Process recording for communication with psychiatric patients techniques for improving skills of communication, in *Recent Advances in Nursing 7: Communication*, (ed. A. Faulkner), Churchill Livingstone, Edinburgh.

Jones, K. (1985) *Designing Your Own Simulations*, Methuen, London.

Jupp, J. and Griffiths, M. (1990) Self-concept changes in shy, socially isolated adolescents following social skills training emphasising role-plays. *Australian Psychologist*, **25**, 165–177.

Jussim, L., Coleman, L. and Nasau, S. (1989) Reactions to interpersonal evaluative feedback. *Journal of Applied Social Psychology*, **19**, 862–884.

Kagan, N. (1980) Influencing human interaction: eighteen years with IPR, in *Psychotherapy Supervision: Theory, Research and Practice*, (ed. A. Hess), John Wiley, New York.

Kagan, C. (ed.) (1985) *Interpersonal Skills in Nursing: Research and Applications*, Croom Helm, London.

Kagan, C., Evans, J. and Kay, B. (1986) *A Manual of Interpersonal Skills for Nurses: An Experiential Approach*, Harper & Row, London.

Kagan, N. and Kagan, H. (1991) Interpersonal process recall, in *Practical Guide to Using Video in the Behavioural Sciences*, (ed. P. Dowrick), John Wiley, New York.

Kahn, R. and Cannell, C. (1957) *The Dynamics of Interviewing*, John Wiley, New York.

Kamal, A. and Blais, C. (1992) Noncontingent positive and negative feedback during maximal exercise. *Perceptual and Motor Skills*, **75**, 203–210.

Kanfer, F. and Gaelick-Buys, L. (1991) Self-management methods, in *Helping People Change: A Textbook of Methods*, 4th edn, (eds F. Kanfer and A. Goldstein), Pergamon, New York.

Kasteler, J., Kane, R., Olsen, D. and Thetford, C. (1976) Issues underlying prevalence of 'doctor shopping' behavior. *Journal of Health and Social Behaviour*, **17**, 328–339.

Kaufman, D. (1984) Professional women: how real are the recent gains?, in *Women: A Feminist Perspective*, (ed. J. Freeman), Mayfield, Palo Alto, CA.

Kauss, D., Robbins, A., Abrass, I. *et al.* (1980) The long-term effectiveness of interpersonal skills training in medical schools. *Journal of Medical Education*, **55**, 595–601.

Keiser, T. and Seeler, J. (1987) Games and simulation, in *Training and Development Handbook: A Guide to Human Resource Development*, (ed. R. Craig), McGraw-Hill, New York.

Kellermann, K. (1992) Communication: inherently strategic and primarily automatic. *Communication Monographs*, **59**, 288–300.

Kelley, H. (1971) *Attribution in Social Interaction*, General Learning Press, Morristown.

Kelly, C., Moran, T and Myatt, P. (1994) Conversion disorder, sexual abuse and interprofessional communication – some lessons to be re-learned. *Irish Journal of Psychological Medicine*, **11**, 135–137.

Kendall, P. (1989) The generalisation and maintenance of behaviour change: comments, considerations and the 'no-cure' criticism. *Behaviour Therapy*, **20**, 357–364.

Kendrick, T. and Freeling, P. (1993) A communication skills course for preclinical students: evaluation of general practice based teaching using group methods. *Medical Education*, **27**, 211–217.

Kernis, M. and Sun, C. R. (1994) Narcissism and reactions to interpersonal feedback. *Journal of Research in Personality*, **28**, 4–13.

Kilkus, S. P. (1993) Assertiveness among professional nurses. *Journal of Advanced Nursing*, **18**, 1324–1330.

Kitching, J. (1986) Communication and the community pharmacist. *Pharmaceutical Journal*, **237**, 449–452.

Kleinke, C. (1986) *Meeting and Understanding People*, Freeman, New York.

Klinzing, D. and Klinzing, D. (1985) *Communication for Allied Health Professionals*, W. C. Brown, Dubuque, IA.

Knapp, M. and Hall, J. (1992) *Nonverbal Communication in Human Interaction*, Holt, Rinehart & Winston, New York.

Knowles, M. (1980) *The Modern Practice of Adult Education*, Association Press, New York.

Knowles, M. (1987) Adult learning, in *Training and Development Handbook: A Guide to Human Resource Development* (ed. R. Craig), McGraw-Hill, New York, pp. 168–179.

Knox, J. and Bouchier, I. (1985) Communication skills teaching, learning and assessment. *Medical Education*, **19**, 285–289.

Kopp, C. and Krakow, J. (1982) *The Child: Development in a Social Context*, Addison-Wesley, Reading, MA.

Korsch, B., Gozzi, E. and Francis, V. (1968) Gaps in doctor–patient communication: doctor–patient interaction and patient satisfaction. *Pediatrics*, **42**, 855–871.

Kotter, J. (1988) *The Leadership Factor*, Free Press, New York.

Kraan, H., Crijnen, A., Zuidweg, J. *et al.* (1989) Evaluating undergraduate training – a checklist for medical interviewing skills, in *Communicating with Medical Patients*, (eds M. Stewart and D. Roter), Sage, Newbury Park, CA.

Kreps, G. (1993) Relational communication in health care, in *Perspectives on Health Communication*, (eds B. C. Thornton and G. L. Kreps), Waveland Press, Illinois.

Kreps, G. and Kunimoto, E. N. (1994) *Effective Communication in Multicultural Health Care Settings*, Sage, Thousand Oaks, CA.

Kreps, G. and Query, J. (1990) Health communication and interpersonal competence, in *Speech Communication: Essays to Commemorate the 75th Anniversary of the Speech Communication Association*, (eds G. Phillips and J. Wood), Southern Illinois University Press, Carbondale and Edwardville, IL.

Kurtz, M. B. (1988) The dual role dilemma, in *New Leadership in Health Care Management: The Physician Executive*, (ed. W. Curry), American College of Physician Executives, Tampa, FL.

Kurtz, P. and Marshall, E. (1982) Evolution of interpersonal skills training, in *Interpersonal Helping Skills*, (eds E. Marshall *et al.*), Jossey-Bass, San Francisco, CA.

Laird, D. (1991) *Approaches to Training and Development*, Addison-Wesley, Reading, MA.

Laker, D. (1990) Dual dimensionality of training transfer. *Human Resource Development Quarterly*, **1**, 209–223.

Lamb, R. (1988) Greeting and parting, in *Eye to Eye: Your Relationships and How They Work*, (ed. P. Marsh), Sidgwick & Jackson, London.

Lambert, B. (1995) Directness and deference in pharmacy students' messages to physicians. *Social Science and Medicine*, **40**, 545–556.

Lang, G. and van der Molen, H. (1990) *Personal Conversations: Roles and Skills for Counsellors*, Routledge, London.

Larsen, K. and Smith, C. (1981) Assessment of nonverbal communication in the patient–physician interview. *Journal of Family Practice*, **12**, 481–488.

Latham, G. (1988) Human resource training and development. *Annual Review of Psychology*, **39**, 545–582.

Law, C. (1991) Individual and group learning, in *Handbook of Training and Development*, (ed. J. Prior), Gower, Aldershot.

Lecca, P. and McNeil, J. (eds) (1985) *Interdisciplinary Team Practice: Issues and Trends*, Praeger, New York.

Lee, J. and Whitford, M. (1992) Effects of performance feedback on teachers' self-evaluations. *Psychological Reports*, **71**, 323–331.

Lee, M., Matsumoto, D., Kobayasahi, M. *et al.* (1992) Cultural influences on noverbal behavior in applied settings, in *Applications of Nonverbal Behavioral Theories and Research*, (ed. R. S. Feldman), Lawrence Erlbaum Associates, Hillsdale, NJ.

Leigh, H. and Reiser, M. (1980) *The Patient: Biological, Psychological, and Social Dimensions of Medical Practice*, Plenum Press, New York.

Leventhal, H. (1970) Findings and theory in the study of fear communications, in *Advances in Experimental Social Psychology*, vol. 5 (ed. L. Berkowitz), Academic Press, New York.

Lewis, J. (1994) Patient views on quality care in general practice: literature review. *Social Science and Medicine*, **39**, 655–670.

Ley, P. (1977) Communicating with the patient, in *Introductory Psychology*, (ed. J. Coleman), Routledge & Kegan Paul, London.

Ley, P. (1982a) Satisfaction, compliance and communication. *British Journal of Clinical Psychology*, **21**, 241–254.

Ley, P. (1982b) Giving information to patients, in *Social Psychology and Behavioral Medicine*, (ed. J. R. Eiser), John Wiley, New York.

Ley, P. (1988) *Communicating with Patients*, Chapman & Hall, London.

Ley, P., Goldman, M., Bradshaw, P., Kincey, J. and Walker, C. (1972) The comprehensibility of some X-ray leaflets. *Journal of the Institute of Health Education*, **10**, 47–53.

Ley, P., Bradshaw, P., Eaves, D. and Walker, C. (1973) A method for increasing patients' recall of information presented by doctors. *Psychological Medicine*, **3**, 217–220.

Lezberg, A. and Fedo, D. (1980) Communication skills and pharmacy education: a case study. *American Journal of Pharmaceutical Education*, **44**, 257–259.

Lierman, B. (1994) How to develop a training simulation. *Training and Development*, **48**, 50–52.

Lillie, F. (1985) The wider social context of interpersonal skills in nursing, in *Interpersonal Skills in Nursing: Research and Applications*, (ed. C. Kagan), Croom Helm, London.

Linstone, H. and Turoff, M. (1975) *The Delphi Method: Techniques and Applications*, Addison-Wesley, Reading, MA.

Livesey, P. (1986) *Partners in Care: The Consultation in General Practice*, Heinemann, London.

Lochman, E. E. (1983) Factors related to patients' satisfaction with their medical care. *Journal of Community Health*, **9**, 91–109.

Locke, E. A. and Latham, G. P. (1990) *A Theory of Goal Setting and Task Performance*, Prentice-Hall, Englewood Cliffs, NJ.

Loftus, E. (1975) Leading questions and the eyewitness report. *Cognitive Psychology*, **7**, 560–572.

Lubbers, C. A. and Roy, S. J. (1990) Communication skills for continuing education in nursing. *Journal of Continuing Education in Nursing*, **21**, 109–112.

McCartan, P. J. and Hargie, O. D. W. (1990) Assessing assertive behaviour in student nurses: a comparison of assertion measures. *Journal of Advanced Nursing*, **15**, 1370–1376.

McCullagh, P. (1986) Model status as a determinant of observational learning and performance. *Journal of Sport Psychology*, **8**, 319–331.

McGarvey, B. and Swallow, D. (1986) *Microteaching in Teacher Education and Training*, Croom Helm, London.

McGhee, A. (1961) *The Patient's Attitude to Nursing Care*, E. & S. Livingstone, Edinburgh.

McGregor, J. (1993) Effectiveness of role playing and anti-racial teaching in reducing student prejudice. *Journal of Educational Research*, **86**, 215–226.

McGuire, W. J. (1981) Theoretical foundations of campaigns, in *Public Communication Campaigns*, (eds R. E. Rice and W. J. Paisley), Sage, Newbury Park, CA.

McIntee, J. and Firth, H. (1984) How to beat the burnout. *Health and Social Services Journal*, 9 February, 166–168.

McKenna, H. (1994) The Delphi technique: a worthwhile research approach for nursing. *Journal of Advanced Nursing*, **19**, 1221–1225.

McKinlay, J. (1972) Some approaches and problems in the study of the use of services: an overview. *Journal of Health and Social Behavior*, **13**, 115–152.

MacLeod Clark, J. (1982) Nurse–patient verbal interaction: an analysis of recorded conversations from selected surgical wards. Unpublished PhD thesis, University of London.

MacLeod Clark, J. (1984) Verbal commmunication in nursing, in *Recent Advances in Nursing 7: Communication*, (ed. A. Faulkner), Churchill Livingstone, Edinburgh.

MacLeod Clark, J. (1985) The development of research in interpersonal skills in nursing, in *Interpersonal Skills in Nursing: Research and Applications*, (ed. C. Kagan), Croom Helm, London.

MacLeod Clark, J. and Faulkner, A. (1987) Communication skills teaching in nurse education, in *Nursing Education: Research and Developments*, (ed. B. Davis), Croom Helm, London.

McManus, I. C., Vincent, C. A., Thom, S. and Kidd, J. (1993) Teaching communication skills to clinical students. *British Medical Journal*, **306**, 1322–1327.

McNeil, B. and Nelson, K. (1991) Meta-analysis of interactive video instruction: a 10 year review of achievement effects. *Journal of Computer Based Instruction*, **18**, 1–6.

McQuellon, R. (1982) Interpersonal process recall, in *Interpersonal Helping Skills*, (eds E. Marshall *et al.*), Jossey-Bass, San Francisco, CA.

Mader, T. E. and Mader, D. C. (1993) *Understanding One Another: Communicating Interpersonally*, William C. Brown, Madison, WI.

Maerker, M., Lisper, H.-O. and Rickberg, S.-E. (1990) Role-play as a method in nursing research. *Journal of Advanced Nursing*, **15**, 180–186.

Magill, R. (1993) *Motor Learning: Concepts and Applications*, W. C. Brown, Dubuque, IA.

Magill, R. (1994) The influence of augmented feedback on skill learning depends on characteristics of the skill and learner. *Quest*, **46**, 31–27.

Maguire, P. (1981) Doctor–patient skills, in *Social Skills and Health*, (ed. M. Argyle), Methuen, London.

Maguire, P. (1984a) Communication skills and patient care, in *Health Care and Human Behaviour*, (eds A. Steptoe and A. Mathews), Academic Press, London.

Maguire, P. (1984b) How we teach interviewing skills. *Medical Teacher*, **6**, 128–133.

Maguire, P. (1985) Deficiencies in key interpersonal skills, in *Interpersonal Skills in Nursing*, (ed. C. Kagan), Croom Helm, London.

Maguire, P. (1986) Social skills training for health professionals, in *Handbook of Social Skills Training*, vol. 2, (eds C. Hollin and P. Trower), Pergamon, Oxford.

Maguire, P., Fairbairn, S. and Fletcher, C. (1986) Consultation skills of young doctors. *British Medical Journal*, **292**, 1573–1578.

Maguire, P., Fairbairn, S. and Fletcher, C. (1989) Consultation skills of young doctors – benefits of undergraduate feedback training in interviewing, in *Communicating with Medical Patients*, (eds M. Stewart and D. Roter), Sage, Newbury Park, CA.

Maguire, P. & Faulkner, A. (1988) Improving the counselling skills of doctors and nurses in cancer care. *British Medical Journal*, **297**, 847–849.

Maguire, P., Roe, P., Goldberg, D. *et al.* (1978) The value of feedback in teaching interviewing skills to medical students. *Psychological Medicine*, **8**, 695–704.

Maguire, P., Tait, A., Brooke, M. and Sellwood, R. (1980a) Emotional aspects of mastectomy: a conspiracy of pretence. *Nursing Mirror*, 10 January, 17–19.

Maguire, P., Tait, A., Brooke, M. *et al.* (1980b) The effect of counselling on the psychiatric morbidity associated with mastectomy. *British Medical Journal*, **281**, 1454–1456.

Makely, S. (1990) Methods for teaching effective patient communication techniques to radiography students. *Radiography Today*, **56**, 14–15.

Marsh, P. (1988) Raising a smile, in *Eye To Eye: Your Relationships and How They Work*, (ed. P. Marsh), Sidgwick & Jackson, London.

Martin, A., Jones, E. and Hearn, G. (1994) Comparing interactive videodisc instruction with traditional methods of social skills training. *Education and Training Technology International*, **31**, 187–195.

Martin, E. and Martin, P. (1984) The reactions of patients to a video camera in the consulting room. *Journal of the Royal College of General Practitioners*, **34**, 607–611.

Martin, E., Russell, D., Goodwin, S. *et al.* (1991) Why patients consult and what happens when they do. *British Medical Journal*, **303**, 289–292.

Marwell, G. and Schmitt, D. (1967a) Compliance-gaining behavior: a synthesis and model. *Sociology Quarterly*, **8**, 317–328.

Marwell, G. and Schmitt, D. (1967b) Dimensions of compliance-gaining behavior: an empirical analysis. *Sociometry*, **30**, 350–364.

Marx, R. (1982) Relapse prevention for managerial training: a model for maintenance of behavioural change. *Academy of Management Review*, **7**, 433–441.

Marx, R. and Ivey, A. (1988) Communication skills programmes that last: face to face and relapse prevention. *International Journal for the Advancement of Counselling*, **11**, 135–151.

Mascelli, J. V. (1965) *The Five C's of Cinematography*, Cine/Graphic Publications, Hollywood, CA.

Maslow, A. (1954) *Motivation and Personality*, Harper & Row, New York.

Mason, H. and Svarstad, B. (1984) Medication counselling behaviors and attitudes of rural community pharmacists. *Drug Intelligence and Clinical Pharmacy*, **18**, 409–414.

Mathews, A. (1993) Biases in processing emotional information. *Psychologist*, **6**, 493–499.

Maxwell, M., Dickson, D. and Saunders, C. (1991) An evaluation of communication skills training for physiotherapy students. *Medical Teacher*, **13**, 333–338.

May, C. (1990) Research on nurse–patient relationships: problems of theory, problems of practice. *Journal of Advanced Nursing*, **15**, 307–315.

Meeuwesen, L., Schaap, C. and van der Staak, C. (1991) Verbal analysis of doctor–patient communication. *Social Science and Medicine*, **32**, 1143–1150.

Menikheim, M. and Ryden, M. (1985) Designing learning to increase competency in interpersonal communication skills. *Journal of Nurse Education*, **24**, 216–218.

Meredith, P. (1993) Patient satisfaction with communication in general surgery. *Social Science and Medicine*, **37**, 591–602.

Metcalfe, D. (1989) Teaching communication skills to medical students, in *Changing Ideas in Health Care*, (eds D. Seedhouse and A. Cribb), John Wiley, New York.

Miles, R. (1987) Experiential learning in the curriculum, in *The Curriculum in Nursing Education*, (eds P. Allan and M. Jolley), Croom Helm, London.

Millar, R., Crute, V. and Hargie, O. (1992) *Professional Interviewing*, Routledge, London.

Miller, S. M., Brody, D. S. and Summerton, J. (1988) Styles of coping with threat: implications for health, *Journal of Personality and Social Psycology*, **54**, 142–148.

Miller, G. and Stiff, J. (1993) *Deceptive Communication*, Sage, Newbury Park.

Miller, G., Boster, F., Roloff, M. and Seibold, D. (1987) MBRS rekindled: some thoughts on compliance gaining in interpersonal settings, in *Interpersonal Processes: New Directions in Communication Research*, (eds M. Roloff and G. Miller), Sage, Beverly Hills, California.

Millis, J. (1975) *Pharmacists for the Future: The Report of the Study Commission on Pharmacy*, Health Administration Press, Ann Arbor, MI.

Mills, G. and Pace, R. (1989) What effects do practice and video feedback have on the development of interpersonal communication skills. *Journal of Business Communication*, **26**, 159–176.

Mishler, E. (1984) *The Discourse of Medicine: Dialectics of Medical Interviews*, Ablex, Norwood, NJ.

Montgomery, C. (1993) *Helping Through Communication: The Practice of Caring*, Sage, Newbury Park, CA.

Moreno, J. (1953) *Who Shall Survive*, Beacon House, Beacon, NY.

Morris, R. (1991) Fear reduction methods, in *Helping People Change*, (eds F. Kanfer and A. Goldstein), Pergamon, New York.

Morris, L. A., Grossman, K., Barkdoll, G. and Gordon, E. (1987) A segmentational analysis of prescription drug information seeking. *Medical Care*, **25**, 953–964.

Morrow, N. (1986) Communication as a focus in pharmacy education and practice. Unpublished PhD thesis, Queen's University, Belfast.

Morrow, N. and Hargie, O. (1985) Interpersonal communication: questioning skills. *Pharmacy Update*, **1**, 255–257.

Morrow, N. and Hargie, O. (1986) Communication as a focus in the continuing education of pharmacists. *Studies in Higher Education*, **11**, 279–288.

Morrow, N. and Hargie, O. (1987a) An investigation of critical incidents in interpersonal communication in pharmacy practice. *Journal of Social and Administrative Pharmacy*, **4**, 112–118.

Morrow, N. and Hargie, O. (1987b) Effectiveness of a communication skills training course in continuing pharmaceutical education in Northern Ireland: a longitudinal study. *American Journal of Pharmaceutical Education*, **51**, 148–152.

Morrow, N. and Hargie, O. (1988a) *Pharmacist–Patient Communication* (an instructor's manual and videotape package), N. C. Morrow and O. D. W. Hargie, Belfast.

Morrow, N. and Hargie, O. (1988b) Effective questioning skills in pharmacy practice, in *The Proprietary Articles Trade Association Official Reference Book*, (ed. A. Balon), Sterling Publications, London.

Morrow, N. and Hargie, O. (1989) A new focus for CST: pharmacy practice as a helping relationship. *Pharmaceutical Journal*, **243**, E16–E18.

Morrow, N. and Hargie, O. (1992) Patient counselling: an investigation of core situations and difficulties in pharmacy practice. *International Journal of Pharmacy Practice*, **1**, 202–205.

Morrow, N. and Hargie, O. (1994) Communication skills and health promotion. *Pharmaceutical Journal*, **253**, 311–313.

Morrow, N. and Hargie, O. (1995) Influencing and persuading skills at the inter-professional interface. *Journal of Continuing Education in the Health Professions*, in press.

Morrow, N., Hargie, O. and Woodman, C. (1993) Consumer perceptions of and attitudes to the advice giving role of community pharmacists. *Pharmaceutical Journal*, **251**, 25–27.

Morrow, N., Hargie, O., Donnelly, H. and Woodman, C. (1993) 'Why do you ask?' A study of questioning behaviour in community pharmacist–client consultations. *International Journal of Pharmacy Practice*, **2**, 90–94.

Morton, T. and Kurtz, P. (1982) Conditions affecting skills learning, in *Interpersonal Helping Skills*, (ed. E. Marshall *et al.*), Jossey-Bass, San Francisco, CA.

Mulac, A. (1974) Effects of three feedback conditions employing videotape and audiotape on acquired speech skill. *Speech Monographs*, **41**, 205–214.

Mulholland, J. (1994) *Handbook of Persuasive Tactics. A Practical Language Guide*, Routledge, London.

Mullan, T. (1986) Generalization in SST. Unpublished MPhil thesis, University of Ulster, Jordanstown.

Mullen, P., Green, L. and Persinger, G. (1985) Clinical trials of patient education for chronic conditions: a comparative meta-analysis of intervention types. *Preventive Medicine*, **14**, 753–781.

Myerscough, P. R. (1989) *Talking With Patients: A Basic Clinical Skills Guide*. Oxford University Press, Oxford.

Napier, R. W. and Gershenfeld, M. K. (1993) *Group: Theory and Experience*, Houghton Mifflin, Boston, MA.

National Board for Nursing, Midwifery and Health Visiting for Northern Ireland (1990) *The Common Foundation Programme in Nursing: Curriculum Requirements and Guidelines*, Circular No. NBNI/90/6/A.

National Health and Medical Research Council (1993) *General Guidelines for Medical Practitioners on Providing Information to Patients*, National Health and Medical Research Council, Canberra.

Neisser, U. (1967) *Cognitive Psychology*, Appleton-Century-Crofts, New York.

Nelson, A., Gold, B., Hutchinson, R. and Benezra, E. (1975) Drug default among schizophrenic patients. *American Journal of Hospital Pharmacy*, **32**, 1237–1242.

Nelson-Jones, R. (1991) *Lifeskills: A Handbook*, Cassell, London.

Nesbitt, M. L. (1990) Failing to communicate. *Journal of the Medical Defence Union*, **6**, 49.

Newell, R. (1994) *Interviewing Skills for Nurses and Other Health Care Professionals. A Structured Approach*, Routledge, London.

Newman, J. and Fuqua, D. (1990) Stability of preferences for microskills across two videotaped clients. *Psychological Reports*, **67**, 1379–1388.

Newstrom, J. (1986) The management of unlearning: exploding the 'clean slate' fallacy. *Training and Development Journal*, **40**, 36–39.

Noble, C. (1991) Are nurses good patient educators? *Journal of Advanced Nursing*, **16**, 1185–1189.

Noe, R. (1986) Trainees' attributes and attitudes: neglected influences on training effectiveness. *Academy of Management Review*, **11**, 736–749.

Noe, R. and Ford, J. (1992) Emerging issues and new directions for training research. *Research in Personnel and Human Resource Management*, **10**, 345–384.

Noe, R. and Schmitt, N. (1986) The influence of trainee attitudes on training effectiveness: test of a model. *Personnel Psychology*, **39**, 497–523.

Noe, R., Sears, J. and Fullenkamp, A. (1990) Relapse training: does it influence trainees' post-training behaviour and cognitive strategies? *Journal of Business and Psychology*, **4**, 317–328.

Norris, J. (1986) Teaching communication skills: effects of two methods of instruction and selected learner characteristics. *Journal of Nurse Education*, **25**, 102–106.

Norton, R. and Mann, R. (1994) *The Relationship Between Patient Satisfaction and Medical Practitioner Service: A National Study of Patient Consumerism among Private Physicians*, Queensland University of Technology, Australia.

Nuffield Committee of Inquiry (1986) *Pharmacy. The Report of the Committee of Inquiry Appointed by the Nuffield Foundation*, Nuffield Foundation, London.

Numann, P. (1988) Our greatest failure. *American Journal of Surgery*, **155**, 212.

O'Connell, M. B. and Johnson, J. F. (1992) Evaluation of medication knowledge in elderly patients. *Annals of Pharmacotherapy*, **17**, 21–25.

O'Dell, S. L. (1991) Producing video modeling tapes, in *Practical Guide to Using Video in the Behavioural Sciences*, (ed. P. Dowrick), John Wiley, New York.

O'Hair, D. and Friedrich, G. W. (1992) *Strategic Communication in Business and the Professions*, Houghton Mifflin, Boston, MA.

Olson, J. and Iwasiw, C. (1987) Effects of a training model on active listening skills of post-RN students. *Journal of Nurse Education*, **26**, 104–107.

Ong, L., de Haes, J., Hoos, A. and Lammes, F. (1995) Doctor–patient communication: a review of the literature. *Social Science and Medicine*, **40**, 903–918.

Oppenheim, A. N. (1992) *Questionnaire Design, Interviewing and Attitude Measurement*, Pinter Publishers, London.

Orr, J. (1992) Assessing individual and community health needs, in *Health Visiting: Towards Community Health Nursing*, (eds K. Luker and J. Orr), Blackwell Scientific, Oxford.

Page, G. and Fielding, D. (1985) Appraising tests. *American Journal of Pharmaceutical Education*, **49**, 80–85.

Parasumaran, A., Zeitholm, V. and Berry, L. (1986) *Servgual: A Multi-item Scale for Measuring Customer Perceptions of Service Quality*, Marketing Science Institute, Working Paper Report No. 86-108, August.

Parathian, A. and Taylor, F. (1993) Can we insulate trainee nurses from exposure to bad practice? A study of role play in communicating bad news to patients. *Journal of Advanced Nursing*, **18**, 801–807.

Parks, M (1994) Communicative competence and interpersonal control, in *Handbook of Interpersonal Communication*, (eds M. Knapp and G. Miller), Sage, Thousand Oaks, CA.

Parrish, J and Babbitt, R. (1991) Video-mediated instruction in medical settings, in *Practical Guide to Using Video in the Behavioural Sciences*, (ed. P. Dowrick), John Wiley, New York.

Parrott, R. (1994) Exploring family practitioners' and patients' information exchange about prescribed medications: implications for practitioners' interviewing and patients' understanding. *Health Communication*, **6**, 267–280.

Parrott, R., Greene, K. and Parker, R. (1992) Negotiating child health care routines during paediatrician–parent consultations. *Journal of Language and Social Psychology*, **11**, 35–46.

Pask, G. (1976) Styles and strategies of learning. *British Journal of Educational Psychology*, **46**, 128–148.

Patterson, C. H. (1986) *Theories of Counseling and Psychotherapy*, Harper & Row, New York.

Pavlov, I. (1927) *Conditioned Reflex*, Dover Reprint, New York.

Pendleton, D., Schofield, T., Tate, P. and Havelock, P. (1984) *The Consultation: An Approach to Learning and Teaching*, Oxford University Press, Oxford.

Perloff, R. (1993) *The Dynamics of Persuasion*, Lawrence Erlbaum Associates, Hillsdale, NJ.

Perry, M. and Furukawa, M. (1986) Modeling methods, in *Helping People Change*, (eds F. Kanfer and A. Goldstein), Pergamon, New York.

Phares, E. J. (1988) *Introduction to Personality*, Scott, Foresman & Co., Glenview, IL.

Pharmaceutical Society of Great Britain (1984) First report of the Working Party on Pharmaceutical Education and Training. *Pharmaceutical Journal*, **232**, 495–508.

Phillips, K. and Fraser, T. (1982) *The Management of Interpersonal Skills Training*, Gower, Aldershot.

Pietrofesa, J., Hoffman, A., Splete, H. and Pinto, D. (1978) *Counselling: Theory, Research and Practice*, Rand McNally, Chicago, IL.

Podell, K. (1975) *Physician Guide to Compliance in Hypertension*, Merck, Rahway, NJ.

Poole, D. and Sanson-Fisher, R. (1981) Long-term effects of empathy training on the interview skills of medical students. *Journal of Patient Counselling and Health Education*, **2**, 125–129.

Pope, B. (1986) *Social Skills Training for Psychiatric Nurses*, Harper & Row, London.

Porritt, L. (1984) *Communication: Choices for Nurses*, Churchill Livingstone, Edinburgh.

Pringle, M., Robins, S. and Brown, G. (1984) Assessing the consultation: methods of observing trainees in general practice. *British Medical Journal*, **288**, 1659–1660.

Pringle, M. and Stewart-Evans, C. (1990) Does awareness of being video recorded affect doctors' consultation behaviour? *British Journal of General Practice*, **40**, 455–458.

Pugh, J. (1995) Groupwork with HIV positive drug misusers in prison. *Irish Journal of Psychological Medicine*, **12**, 12–16.

Quigley, B. and Nyquist, J. (1992) Using video technology to provide feedback to students in performance courses. *Communication Education*, **41**, 324–334.

Rabin, C. and Zelner, D. (1992) The role of assertiveness in clarifying roles and strengthening job satisfaction of social workers in mulidisciplinary mental health settings. *British Journal of Social Work*, **22**, 17–32.

Rakos, R. (1986) Asserting and confronting, in *A Handbook of Communication Skills*, (ed. O. Hargie), Croom Helm, London.

Rakos, R. (1991) *Assertive Behavior: Research, Theory and Training*, Routledge, London.

Rapport, H. (1983) A methodology for the identification and assessment of health planning goals: application to pharmacy services. *Journal of Social and Administrative Pharmacy*, **1**, 161–171.

Rasinski, D. (1993) Cross-cultural concerns and communication in health care, in *Perspectives on Health Communication*, (eds B. Thornton and G. Kreps), Waveland Press, Illinois.

Raven, B. and Haley, R. (1982) Social influence and compliance of hospital nurses with infection control policies, in *Social Psychology and Behavioral Medicine*, (ed. J. Eiser), John Wiley, Chichester.

Raven, B. and Rubin, J. (1983) *Social Psychology*, 2nd edn, John Wiley, New York.

Ray, E. (ed.) (1993) *Case Studies in Health Communication*, Lawrence Erlbaum Associates, Hillsdale, NJ.

Reardon, K. (1991) *Persuasion in Practice*, Sage, Newbury Park, CA.

Rees, A. M. (1993) Communication in the physician–patient relationship. *Bulletin of the Medical Library Association*, **81**, 1–10.

Rhys, S. (1992) Training student health visitors in helping skills, in *Experiential Training: Practical Guidelines*, (ed. T. Hobbs), Routledge, London.

Richardson, S., Dohrenwend, N. and Klein, D. (1965) *Interviewing: Its Forms and Functions*, Basic Books, New York.

Ridderikhoff, J. (1993). Information exchange in a patient physician encounter. A quantitative approach. *Methods in Information and Medicine*, **32**, 73–78.

Ridge, A. (1993) A perspective of listening skills, in *Perspectives on Listening*, (eds A. Wolvin and C. Coakley), Ablex, Norwood, NJ.

Riggio, R. (1992) Social interaction skills and nonverbal behavior, in *Applications of Nonverbal Behavioral Theories and Research*, (ed. R. Feldman), Lawrence Erlbaum Associates, Hillsdale, NJ.

Roffers, T., Cooper, B. and Sultanoff, S. (1988) Can counsellor trainees apply their skills in actual client interviews? *Journal of Counselling and Development*, **66**, 385–388.

Rogers, C. (1951) *Client-Centred Therapy*, Houghton Mifflin, Boston, MA.

Rogers, C. (1975) Empathic: an unappreciated way of being. *Counselling Psychologist*, **5**, 2–10.

Rogers, R. (1984) Changing health-related attitudes and behavior: the role of preventive health psychology, in *Social Perception in Clinical and Counseling Psychology*, vol. 2, (eds J. Harvev, J. Maddux, R. McGlynn and D. Stoltenberg), Texas Tech. University Press, Lubbock, TX.

Rose, Y. and Tryon, W. (1979) Judgements of assertion behavior as a function of speech, loudness, latency, content, gestures, inflection and sex. *Behavior Modification*, **3**, 112–123.

Rosenberg, M., Nelson, C. and Vivekanathan, P. (1968) A multidimensional approach to the structure of personality impression. *Journal of Personality and Social Psychology*, **9**, 283–294.

Rosenfarb, I., Hayes, S. and Linehan, M. (1989) Instructions and experiential feedback in the treatment of social skills deficits in adults. *Psychotherapy*, **26**, 242–251.

Roser, C. and Thompson, M. (1995) Fear appeals and the formation of active publics. *Journal of Communication*, **45**, 103–121.

Ross, F. M., Bower, P. J. and Sibbald, B. S. (1994) Practice nurses: characteristics, workload and training needs *British Journal of General Practice*, **44**, 15–18.

Roter, D. (1977) Patient participation in the patient–provider interaction: the effects of patient question asking on the quality of interaction satisfaction and compliance. *Health Education Monographs*, **5**, 281–315.

Roter, D. (1989) Which facets of communication have strong effects on outcome?, in *Communicating with Medical Students*, (eds M. Stewart and D. Roter), Sage, Newbury Park, CA.

Roter, D. L. and Hall, J. A. (1989) Studies of doctor–patient interaction. *Annual Review of Public Health*, **10**, 163–180.

Roter, D., Lipkin, M. and Korsgaard, A. (1991) Sex differences in patients' and physicians' communication during primary care medical visits. *Medical Care*, **29**, 1083–1093.

Rowland, N., Irving, J. and Maynard, A. (1989) Can general practitioners counsel? *Journal of the Royal College of General Practitioners*, **39**, 118–120.

Rowland, P. and Stuessy, C. (1987) Effects of modes of computer-assisted instruction on conceptual understanding and achievement of college students exhibiting individual differences in learning: a pilot study. Paper presented at the annual meeting of the National Association for Research in Science Teaching, Washington, DC, April.

Royal College of General Practitioners Working Party (1972) *The Future General Practitioner*, Royal College of General Practitioners, London.

Royal Pharmaceutical Society of Great Britain (1992) *Report of the Joint Working Party on the Future Role of the Community Pharmaceutical Services*, Royal Pharmaceutical Society of Great Britain, London.

Royal Pharmaceutical Society of Great Britain (1995) *Medicines, Ethics and Practice. A Guide for Pharmacists*, Royal Pharmaceutical Society of Great Britain, London.

Rozelle, R., Druckman, D. and Baxter, J. (1997) Nonverbal communication, in *A Handbook of Communication Skills*, 2nd edn, (ed. O. Hargie), Routledge, London.

Rubin, J. (1984) Introduction, in *Group Decision Making*, (ed. W. C. Swap), Sage, Beverly Hills, CA.

Rubin, R. (1990) Communication competence, in *Speech Communication: Essays to Commemorate the 75th Anniversary of the Speech Communication Association*, (eds G. Phillips and J. Wood), Southern Illinois University Press, Carbondale and Edwardville, IL.

Sailor, W., Goetz, l., Anderson, J. *et al.* (1988) Research on community intensive instruction as a model for building functional, generalized skills, in *Generalization and Maintenance*, (eds R. Horner, G. Dunlap and R. Koegel), Brooks, Baltimore, MD.

Saks, M. J. and Krupat, E. (1988) *Social Psychology and its Applications*, Harper & Row, New York.

Sampson, E. E. and Marthas, M. (1981) *Group Process for the Health Professions*, John Wiley, New York.

Sanders, M. (1982) The effects of instructions, feedback and cueing procedures in behavioural parent training. *Australian Journal of Psychology*, **34**, 53–69.

Sanson-Fisher, R., Redman, R., Walsh, R. *et al.* (1991) Training medical practitioners in information transfer skills: the new challenge. *Medical Education*, **25**, 322–333.

Saunders, C. (1986) Opening and closing, in *A Handbook of Communication Skills*, (ed. O. Hargie), Croom Helm, London.

Saunders, C. and Caves, R. (1986) An empirical approach to the identification of communication skills with reference to speech therapy. *Journal of Further and Higher Education*, **10**, 29–44.

Scheflen, A. (1974) *How Behaviour Means*, Anchor, Garden City, NJ.

Schneider, D. E. and Tucker, R. (1992) Measuring communicative satisfaction in doctor–patient relations: the Doctor–Patient Inventory. *Health Communication*, **4**, 19–28.

Schofield, T. and Arntson, P. (1989) A model for teaching doctor–patient communication during residency, in *Communicating with Medical Patients*, (eds M. Stewart and D. Roter), Sage, Newbury Park CA.

Schommer, J. (1994) Effects of interrole congruence on pharmacist–patient communication. *Health Communication*, **6**, 297–309.

Schroeder, J., Dyer, F., Czemy, P. *et al.* (1986) Videodisc interpersonal skills training and assessment: overview and findings, vol. 1. *US Army Research Institute for the Behavioural Sciences Report*, January, RPT 703.

Seale, C. (1992) Community nurses and the care of the dying. *Social Science and Medicine*, **34**, 375–382.

Seibold, D. R., Cantrill, J. G. and Meyers, R. A. (1994) Communication and interpersonal influence, in *Handbook of Interpersonal Communication*, (eds M. Knapp and G. Miller), Sage, Thousand Oaks, CA.

Sellick, K. (1991) Nurses' interpersonal behaviours and the development of helping skills. *International Journal of Nursing Studies*, **28**, 3–11.

Serna, L. Schumaker, J. and Sheldon, L. (1992) A comparison of the effects of feedback procedures on college student performance on written essay papers. *Behaviour Modification*, **16**, 64–81.

Servant, J. and Matheson, J. (1986) Video recording in general practice: the patients do mind. *Journal of the Royal College of General Practitioners*, **36**, 555–556.

Sharf, B. (1993) Reading the vital signs: research in health care communication. *Communication Monographs*, **60**, 35–41.

Shaw, M. E. (1976) *Group Dynamics: The Psychology of Small Group Behavior*, McGraw-Hill, New York.

Sheppe, W. and Stevenson, I. (1963) Techniques of interviewing, in *The Psychological Basis of Medical Practice*, (eds H. Lief, F. Lief and N. Lief), Hoeber, New York.

Sherbourne, C., Hays, R., Ordway, L. *et al.* (1992) Antecedents of adherence to medical recommendations: results from the medical outcomes study. *Journal of Behavioural Medicine*, **15**, 447–468.

Shooter, M. (1992) Coping with death: workshops for those helping with the dying and bereaved, in *Experiential Training: Practical Guidelines*, (ed. T. Hobbs), Routledge, London.

Shorter, E. (1985) *Bedside Manners*, Viking Penguin, New York.

Shuy, R. (1983) Three types of interference to an effective exchange of information in the medical interview, in *Social Organisation of Doctor–Patient Communication*, (eds S. Fisher and A. Todd), Center for Applied Linguistics, Washington, DC.

Simpson, M., Buckman, R., Stewart, M. *et al.* (1991) Doctor–patient communication: the Toronto consensus statement. *British Medical Journal*, **303**, 1385–1387.

Sines, D. (1988) Maintaining an ordinary life, in *Towards Integration: Comprehensive Services for People with Mental Handicaps*, (ed. D. Sines), Harper & Row, London.

Singleton, S. J. (1983) The hospital doctor, in *Social Skills*, (ed. W. T. Singleton), MTP Press, Lancaster.

Skinner, B. (1953) *Science and Human Behaviour*, Appleton-Century-Crofts, New York.

Skinner, B. (1969) *Contingencies of Reinforcement*, Collier Macmillan, London.

Skinner, B. (1971) How to teach animals, in *Contemporary Psychology*, (ed. R. Atkinson), Freeman, San Francisco, CA.

Skinner, B. (1976) *About Behaviourism*, Vintage Books, New York.

Skipper, M. (1992) Communication processes and their effectiveness in the management and treatment of dysphagia. Unpublished DPhil thesis, University of Ulster, Jordanstown.

Slater, J. (1990) Effecting personal effectiveness: assertiveness training for nurses. *Journal of Advanced Nursing*, **15**, 337–356.

Sleight, P. (1995) Teaching communication skills: part of medical education? *Journal of Human Hypertension*, **9**, 67–69.

Sloan, D., Donnelly, M., Johnson, S. *et al.* (1994) Assessing surgical residents' and medical students' interpersonal skills. *Journal of Surgical Research*, **57**, 613–618.

Smith, V. (1986) Listening, in *A Handbook of Communication Skills*, (ed. O. Hargie), Croom Helm, London.

Smith, F. (1992a) A study of the advisory and health promotion activity of community pharmacists. *Health Education Journal*, **51**, 68–71.

Smith, F. (1992b). Community pharmacists and health promotion: a study of consultations between pharmacists and clients. *Health Promotion International*, **7**, 249–255.

Smith, V. and Bass, T. (1982) *Communication for the Health Care Team*, Harper & Row, London.

Snyder, M. (1987) *Public Appearances, Private Realities: The Psychology of Self-monitoring*, Freeman, New York.

Sorenson, R. and Pickett, T. (1986) A test of two teaching strategies designed to improve interview effectiveness: rating behaviour and videotape feedback. *Communication Education*, **35**, 13–22.

Speedie, S. (1985) Reliability: the accuracy of a test. *American Journal of Pharmaceutical Education*, **49**, 76–79.

Spitzberg, B. and Cupach, W. (1989) *Handbook of Interpersonal Competence Research*, Springer-Verlag, New York.

Stiles, W. and Putnam, S. (1989) Analysis of verbal and nonverbal behaviour in doctor–patient encounters, in *Communicating with Medical Patients*, (eds M. Stewart and D. Roter), Sage, Newbury Park, CA.

Stimson, G. and Webb, B. (1975) *Going to the Doctor*, Routledge & Kegan Paul, London.

Stokes, T. and Baer, D. (1977) A implicit technology of generalisation. *Journal of Applied Behaviour Analysis*, **10**, 349–367.

Stokes, T. and Osnes, P. (1988) The developing applied technology of generalisation. *Journal of Applied Behaviour Analysis*, **10**, 349–367.

Street, R. L. (1992) Analyzing communication in medical consultations. Do behavioural measures correspond to patients' perceptions? *Medical Care*, **30**, 976–988.

Stricker, G. and Fisher, M. (eds) (1990) *Self-disclosure in the Therapeutic Relationship*, Plenum Press, New York.

Stroebe, W. (1994) Why groups are less effective than their members: on personality losses in idea-generating groups. *BPS Social Psychology Section Newsletter*, **31**, 4–20.

Sutherland, H., Lochwood, G., Tritchler, D. *et al.* (1991) Communicating problematic information to cancer patients: is there 'noise' on the line? *Social Science and Medicine*, **32**, 725–731.

Sutton, S. (1982) Fear-arousing communications: a critical examination of theory and research, in *Social Psychology and Behavioral Medicine*, (ed. J. Eiser), John Wiley, Chichester.

Swann, W., Krull, D., Wenzlaff, R. and Pelham, B. (1992) Allure of negative feedback: self-verification strivings among depressed persons. *Journal of Abnormal Psychology*, **101**, 293–306.

Swanson, D. B. and Stillman, P. L. (1990) Use of standardized patients for teaching and assessing clinical skills. *Evaluation and the Health Professions*, **13**, 79–103.

Swap, W. C. (1984) Destructive effects of groups on individuals, in *Group Decision Making*, (ed. W. C. Swap), Sage, Beverly Hills, CA.

Tahka, V. (1984) *The Patient–Doctor Relationship*, ADIS Health Science Press, Sydney.

Talbot, C. (1992) Evaluation and validation: a mixed approach. *Journal of European Industrial Training*, **16**, 22–32.

Tannenbaum, S. and Yukl, G. (1992) Training and development in work organisations. *Annual Review of Psychology*, **43**, 399–441.

Ter Horst, G., Leeds, J. and Hoogstraten, J. (1984) Effectiveness of communication skills training for dental students. *Psychology Reports*, **55**, 7–11.

Thatcher, D. (1990) A consideration of the use of simulation for the promotion of empathy in the training for the caring professions – ME-THE-SLOW LEARNER: a case study. *Simulation and Gaming*, **21**, 248–255.

Thomas, P. (1993) An exploration of patients' perceptions of counselling with particular reference to counselling within general practice. *Counselling*, **4**, 24–30.

Thomlinson, D. (1991) Intercultural listening, in *Listening in Everyday Life*, (eds D. Borisoff and M. Purdy), University of America Press, Maryland.

Thompson, T. (1990) Patient health care: issues in interpersonal communication, in *Communication and Health: Systems and Applications*, (eds E. Ray and L. Donohew), Lawrence Erlbaum Associates, Hillsdale, NJ.

Thompson, A. N. (1992) Can communication skills be assessed independently of their context? *Medical Education*, **26**, 364–367.

Thompson, T. (1994) Interpersonal communication and health care, in *Handbook of Interpersonal Communication*, (eds M. Knapp and G. Miller), Sage, Thousand Oaks, CA.

Thompson, J. and Anderson, J. (1982) Patient preferences and the bedside manner. *Medical Education*, **16**, 17–21.

Thorndike, E. and Woodworth, R. (1901) The influence of improvement in one mental function upon the efficiency of other functions. *Psychology Review*, **8**, 247–261.

Thornquist, E. (1992) Examination and communication: a study of first encounters between patients and physiotherapists. *Family Practice*, **9**, 195–202.

Tickle-Degnen, L. and Rosenthal, R. (1992) Nonverbal aspects of therapeutic rapport, in *Applications of Nonverbal Behavioral: Theories and Research*, (ed. R. Feldman), Lawrence Erlbaum Associates, Hillsdale, NJ.

Tittmar, H., Hargie, O. and Dickson, D. (1978) The moulding of health visitors: the evolved role played by mini-training. *Health Visitor Journal*, **51**, 130–136.

Tourish, D. and Hargie, O. (1993) Quality assurance and internal organizational communications. *International Journal of Health Care Quality Assurance*, **6**, 22–28.

Trimboli, A. and Walker, M. (1993) The CAST Test of nonverbal sensitivity. *Journal of Language and Social Psychology*, **12**, 49–65.

Truax, C. (1966) Reinforcement and non-reinforcement in Rogerian psychotherapy. *Journal of Abnormal Psychology*, **71**, 1–9.

Tubbs, S. L. (1995) *A Systems Approach to Small Group Interaction*, 5th edn, McGraw Hill, New York.

Turner, J. C. (1991) *Social Influence*, Open University Press, Buckingham.

UKCC (1986) *Project 2000: A New Preparation for Practice*, UKCC, London.

van Ments, M. (1983) *The Effective Use of Role-Play: A Handbook for Teachers and Trainers*, Kogan Page, London.

Verby, J., Holden, P. and Davis, R. (1979) Peer review of consultations in primary care: the use of audiovisual recordings. *British Medical Journal*, **280**, 1686–1688.

Verhaak, P. F. (1988) Detection of psychologic complaints by general practitioners. *Medical Care*, **26**, 1009–1020.

Waitzkin, H. (1984) Doctor–patient communication: clinical implications of social scientific research. *Journal of the American Medical Association*, **252**, 2441–2446.

Waitzkin, H. (1985) Information giving in medical care. *Journal of Health and Social Behavior*, **26**, 81–101.

Walsh, P. and Green, J. (1982) Pathways to impact evaluation in continuing education in the health professions. *Journal of Allied Health*, **11**, 115–123.

Walton, L. and MacLeod Clark, J. (1986) Making contact. *Nursing Times*, **82**, 28–32.

Watson, J. (1988) New dimensions of human caring theory. *Nursing Science Quarterly*, **1**, 175–181.

Watzlawick, P., Beavin, J. and Jackson, D. (1967), *Pragmatics of Human Communication*, W. W. Norton, New York.

Weiner, M. (1980) Personal openness with patients: help or hindrance. *Texas Medicine*, **76**, 60–62.

Weinman, J. (1984) A modified essay question evaluation of pre-clinical teaching of communication skills. *Medical Education*, **18**, 164–167.

Weldon, E. and Weingart, L. (1993) Group goals and group performance. *British Journal of Social Psychology*, **32**, 307–334.

Wessler, R. (1984) Cognitive–social psychological theories and social skills: a review, in *Radical Approaches to Social Skills Training*, (ed. P. Trower), Croom Helm, London.

West, C. (1983) Ask me no questions . . . an analysis of questions and replies, in *The Social Organization of Doctor–Patient Communication*, (eds S. Fisher and A. Todd), Center for Applied Linguistics, Washington, DC.

Wetchler, J. and Vaughan, K. (1991) Perceptions of primary supervisors' interpersonal skills: a critical incident analysis. *Contemporary Family Therapy*, **13**, 61–68.

Wetzel, C., Radtke, P. and Stern, H. (1994) *Instructional Effectiveness of Video Media*, Lawrence Erlbaum Associates, Hillsdale, NJ.

Wexley, K. (1984) Personnel training. *Annual Review of Psychology*, **35**, 519–551.

Whitcher, S. and Fisher, J. (1979) Multi-dimensional reactions to therapeutic touch in a hospital setting. *Journal of Personality and Social Psychology*, **37**, 87–96.

White, K. (1988) *The Task of Medicine*, The Henry J. Kaiser Foundation, Menlo Park, CA.

White, J., Levinson, W. and Roter, D. (1994) 'Oh by the way. . .': the closing moments of the medical visit. *Journal of General and Internal Medicine*, **9**, 24–28.

White, B. and Sanders, S. (1986) The influence on patients' pain intensity ratings of antecedent reinforcement of pain talk or well talk. *Journal of Behavior Therapy and Experimental Psychiatry*, **17**, 155–159.

Whitehouse, C. (1991) The teaching of communication skills in United Kingdom medical schools. *Medical Education*, **25**, 311–318.

Whittington, D. (1986) Chairmanship, in *A Handbook of Communication Skills*, (ed. O. Hargie), Croom Helm, London.

Wiederholt, J. B., Clarridge, B. R. and Svarstad, B. L. (1992) Verbal consultation regarding prescription drugs: findings from a statewide study. *Medical Care*, **30**, 159–173.

Wilke, H. A. M. and Meertens, R. W. (1994) *Group Performance*, Routledge, London.

Wilkinson, S. (1991) Factors which influence how nurses communicate with cancer patients. *Journal of Advanced Nursing*, **16**, 677–688.

Wilkinson, J. (1995) Direct observation, in *Research Methods in Psychology*, (eds G. Breakwell, S. Hammond, and C. Fife-Schaw), Sage, London.

Williams, T., Thayer, P. and Pond, S. (1991) Test of a model of motivation influences on reactions to training and learning. Paper presented at the 6th Annual Conference of the Society of Industrial and Organisational Psychology, St Louis, MO.

Wilmot, W. (1987) *Dyadic Communication*, Random House, New York.

Wilmot, W. (1995) *Relational Communication*, McGraw-Hill, New York.

Wilson, L. K. and Gallois, C. (1993) *Assertion and its Social Context*, Pergamon, Oxford.

Wlodkowski, R. (1985) *Enhancing Adult Motivation to Learn*, Jossey-Bass, San Francisco, CA.

Wohlking, W. and Gill, P. (1980) *Role Playing*, Educational Technology Publications, Englewood Cliffs, NJ.

Wolff, F., Marsnik, N., Tacey, W. and Nichols, R. (1983) *Perceptive Listening*, Holt, Rinehart & Winston, New York.

Wolinsky, J. (1983) Research crumbles stereotypes of age. *APA Monitor*, **14**, 26–28.

Wolvin, A. and Coakley, C. (eds) (1993) *Perspectives on Listening*, Ablex, Norwood, NJ.

Woolfe (1992) Coping with stress, in *Experiential Training: Practical Guidelines*, (ed. T. Hobbs), Routledge, London.

Worchel, S., Wood, W. and Simpson, J. (eds) (1993) *Group Process and Productivity*, Sage, Beverly Hills, CA.

Wrate, R. M. and Masterson, G. (1990) Teaching medical students about doctor–patient consultations. Paper presented at the International Conference on Communication in Health Care, St Catherine's College, Oxford.

Yager, G. and Beck, T. (1985) Beginning practicum: it only hurt until I laughed. *Counsellor Education and Supervision*, **25**, 149–156.

Yank, G. R., Barber, J. W. and Spradlin, W. W. (1994) Mental health treatment teams and leadership: a systems model. *Behavioral Science*, **39**, 293–310.

Yoder, D., Hugenberg, L. and Wallace, S. (1993) *Creating Competent Communication*, W. C. Brown, Dubuque, IA.

Zebrowitz, L. A. (1990) *Social Perception*, Open University, Milton Keynes.

Zimbardo, P. and Leippe, M. (1991) *The Psychology of Attitude Change and Social Influence*, McGraw-Hill, New York.

Author index

Subject index